THE OFFICIAL
PATIENT'S SOURCEBOOK
on

COCAINE
DEPENDENCE

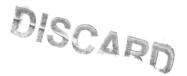

JAMES N. PARKER, M.D.
AND PHILIP M. PARKER, PH.D., EDITORS

ICON Health Publications
ICON Group International, Inc.
4370 La Jolla Village Drive, 4th Floor
San Diego, CA 92122 USA

Printed in the United States of America.

Last digit indicates print number: 10 9 8 7 6 4 5 3 2 1

Publisher, Health Care: Philip Parker, Ph.D.
Editor(s): James Parker, M.D., Philip Parker, Ph.D.

Publisher's note: The ideas, procedures, and suggestions contained in this book are not intended as a substitute for consultation with your physician. All matters regarding your health require medical supervision. As new medical or scientific information becomes available from academic and clinical research, recommended treatments and drug therapies may undergo changes. The authors, editors, and publisher have attempted to make the information in this book up to date and accurate in accord with accepted standards at the time of publication. The authors, editors, and publisher are not responsible for errors or omissions or for consequences from application of the book, and make no warranty, expressed or implied, in regard to the contents of this book. Any practice described in this book should be applied by the reader in accordance with professional standards of care used in regard to the unique circumstances that may apply in each situation, in close consultation with a qualified physician. The reader is advised to always check product information (package inserts) for changes and new information regarding dose and contraindications before taking any drug or pharmacological product. Caution is especially urged when using new or infrequently ordered drugs, herbal remedies, vitamins and supplements, alternative therapies, complementary therapies and medicines, and integrative medical treatments.

Cataloging-in-Publication Data

Parker, James N., 1961-
Parker, Philip M., 1960-

        The Official Patient's Sourcebook on Cocaine Dependence: Revised and Updated for the Internet Age/James N. Parker and Philip M. Parker, editors
                        p.   cm.
        Includes bibliographical references, glossary and index.
        ISBN: 0-497-00955-2
        1. Cocaine Dependence-Popular works.   I. Title.

Disclaimer

This publication is not intended to be used for the diagnosis or treatment of a health problem or as a substitute for consultation with licensed medical professionals. It is sold with the understanding that the publisher, editors, and authors are not engaging in the rendering of medical, psychological, financial, legal, or other professional services.

References to any entity, product, service, or source of information that may be contained in this publication should not be considered an endorsement, either direct or implied, by the publisher, editors or authors. ICON Group International, Inc., the editors, or the authors are not responsible for the content of any Web pages nor publications referenced in this publication.

Copyright Notice

Dedication

To the healthcare professionals dedicating their time and efforts to the study of cocaine dependence.

Acknowledgements

The collective knowledge generated from academic and applied research summarized in various references has been critical in the creation of this sourcebook which is best viewed as a comprehensive compilation and collection of information prepared by various official agencies which directly or indirectly are dedicated to cocaine dependence. All of the *Official Patient's Sourcebooks* draw from various agencies and institutions associated with the United States Department of Health and Human Services, and in particular, the Office of the Secretary of Health and Human Services (OS), the Administration for Children and Families (ACF), the Administration on Aging (AOA), the Agency for Healthcare Research and Quality (AHRQ), the Agency for Toxic Substances and Disease Registry (ATSDR), the Centers for Disease Control and Prevention (CDC), the Food and Drug Administration (FDA), the Healthcare Financing Administration (HCFA), the Health Resources and Services Administration (HRSA), the Indian Health Service (IHS), the institutions of the National Institutes of Health (NIH), the Program Support Center (PSC), and the Substance Abuse and Mental Health Services Administration (SAMHSA). In addition to these sources, information gathered from the National Library of Medicine, the United States Patent Office, the European Union, and their related organizations has been invaluable in the creation of this sourcebook. Some of the work represented was financially supported by the Research and Development Committee at INSEAD. This support is gratefully acknowledged. Finally, special thanks are owed to Tiffany Freeman for her excellent editorial support.

About the Editors

James N. Parker, M.D.

Dr. James N. Parker received his Bachelor of Science degree in Psychobiology from the University of California, Riverside and his M.D. from the University of California, San Diego. In addition to authoring numerous research publications, he has lectured at various academic institutions. Dr. Parker is the medical editor for the *Official Patient's Sourcebook* series published by ICON Health Publications.

Philip M. Parker, Ph.D.

Philip M. Parker is the Eli Lilly Chair Professor of Innovation, Business and Society at INSEAD (Fontainebleau, France and Singapore). Dr. Parker has also been Professor at the University of California, San Diego and has taught courses at Harvard University, the Hong Kong University of Science and Technology, the Massachusetts Institute of Technology, Stanford University, and UCLA. Dr. Parker is the associate editor for the *Official Patient's Sourcebook* series published by ICON Health Publications.

About ICON Health Publications

In addition to cocaine dependence, *Official Patient's Sourcebooks* are available for the following related topics:

- The Official Patient's Sourcebook on Alcoholism
- The Official Patient's Sourcebook on Anabolic Steroid Dependence
- The Official Patient's Sourcebook on Club Drug Dependence
- The Official Patient's Sourcebook on Dextromethorphan Dependence
- The Official Patient's Sourcebook on Dissociative Drug Dependence
- The Official Patient's Sourcebook on GHB Dependence
- The Official Patient's Sourcebook on Hepatitis C
- The Official Patient's Sourcebook on Heroin Dependence
- The Official Patient's Sourcebook on Inhalants Dependence
- The Official Patient's Sourcebook on Ketamine Dependence
- The Official Patient's Sourcebook on LSD Dependence
- The Official Patient's Sourcebook on Marijuana Dependence
- The Official Patient's Sourcebook on MDMA Dependence
- The Official Patient's Sourcebook on Methamphetamine Dependence
- The Official Patient's Sourcebook on Nicotine Dependence
- The Official Patient's Sourcebook on PCP Dependence
- The Official Patient's Sourcebook on Prescription CNS Depressants Dependence
- The Official Patient's Sourcebook on Prescription Drug Dependence
- The Official Patient's Sourcebook on Prescription Opioids Dendedence
- The Official Patient's Sourcebook on Prescription Stimulants Dependence
- The Official Patient's Sourcebook on Rohypnol Dependence

To discover more about ICON Health Publications, simply check with your preferred online booksellers, including Barnes&Noble.com and Amazon.com which currently carry all of our titles. Or, feel free to contact us directly for bulk purchases or institutional discounts:

ICON Group International, Inc.
4370 La Jolla Village Drive, Fourth Floor
San Diego, CA 92122 USA
Fax: 858-546-4341
Web site: **www.icongrouponline.com/health**

Table of Contents

INTRODUCTION 1
    Overview 1
    Organization 3
    Scope 3
    Moving Forward 4

PART I: THE ESSENTIALS 7

CHAPTER 1. THE ESSENTIALS ON COCAINE DEPENDENCE:
GUIDELINES 9
    Overview 9
    What Is Cocaine? 12
    What Is Crack? 13
    What Is the Scope of Cocaine Use in the United States? 14
    How Is Cocaine Used? 15
    How Does Cocaine Produce Its Effects? 15
    What Are the Short-Term Effects of Cocaine Use? 17
    What Are the Long-Term Effects of Cocaine Use? 18
    What Are the Medical Complications of Cocaine Abuse? 18
    What Is the Effect of Maternal Cocaine Use? 20
    What Treatments Are Effective for Cocaine Abusers? 21
    Crack and Cocaine INFOFAX 24
    Health Hazards 25
    Treatment 26
    Extent of Use 26
    More Guideline Sources 28
    Vocabulary Builder 35
CHAPTER 2. SEEKING GUIDANCE 37
    Overview 37
    Finding Associations 37
    Finding Drug Treatment and Alcohol Abuse Treatment Programs 39
    Finding Doctors 40
    Selecting Your Doctor 41
    Working with Your Doctor 42
    Broader Health-Related Resources 43

**PART II: ADDITIONAL RESOURCES AND
ADVANCED MATERIAL** 45

CHAPTER 3. STUDIES ON COCAINE DEPENDENCE 47
    Overview 47
    The Combined Health Information Database 47
    Federally Funded Research on Cocaine Dependence 52

E-Journals: PubMed Central 137
The National Library of Medicine: PubMed 137
Vocabulary Builder 181

CHAPTER 4. PATENTS ON COCAINE DEPENDENCE 187
Overview 187
Patent Applications on Cocaine Dependence 188
Keeping Current 192

CHAPTER 5. BOOKS ON COCAINE DEPENDENCE 193
Overview 193
Book Summaries: Federal Agencies 193
Book Summaries: Online Booksellers 194
Chapters on Cocaine Dependence 208
General Home References 208
Vocabulary Builder 209

CHAPTER 6. PERIODICALS AND NEWS ON COCAINE DEPENDENCE 211
Overview 211
News Services and Press Releases 211
Academic Periodicals covering Cocaine Dependence 216

CHAPTER 7. PHYSICIAN GUIDELINES AND DATABASES 223
Overview 223
NIH Guidelines 223
NIH Databases 224
Other Commercial Databases 227

CHAPTER 8. DISSERTATIONS ON COCAINE DEPENDENCE...............229
Overview 229
Dissertations on Cocaine Dependence 229
Keeping Current 235
Vocabulary Builder 236

PART III. APPENDICES 237

APPENDIX A. RESEARCHING YOUR MEDICATIONS 239
Overview 239
Your Medications: The Basics 239
Learning More about Your Medications 241
Commercial Databases 242
Researching Orphan Drugs 243
Contraindications and Interactions (Hidden Dangers) 245
A Final Warning 246
General References 247
Vocabulary Builder 248

APPENDIX B. RESEARCHING NUTRITION 249
Overview 249
Food and Nutrition: General Principles 249

Finding Studies on Cocaine Dependence 254
Federal Resources on Nutrition..259
Additional Web Resources..260
APPENDIX C. FINDING MEDICAL LIBRARIES 263
Overview 263
Preparation 263
Finding a Local Medical Library...264
Medical Libraries in the U.S. and Canada 264
APPENDIX D. PRINCIPLES OF DRUG ADDICTION TREATMENT 271
Overview 271
Principles of Effective Treatment 271
What Is Drug Addiction?..274
Frequently Asked Questions 275
Drug Addiction Treatment in the United States 282
General Categories of Treatment Programs 283
Treating Criminal Justice-Involved Drug Abusers and Addicts......................286
Scientifically-Based Approaches to Drug Addiction Treatment......................287
Resources 295
Selected NIDA Educational Resources on Drug Addiction Treatment............296

ONLINE GLOSSARIES...301
Online Dictionary Directories 303

COCAINE DEPENDENCE GLOSSARY 305
General Dictionaries and Glossaries 310

INDEX 313

INTRODUCTION

Overview

Dr. C. Everett Koop, former U.S. Surgeon General, once said, "The best prescription is knowledge."[1] The Agency for Healthcare Research and Quality (AHRQ) of the National Institutes of Health (NIH) echoes this view and recommends that every patient incorporate education into the treatment process. According to the AHRQ:

> Finding out more about your condition is a good place to start. By contacting groups that support your condition, visiting your local library, and searching on the Internet, you can find good information to help guide your treatment decisions. Some information may be hard to find—especially if you don't know where to look.[2]

As the AHRQ mentions, finding the right information is not an obvious task. Though many physicians and public officials had thought that the emergence of the Internet would do much to assist patients in obtaining reliable information, in March 2001 the National Institutes of Health issued the following warning:

> The number of Web sites offering health-related resources grows every day. Many sites provide valuable information, while others may have information that is unreliable or misleading.[3]

---

[1] Quotation from **http://www.drkoop.com**.
[2] The Agency for Healthcare Research and Quality (AHRQ):
http://www.ahcpr.gov/consumer/diaginfo.htm.
[3] From the NIH, National Cancer Institute (NCI):
http://cancertrials.nci.nih.gov/beyond/evaluating.html.

Since the late 1990s, physicians have seen a general increase in patient Internet usage rates. Patients frequently enter their doctor's offices with printed Web pages of home remedies in the guise of latest medical research. This scenario is so common that doctors often spend more time dispelling misleading information than guiding patients through sound therapies. *The Official Patient's Sourcebook on Cocaine Dependence* has been created for patients who have decided to make education and research an integral part of the treatment process. The pages that follow will tell you where and how to look for information covering virtually all topics related to cocaine dependence, from the essentials to the most advanced areas of research.

The title of this book includes the word "official." This reflects the fact that the sourcebook draws from public, academic, government, and peer-reviewed research. Selected readings from various agencies are reproduced to give you some of the latest official information available to date on cocaine dependence.

Given patients' increasing sophistication in using the Internet, abundant references to reliable Internet-based resources are provided throughout this sourcebook. Where possible, guidance is provided on how to obtain free-of-charge, primary research results as well as more detailed information via the Internet. E-book and electronic versions of this sourcebook are fully interactive with each of the Internet sites mentioned (clicking on a hyperlink automatically opens your browser to the site indicated). Hard copy users of this sourcebook can type cited Web addresses directly into their browsers to obtain access to the corresponding sites. Since we are working with ICON Health Publications, hard copy *Sourcebooks* are frequently updated and printed on demand to ensure that the information provided is current.

In addition to extensive references accessible via the Internet, every chapter presents a "Vocabulary Builder." Many health guides offer glossaries of technical or uncommon terms in an appendix. In editing this sourcebook, we have decided to place a smaller glossary within each chapter that covers terms used in that chapter. Given the technical nature of some chapters, you may need to revisit many sections. Building one's vocabulary of medical terms in such a gradual manner has been shown to improve the learning process.

We must emphasize that no sourcebook on cocaine dependence should affirm that a specific diagnostic procedure or treatment discussed in a research study, patent, or doctoral dissertation is "correct" or your best option. This sourcebook is no exception. Each patient is unique. Deciding on appropriate options is always up to the patient in consultation with their physician and healthcare providers.

Organization

This sourcebook is organized into three parts. Part I explores basic techniques to researching cocaine dependence (e.g. finding guidelines on diagnosis, treatments, and prognosis), followed by a number of topics, including information on how to get in touch with organizations, associations, or other patient networks dedicated to cocaine dependence. It also gives you sources of information that can help you find a doctor in your local area specializing in treating cocaine dependence. Collectively, the material presented in Part I is a complete primer on basic research topics for patients with cocaine dependence.

Part II moves on to advanced research dedicated to cocaine dependence. Part II is intended for those willing to invest many hours of hard work and study. It is here that we direct you to the latest scientific and applied research on cocaine dependence. When possible, contact names, links via the Internet, and summaries are provided. It is in Part II where the vocabulary process becomes important as authors publishing advanced research frequently use highly specialized language. In general, every attempt is made to recommend "free-to-use" options.

Part III provides appendices of useful background reading for all patients with cocaine dependence or related disorders. The appendices are dedicated to more pragmatic issues faced by many patients with cocaine dependence. Accessing materials via medical libraries may be the only option for some readers, so a guide is provided for finding local medical libraries which are open to the public. Part III, therefore, focuses on advice that goes beyond the biological and scientific issues facing patients with cocaine dependence.

Scope

While this sourcebook covers cocaine dependence, your doctor, research publications, and specialists may refer to your condition using a variety of terms. Therefore, you should understand that cocaine dependence is often considered a synonym or a condition closely related to the following:

- Cocaine
- Cocaine Abuse

- Cocaine Addiction
- Cocaine Hydrochloride Abuse
- Cocaine Hydrochloride Addiction
- Cocaine Hydrochloride Dependence
- Cocaine Intoxication
- Cocainism
- Intoxication with Cocaine

In addition to synonyms and related conditions, physicians may refer to cocaine dependence using certain coding systems. The International Classification of Diseases, 9th Revision, Clinical Modification (ICD-9-CM) is the most commonly used system of classification for the world's illnesses. Your physician may use this coding system as an administrative or tracking tool. The following classification is commonly used for cocaine dependence:[4]

- 304.2 cocaine dependence
- 305.6 cocaine abuse

For the purposes of this sourcebook, we have attempted to be as inclusive as possible, looking for official information for all of the synonyms relevant to cocaine dependence. You may find it useful to refer to synonyms when accessing databases or interacting with healthcare professionals and medical librarians.

Moving Forward

Since the 1980s, the world has seen a proliferation of healthcare guides covering most illnesses. Some are written by patients or their family members. These generally take a layperson's approach to understanding and coping with an illness or disorder. They can be uplifting, encouraging, and highly supportive. Other guides are authored by physicians or other healthcare providers who have a more clinical outlook. Each of these two styles of guide has its purpose and can be quite useful.

---

[4] This list is based on the official version of the World Health Organization's 9th Revision, International Classification of Diseases (ICD-9). According to the National Technical Information Service, "ICD-9CM extensions, interpretations, modifications, addenda, or errata other than those approved by the U.S. Public Health Service and the Health Care Financing Administration are not to be considered official and should not be utilized. Continuous maintenance of the ICD-9-CM is the responsibility of the federal government."

As editors, we have chosen a third route. We have chosen to expose you to as many sources of official and peer-reviewed information as practical, for the purpose of educating you about basic and advanced knowledge as recognized by medical science today. You can think of this sourcebook as your personal Internet age reference librarian.

Why "Internet age"? All too often, patients diagnosed with cocaine dependence will log on to the Internet, type words into a search engine, and receive several Web site listings which are mostly irrelevant or redundant. These patients are left to wonder where the relevant information is, and how to obtain it. Since only the smallest fraction of information dealing with cocaine dependence is even indexed in search engines, a non-systematic approach often leads to frustration and disappointment. With this sourcebook, we hope to direct you to the information you need that you would not likely find using popular Web directories. Beyond Web listings, in many cases we will reproduce brief summaries or abstracts of available reference materials. These abstracts often contain distilled information on topics of discussion.

While we focus on the more scientific aspects of cocaine dependence, there is, of course, the emotional side to consider. Later in the sourcebook, we provide a chapter dedicated to helping you find peer groups and associations that can provide additional support beyond research produced by medical science. We hope that the choices we have made give you the most options available in moving forward. In this way, we wish you the best in your efforts to incorporate this educational approach into your treatment plan.

The Editors

PART I: THE ESSENTIALS

ABOUT PART I

Part I has been edited to give you access to what we feel are "the essentials" on cocaine dependence. The essentials of a disease typically include the definition or description of the disease, a discussion of who it affects, the signs or symptoms associated with the disease, tests or diagnostic procedures that might be specific to the disease, and treatments for the disease. Your doctor or healthcare provider may have already explained the essentials of cocaine dependence to you or even given you a pamphlet or brochure describing cocaine dependence. Now you are searching for more in-depth information. As editors, we have decided, nevertheless, to include a discussion on where to find essential information that can complement what your doctor has already told you. In this section we recommend a process, not a particular Web site or reference book. The process ensures that, as you search the Web, you gain background information in such a way as to maximize your understanding.

CHAPTER 1. THE ESSENTIALS ON COCAINE DEPENDENCE: GUIDELINES

Overview

Official agencies, as well as federally funded institutions supported by national grants, frequently publish a variety of guidelines on cocaine dependence. These are typically called "Fact Sheets" or "Guidelines." They can take the form of a brochure, information kit, pamphlet, or flyer. Often they are only a few pages in length. The great advantage of guidelines over other sources is that they are often written with the patient in mind. Since new guidelines on cocaine dependence can appear at any moment and be published by a number of sources, the best approach to finding guidelines is to systematically scan the Internet-based services that post them.

The National Institutes of Health (NIH)[5]

The National Institutes of Health (NIH) is the first place to search for relatively current patient guidelines and fact sheets on cocaine dependence. Originally founded in 1887, the NIH is one of the world's foremost medical research centers and the federal focal point for medical research in the United States. At any given time, the NIH supports some 35,000 research grants at universities, medical schools, and other research and training institutions, both nationally and internationally. The rosters of those who have conducted research or who have received NIH support over the years include the world's most illustrious scientists and physicians. Among them are 97 scientists who have won the Nobel Prize for achievement in medicine.

---

[5] Adapted from the NIH: **http://www.nih.gov/about/NIHoverview.html**.

There is no guarantee that any one Institute will have a guideline on a specific disease, though the National Institutes of Health collectively publish over 600 guidelines for both common and rare diseases. The best way to access NIH guidelines is via the Internet. Although the NIH is organized into many different Institutes and Offices, the following is a list of key Web sites where you are most likely to find NIH clinical guidelines and publications dealing with cocaine dependence and associated conditions:

- Office of the Director (OD); guidelines consolidated across agencies available at **http://www.nih.gov/health/consumer/conkey.htm**

- National Library of Medicine (NLM); extensive encyclopedia (A.D.A.M., Inc.) with guidelines available at **http://www.nlm.nih.gov/medlineplus/healthtopics.html**

- National Institute on Drug Abuse (NIDA); guidelines on abused drugs at **http://www.nida.nih.gov/DrugAbuse.html**

Among these, the National Institute on Drug Abuse is particularly noteworthy.[6] NIDA was established in 1974, and in October 1992 it became part of the National Institutes of Health, Department of Health and Human Services. The Institute is organized into divisions and offices, each of which plays an important role in programs of drug abuse research. NIDA's mission is to lead the Nation in bringing the power of science to bear on drug abuse and addiction. This charge has two critical components. The first is the strategic support and conduct of research across a broad range of disciplines. The second is to ensure the rapid and effective dissemination and use of the results of that research to significantly improve drug abuse and addiction prevention, treatment, and policy.

NIDA supports over 85 percent of the world's research on the health aspects of drug abuse and addiction. NIDA supported science addresses the most fundamental and essential questions about drug abuse, ranging from the molecule to managed care, and from DNA to community outreach research. NIDA is not only seizing upon unprecedented opportunities and technologies to further understanding of how drugs of abuse affect the brain and behavior, but also working to ensure the rapid and effective transfer of scientific data to policy makers, drug abuse practitioners, other health care practitioners and the general public. The NIDA web page is an important part of this effort (**http://www.nida.nih.gov/**). Before citing NIDA's most

---

[6] The section is reproduced or adapted from the NIDA: **http://www.nida.nih.gov/NIDAWelcome.html#Mission**. For the remainder of this book, "adapted" signifies attributed "reproduction" with formatting and other minimal editorial changes.

recent guideline on cocaine dependence, the discussion below reproduces NIDA's general overview of drug abuse and addiction.

Understanding Drug Abuse and Addiction[7]

Many people view drug abuse and addiction as strictly a social problem. Parents, teens, older adults, and other members of the community tend to characterize people who take drugs as morally weak or as having criminal tendencies. They believe that drug abusers and addicts should be able to stop taking drugs if they are willing to change their behavior.

These myths have not only stereotyped those with drug-related problems, but also their families, their communities, and the health care professionals who work with them. Drug abuse and addiction comprise a public health problem that affects many people and has wide-ranging social consequences. It is NIDA's goal to help the public replace its myths and long-held mistaken beliefs about drug abuse and addiction with scientific evidence that addiction is a chronic, relapsing, and treatable disease.

Addiction *does* begin with drug abuse when an individual makes a conscious choice to use drugs, but addiction is not just "a lot of drug use." Recent scientific research provides overwhelming evidence that not only do drugs interfere with normal brain functioning creating powerful feelings of pleasure, but they also have long-term effects on brain metabolism and activity. At some point, changes occur in the brain that can turn drug abuse into addiction, a chronic, relapsing illness. Those addicted to drugs suffer from a compulsive drug craving and usage and cannot quit by themselves. Treatment is necessary to end this compulsive behavior.

A variety of approaches are used in treatment programs to help patients deal with these cravings and possibly avoid drug relapse. NIDA research shows that addiction is clearly treatable. Through treatment that is tailored to individual needs, patients can learn to control their condition and live relatively normal lives.

Treatment can have a profound effect not only on drug abusers, but on society as a whole by significantly improving social and psychological functioning, decreasing related criminality and violence, and reducing the spread of AIDS. It can also dramatically reduce the costs to society of drug abuse.

---

[7] Adapted from **http://165.112.78.61/Infofax/understand.html**.

Understanding drug abuse also helps in understanding how to prevent use in the first place. Results from NIDA-funded prevention research have shown that comprehensive prevention programs that involve the family, schools, communities, and the media are effective in reducing drug abuse. It is necessary to keep sending the message that it is better to not start at all than to enter rehabilitation if addiction occurs.

A tremendous opportunity exists to effectively change the ways in which the public understands drug abuse and addiction because of the wealth of scientific data NIDA has amassed. Overcoming misconceptions and replacing ideology with scientific knowledge is the best hope for bridging the "great disconnect" - the gap between the public perception of drug abuse and addiction and the scientific facts.

The National Institutes of Health has recently published the following guideline for cocaine dependence:

What Is Cocaine?[8]

Cocaine is a powerfully addictive stimulant that directly affects the brain. Cocaine has been labeled the drug of the 1980s and '90s, because of its extensive popularity and use during this period. However, cocaine is not a new drug. In fact, it is one of the oldest known drugs. The pure chemical, cocaine hydrochloride, has been an abused substance for more than 100 years, and coca leaves, the source of cocaine, have been ingested for thousands of years.

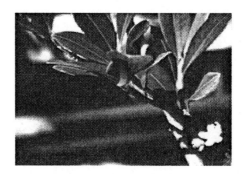

---

[8] Adapted from The National Institute on Drug Abuse:
http://165.112.78.61/ResearchReports/Cocaine/cocaine.html.

Pure cocaine was first extracted from the leaf of the *Erythroxylon* coca bush, which grows primarily in Peru and Bolivia, in the mid-19th century. In the early 1900s, it became the main stimulant drug used in most of the tonics/elixirs that were developed to treat a wide variety of illnesses. Today, cocaine is a Schedule II drug, meaning that it has high potential for abuse, but can be administered by a doctor for legitimate medical uses, such as a local anesthetic for some eye, ear, and throat surgeries.

There are basically two chemical forms of cocaine: the hydrochloride salt and the "freebase." The hydrochloride salt, or powdered form of cocaine, dissolves in water and, when abused, can be taken intravenously (by vein) or intranasally (in the nose). Freebase refers to a compound that has not been neutralized by an acid to make the hydrochloride salt. The freebase form of cocaine is smokable.

Cocaine is generally sold on the street as a fine, white, crystalline powder, known as "coke," "C," "snow," "flake," or "blow." Street dealers generally dilute it with such inert substances as cornstarch, talcum powder, and/or sugar, or with such active drugs as procaine (a chemically-related local anesthetic) or with such other stimulants as amphetamines.

What Is Crack?

Crack is the street name given to the freebase form of cocaine that has been processed from the powdered cocaine hydrochloride form to a smokable substance. The term "crack" refers to the crackling sound heard when the mixture is smoked. Crack cocaine is processed with ammonia or sodium bicarbonate (baking soda) and water, and heated to remove the hydrochloride.

Because crack is smoked, the user experiences a high in less than 10 seconds. This rather immediate and euphoric effect is one of the reasons that crack became enormously popular in the mid 1980s. Another reason is that crack is inexpensive both to produce and to buy.

What Is the Scope of Cocaine Use in the United States?

Trends in 30-Day Prevalence of Cocaine Abuse among Eighth, Tenth, and Twelfth Graders, 1991-1998

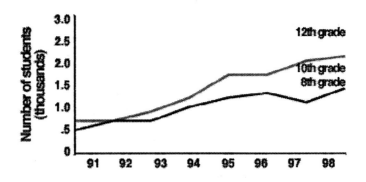

In 1997, an estimated 1.5 million Americans (0.7 percent of those age 12 and older) were current cocaine users, according to the 1997 National Household Survey on Drug Abuse (NHSDA). This number has not changed significantly since 1992, although it is a dramatic decrease from the 1985 peak of 5.7 million cocaine users(3 percent of the population). Based upon additional data sources that take into account users underrepresented in the NHSDA, the Office of National Drug Control Policy estimates the number of chronic cocaine users at 3.6 million.

Adults 18 to 25 years old have a higher rate of current cocaine use than those in any other age group. Overall, men have a higher rate of current cocaine use than do women. Also, according to the 1997 NHSDA, rates of current cocaine use were 1.4 percent for African Americans, 0.8 percent for Hispanics, and 0.6 percent for Caucasians.

Crack cocaine remains a serious problem in the United States. The NHSDA estimated the number of current crack users to be about 604,000 in 1997, which does not reflect any significant change since 1988.

The 1998 Monitoring the Future Survey, which annually surveys teen attitudes and recent drug use, reports that lifetime and past-year use of crack increased among eighth graders to its highest levels since 1991, the first year data were available for this grade. The percentage of eighth graders reporting crack use at least once in their lives increased from 2.7 percent in 1997 to 3.2 percent in 1998. Past-year use of crack also rose slightly among this group, although no changes were found for other grades.

Data from the Drug Abuse Warning Network (DAWN) showed that cocaine-related emergency room visits, after increasing 78 percent between 1990 and 1994, remained level between 1994 and 1996, with 152,433 cocaine-related episodes reported in 1996.

How Is Cocaine Used?

The principal routes of cocaine administration are oral, intranasal, intravenous, and inhalation. The slang terms for these routes are, respectively, "chewing," "snorting," "mainlining," "injecting," and "smoking" (including freebase and crack cocaine). Snorting is the process of inhaling cocaine powder through the nostrils, where it is absorbed into the bloodstream through the nasal tissues. Injecting releases the drug directly into the bloodstream, and heightens the intensity of its effects. Smoking involves the inhalation of cocaine vapor or smoke into the lungs, where absorption into the bloodstream is as rapid as by injection. The drug can also be rubbed onto mucous tissues. Some users combine cocaine powder or crack with heroin in a "speedball."

Cocaine use ranges from occasional use to repeated or compulsive use, with a variety of patterns between these extremes. There is no safe way to use cocaine. Any route of administration can lead to absorption of toxic amounts of cocaine, leading to acute cardiovascular or cerebrovascular emergencies that could result in sudden death. Repeated cocaine use by any route of administration can produce addiction and other adverse health consequences.

How Does Cocaine Produce Its Effects?

A great amount of research has been devoted to understanding the way cocaine produces its pleasurable effects, and the reasons it is so addictive. One mechanism is through its effects on structures deep in the brain. Scientists have discovered regions within the brain that, when stimulated, produce feelings of pleasure. One neural system that appears to be most affected by cocaine originates in a region, located deep within the brain, called the ventral tegmental area (VTA). Nerve cells originating in the VTA extend to the region of the brain known as the nucleus accumbens, one of the brain's key pleasure centers. In studies using animals, for example, all types of pleasurable stimuli, such as food, water, sex, and many drugs of abuse, cause increased activity in the nucleus accumbens.

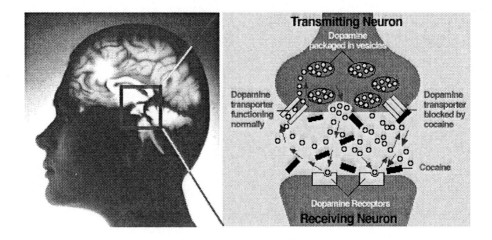

Cocaine in the Brain

In the normal communication process, dopamine is released by a neuron into the synapse, where it can bind with dopamine receptors on neighboring neurons. Normally dopamine is then recycled back into the transmitting neuron by a specialized protein called the dopamine transporter. If cocaine is present, it attaches to the dopamine transporter and blocks the normal recycling process, resulting in a build-up of dopamine in the synapse which contributes to the pleasurable effects of cocaine.

Researchers have discovered that, when a pleasurable event is occurring, it is accompanied by a large increase in the amounts of dopamine released in the nucleus accumbens by neurons originating in the VTA. In the normal communication process, dopamine is released by a neuron into the synapse (the small gap between two neurons), where it binds with specialized proteins (called dopamine receptors) on the neighboring neuron, thereby sending a signal to that neuron. Drugs of abuse are able to interfere with this normal communication process. For example, scientists have discovered that cocaine blocks the removal of dopamine from the synapse, resulting in an accumulation of dopamine. This buildup of dopamine causes continuous stimulation of receiving neurons, probably resulting in the euphoria commonly reported by cocaine abusers.

As cocaine abuse continues, tolerance often develops. This means that higher doses and more frequent use of cocaine are required for the brain to register the same level of pleasure experienced during initial use. Recent studies have shown that, during periods of abstinence from cocaine use, the memory of the euphoria associated with cocaine use, or mere exposure to cues associated with drug use, can trigger tremendous craving and relapse to drug use, even after long periods of abstinence.

What Are the Short-Term Effects of Cocaine Use?

- Increased energy
- Decreased appetite
- Mental alertness
- Increased heart rate and blood pressure
- Constricted blood vessels
- Increased temperature
- Dilated pupils

Cocaine's effects appear almost immediately after a single dose, and disappear within a few minutes or hours. Taken in small amounts (up to 100 mg), cocaine usually makes the user feel euphoric, energetic, talkative, and mentally alert, especially to the sensations of sight, sound, and touch. It can also temporarily decrease the need for food and sleep. Some users find that the drug helps them to perform simple physical and intellectual tasks more quickly, while others can experience the opposite effect.

The duration of cocaine's immediate euphoric effects depends upon the route of administration. The faster the absorption, the more intense the high. Also, the faster the absorption, the shorter the duration of action. The high from snorting is relatively slow in onset, and may last 15 to 30 minutes, while that from smoking may last 5 to 10 minutes.

The short-term physiological effects of cocaine include constricted blood vessels; dilated pupils; and increased temperature, heart rate, and blood pressure. Large amounts (several hundred milligrams or more) intensify the user's high, but may also lead to bizarre, erratic, and violent behavior. These users may experience tremors, vertigo, muscle twitches, paranoia, or, with repeated doses, a toxic reaction closely resembling amphetamine poisoning. Some users of cocaine report feelings of restlessness, irritability, and anxiety. In rare instances, sudden death can occur on the first use of cocaine or unexpectedly thereafter. Cocaine-related deaths are often a result of cardiac arrest or seizures followed by respiratory arrest.

What Are the Long-Term Effects of Cocaine Use?

- Addiction
- Irritability and mood disturbances
- Restlessness
- Paranoia
- Auditory hallucinations

Cocaine is a powerfully addictive drug. Once having tried cocaine, an individual may have difficulty predicting or controlling the extent to which he or she will continue to use the drug. Cocaine's stimulant and addictive effects are thought to be primarily a result of its ability to inhibit the reabsorption of dopamine by nerve cells. Dopamine is released as part of the brain's reward system, and is either directly or indirectly involved in the addictive properties of every major drug of abuse.

An appreciable tolerance to cocaine's high may develop, with many addicts reporting that they seek but fail to achieve as much pleasure as they did from their first experience. Some users will frequently increase their doses to intensify and prolong the euphoric effects. While tolerance to the high can occur, users can also become more sensitive (sensitization) to cocaine's anesthetic and convulsant effects, without increasing the dose taken. This increased sensitivity may explain some deaths occurring after apparently low doses of cocaine.

Use of cocaine in a binge, during which the drug is taken repeatedly and at increasingly high doses, leads to a state of increasing irritability, restlessness, and paranoia. This may result in a full-blown paranoid psychosis, in which the individual loses touch with reality and experiences auditory hallucinations.

What Are the Medical Complications of Cocaine Abuse?

- Cardiovascular effects
- Disturbances in heart rhythm
- Heart attacks
- Respiratory effects
- Chest pain
- Respiratory failure

- Neurological effects
- Strokes
- Seizures and headaches
- Gastrointestinal complications
- Abdominal pain
- Nausea

There are enormous medical complications associated with cocaine use. Some of the most frequent complications are cardiovascular effects, including disturbances in heart rhythm and heart attacks; such respiratory effects as chest pain and respiratory failure; neurological effects, including strokes, seizure, and headaches; and gastrointestinal complications, including abdominal pain and nausea.

Cocaine use has been linked to many types of heart disease. Cocaine has been found to trigger chaotic heart rhythms, called ventricular fibrillation; accelerate heartbeat and breathing; and increase blood pressure and body temperature. Physical symptoms may include chest pain, nausea, blurred vision, fever, muscle spasms, convulsions and coma.

Different routes of cocaine administration can produce different adverse effects. Regularly snorting cocaine, for example, can lead to loss of sense of smell, nosebleeds, problems with swallowing, hoarseness, and an overall irritation of the nasal septum, which can lead to a chronically inflamed, runny nose. Ingested cocaine can cause severe bowel gangrene, due to reduced blood flow. And, persons who inject cocaine have puncture marks and "tracks," most commonly in their forearms. Intravenous cocaine users may also experience an allergic reaction, either to the drug, or to some additive in street cocaine, which can result, in severe cases, in death. Because cocaine has a tendency to decrease food intake, many chronic cocaine users lose their appetites and can experience significant weight loss and malnourishment.

Research has revealed a potentially dangerous interaction between cocaine and alcohol. Taken in combination, the two drugs are converted by the body to cocaethylene. Cocaethylene has a longer duration of action in the brain and is more toxic than either drug alone. While more research needs to be done, it is noteworthy that the mixture of cocaine and alcohol is the most common two-drug combination that results in drug-related death.

Are Cocaine Abusers at Risk for Contracting HIV/AIDS and Hepatitis B and C?

Yes. Cocaine abusers, especially those who inject, are at increased risk for contracting such infectious diseases as human immunodeficiency virus (HIV/AIDS) and hepatitis. In fact, use and abuse of illicit drugs, including crack cocaine, have become the leading risk factors for new cases of HIV. Drug abuse-related spread of HIV can result from direct transmission of the virus through the sharing of contaminated needles and paraphernalia between injecting drug users. It can also result from indirect transmission, such as an HIV-infected mother transmitting the virus perinatally to her child. This is particularly alarming, given that more than 60 percent of new AIDS cases are women. Research has also shown that drug use can interfere with judgment about risk-taking behavior, and can potentially lead to reduced precautions about having sex, the sharing of needles and injection paraphernalia, and the trading of sex for drugs, by both men and women.

Additionally, hepatitis C is spreading rapidly among injection drug users; current estimates indicate infection rates of 65 to 90 percent in this population. At present, there is no vaccine for the hepatitis C virus, and the only treatment is expensive, often unsuccessful, and may have serious side effects.

What Is the Effect of Maternal Cocaine Use?

The full extent of the effects of prenatal drug exposure on a child is not completely known, but many scientific studies have documented that babies born to mothers who abuse cocaine during pregnancy are often prematurely delivered, have low birth weights and smaller head circumferences, and are often shorter in length.

Estimating the full extent of the consequences of maternal drug abuse is difficult, and determining the specific hazard of a particular drug to the unborn child is even more problematic, given that, typically, more than one substance is abused. Such factors as the amount and number of all drugs abused; inadequate prenatal care; abuse and neglect of the children, due to the mother's lifestyle; socio-economic status; poor maternal nutrition; other health problems; and exposure to sexually transmitted diseases, are just some examples of the difficulty in determining the direct impact of perinatal cocaine use, for example, on maternal and fetal outcome.

Many may recall that "crack babies," or babies born to mothers who used cocaine while pregnant, were written off by many a decade ago as a lost generation. They were predicted to suffer from severe, irreversible damage, including reduced intelligence and social skills. It was later found that this was a gross exaggeration. Most crack-exposed babies appear to recover quite well. However, the fact that most of these children appear normal should not be over-interpreted as a positive sign. Using sophisticated technologies, scientists are now finding that exposure to cocaine during fetal development may lead to subtle, but significant, deficits later, especially with behaviors that are crucial to success in the classroom, such as blocking out distractions and concentrating for long periods of time.

What Treatments Are Effective for Cocaine Abusers?

There has been an enormous increase in the number of people seeking treatment for cocaine addiction during the 1980s and 1990s. Treatment providers in most areas of the country, except in the West and Southwest, report that cocaine is the most commonly cited drug of abuse among their clients. The majority of individuals seeking treatment smoke crack, and are likely to be poly-drug users, or users of more than one substance. The widespread abuse of cocaine has stimulated extensive efforts to develop treatment programs for this type of drug abuse. Cocaine abuse and addiction is a complex problem involving biological changes in the brain as well as a myriad of social, familial, and environmental factors. Therefore, treatment of cocaine addiction is complex, and must address a variety of problems. Like any good treatment plan, cocaine treatment strategies need to assess the psychobiological, social, and pharmacological aspects of the patient's drug abuse.

Pharmacological Approaches

There are no medications currently available to treat cocaine addiction specifically. Consequently, NIDA is aggressively pursuing the identification and testing of new cocaine treatment medications. Several newly emerging compounds are being investigated to assess their safety and efficacy in treating cocaine addiction. For example, one of the most promising anti-cocaine drug medications to date, selegeline, is being taken into multi-site phase III clinical trials in 1999. These trials will evaluate two innovative routes of selegeline administration: a transdermal patch and a time-released pill, to determine which is most beneficial. Disulfiram, a medication that has been used to treat alcoholism, has also been shown, in clinical studies, to be effective in reducing cocaine abuse. Because of mood changes experienced during the early stages of cocaine abstinence, antidepressant drugs have been shown to be of some benefit. In addition to the problems of treating addiction, cocaine overdose results in many deaths every year, and medical treatments are being developed to deal with the acute emergencies resulting from excessive cocaine abuse.

Behavioral Interventions

Many behavioral treatments have been found to be effective for cocaine addiction, including both residential and outpatient approaches. Indeed, behavioral therapies are often the only available, effective treatment approaches to many drug problems, including cocaine addiction, for which there is, as yet, no viable medication. However, integration of both types of treatments is ultimately the most effective approach for treating addiction. It is important to match the best treatment regimen to the needs of the patient. This may include adding to or removing from an individual's treatment regimen a number of different components or elements. For example, if an individual is prone to relapses, a relapse component should be added to the program.

A behavioral therapy component that is showing positive results in many cocaine-addicted populations, is contingency management. Contingency management uses a voucher-based system to give positive rewards for staying in treatment and remaining cocaine free. Based on drug-free urine tests, the patients earn points, which can be exchanged for items that encourage healthy living, such as joining a gym, or going to a movie and dinner.

Cognitive-behavioral therapy is another approach. Cognitive-behavioral coping skills treatment, for example, is a short-term, focused approach to helping cocaine-addicted individuals become abstinent from cocaine and other substances. The underlying assumption is that learning processes play an important role in the development and continuation of cocaine abuse and dependence. The same learning processes can be employed to help individuals reduce drug use. This approach attempts to help patients to recognize, avoid, and cope; i.e., recognize the situations in which they are most likely to use cocaine, avoid these situations when appropriate, and cope more effectively with a range of problems and problematic behaviors associated with drug abuse. This therapy is also noteworthy because of its compatibility with a range of other treatments patients may receive, such as pharmacotherapy.

Therapeutic communities, or residential programs with planned lengths of stay of 6 to 12 months, offer another alternative to those in need of treatment for cocaine addiction. Therapeutic communities are often comprehensive, in that they focus on the resocialization of the individual to society, and can include on-site vocational rehabilitation and other supportive services. Therapeutic communities typically are used to treat patients with more severe problems, such as co-occurring mental health problems and criminal involvement.

Where Can I Get Further Scientific Information about Cocaine Addiction?

To learn more about cocaine and other drugs of abuse, contact the National Clearinghouse for Alcohol and Drug Information (NCADI) at 1-800-729-6686. Information specialists are available to assist you in locating needed information and resources.

Fact sheets on the health effects of drug abuse and other topics can be ordered free of charge, in English and Spanish, by calling NIDA INFOFAX at 1-888-NIH-NIDA (1-888-644-6432), or for hearing impaired persons, 1-888-TTY-NIDA (1-888-889-6432).

Information can also be accessed through the NIDA World Wide Web site (**http://www.nida.nih.gov/**)   or   the   NCADI   Web   site (**http://www.health.org/**).

NIDA's Therapy Manuals series presents clear, helpful information to aid drug treatment practitioners in providing the best possible care. The therapies presented in the manuals exemplify the best of what is currently known about treating cocaine addiction. The first three manuals in the series are:

- Manual 1: A Cognitive-Behavioral Approach: Treating Cocaine Addiction: **http://165.112.78.61/TXManuals/CBT/CBT1.html**

- Manual 2: A Community Reinforcement Plus Vouchers Approach: Treating Cocaine Addiction: **http://165.112.78.61/TXManuals/CRA/CRA1.html**

- Manual 3: An Individual Drug Counseling Approach to Treat Cocaine Addiction: The Collaborative Cocaine Treatment Study Model: **http://165.112.78.61/TXManuals/IDCA/IDCA1.html**

In addition to the guideline above, NIDA also publishes shorter guidelines in the form of INFOFAXs. The INFOFAX below is one recently dedicated to crack and cocaine:

Crack and Cocaine INFOFAX[9]

Cocaine is a powerfully addictive drug of abuse. Once having tried cocaine, an individual cannot predict or control the extent to which he or she will continue to use the drug.

The major routes of administration of cocaine are sniffing or snorting, injecting, and smoking (including free-base and crack cocaine). Snorting is the process of inhaling cocaine powder through the nose where it is absorbed into the bloodstream through the nasal tissues. Injecting is the act of using a needle to release the drug directly into the bloodstream. Smoking involves inhaling cocaine vapor or smoke into the lungs where absorption into the bloodstream is as rapid as by injection.

"Crack" is the street name given to cocaine that has been processed from cocaine hydrochloride to a free base for smoking. Rather than requiring the more volatile method of processing cocaine using ether, crack cocaine is processed with ammonia or sodium bicarbonate (baking soda) and water and heated to remove the hydrochloride, thus producing a form of cocaine that can be smoked. The term "crack" refers to the crackling sound heard when the mixture is smoked (heated), presumably from the sodium bicarbonate.

There is great risk whether cocaine is ingested by inhalation (snorting), injection, or smoking. It appears that compulsive cocaine use may develop even more rapidly if the substance is smoked rather than snorted. Smoking allows extremely high doses of cocaine to reach the brain very quickly and brings an intense and immediate high. The injecting drug user is at risk for transmitting or acquiring HIV infection/AIDS if needles or other injection equipment are shared.

---

[9] Adapted from **http://165.112.78.61/Infofax/cocaine.html**.

Health Hazards

Cocaine is a strong central nervous system stimulant that interferes with the reabsorption process of dopamine, a chemical messenger associated with pleasure and movement. Dopamine is released as part of the brain's reward system and is involved in the high that characterizes cocaine consumption. Physical effects of cocaine use include constricted peripheral blood vessels, dilated pupils, and increased temperature, heart rate, and blood pressure. The duration of cocaine's immediate euphoric effects, which include hyper-stimulation, reduced fatigue, and mental clarity, depends on the route of administration. The faster the absorption, the more intense the high. On the other hand, the faster the absorption, the shorter the duration of action. The high from snorting may last 15 to 30 minutes, while that from smoking may last 5 to 10 minutes. Increased use can reduce the period of stimulation.

Some users of cocaine report feelings of restlessness, irritability, and anxiety. An appreciable tolerance to the high may be developed, and many addicts report that they seek but fail to achieve as much pleasure as they did from their first exposure. Scientific evidence suggests that the powerful neuropsychologic reinforcing property of cocaine is responsible for an individual's continued use, despite harmful physical and social consequences. In rare instances, sudden death can occur on the first use of cocaine or unexpectedly thereafter. However, there is no way to determine who is prone to sudden death.

High doses of cocaine and/or prolonged use can trigger paranoia. Smoking crack cocaine can produce a particularly aggressive paranoid behavior in users. When addicted individuals stop using cocaine, they often become depressed. This also may lead to further cocaine use to alleviate depression. Prolonged cocaine snorting can result in ulceration of the mucous membrane of the nose and can damage the nasal septum enough to cause it to collapse. Cocaine-related deaths are often a result of cardiac arrest or seizures followed by respiratory arrest.

Added Danger: Cocaethylene

When people mix cocaine and alcohol consumption, they are compounding the danger each drug poses and unknowingly forming a complex chemical experiment within their bodies. NIDA-funded researchers have found that the human liver combines cocaine and alcohol and manufactures a third substance, cocaethylene, that intensifies cocaine's euphoric effects, while possibly increasing the risk of sudden death.

Treatment

The widespread abuse of cocaine has stimulated extensive efforts to develop treatment programs for this type of drug abuse.

NIDA's top research priority is to find a medication to block or greatly reduce the effects of cocaine, to be used as one part of a comprehensive treatment program. NIDA-funded researchers are also looking at medications that help alleviate the severe craving that people in treatment for cocaine addiction often experience. Several medications are currently being investigated to test their safety and efficacy in treating cocaine addiction.

In addition to treatment medications, behavioral interventions, particularly cognitive behavioral therapy, can be effective in decreasing drug use by patients in treatment for cocaine abuse. Providing the optimal combination of treatment services for each individual is critical to successful treatment outcome.

Extent of Use

Monitoring the Future Study (MTF)

MTF is an annual survey on drug use and related attitudes of America's adolescents that began in 1975. The survey is conducted by the University of Michigan's Institute for Social Research and is funded by NIDA. Copies of the latest survey are available from the National Clearinghouse for Alcohol and Drug Information at 1-800-729-6686 The MTF assesses the extent of drug use among adolescents and young adults across the country.

The proportion of high school seniors who have used cocaine at least once in their lifetimes has increased from a low of 5.9 percent in 1994 to 9.8 percent in 1999. However, this is lower than its peak of 17.3 percent in 1985. Current (past month) use of cocaine by seniors decreased from a high of 6.7 percent in 1985 to 2.6 percent in 1999. Also in 1999, 7.7 percent of 10th-graders had tried cocaine at least once, up from a low of 3.3 percent in 1992. The percentage of 8th-graders who had ever tried cocaine has increased from a low of 2.3 percent in 1991 to 4.7 percent in 1999.

Of college students 1 to 4 years beyond high school, in 1995, 3.6 percent had used cocaine within the past year, and 0.7 percent had used cocaine in the past month.

Cocaine Use by Students, 1999: Monitoring the Future Study

	8th-Graders	10th-Graders	12th-Graders
Ever Used	4.7%	7.7%	9.8%
Used in Past Year	2.7	4.9	6.2
Used in Past Month	1.3	1.8	2.6

Community Epidemiology Work Group (CEWG)

CEWG is a NIDA-sponsored network of researchers from 20 major U.S. metropolitan areas and selected foreign countries who meet semiannually to discuss the current epidemiology of drug abuse. Although demographic data continue to show most cocaine users as older, inner-city crack addicts, isolated field reports indicate new groups of users: teenagers smoking crack with marijuana in some cities; Hispanic crack users in Texas; and in the Atlanta area, middle-class suburban users of cocaine hydrochloride and female crack users in their thirties with no prior drug history.

National Household Survey on Drug Abuse (NHSDA)

NHSDA is an annual survey conducted by the Substance Abuse and Mental Health Services Administration. Copies of the latest survey are available from the National Clearinghouse for Alcohol and Drug Information at 1-800-729-6686. In 1998, about 1.7 million Americans were current (at least once per month) cocaine users. This is about 0.8 percent of the population age 12 and older; about 437,000 of these used crack. The rate of current cocaine use in 1998 was highest among Americans ages 18 to 25 (2.0 percent). The rate of use for this age group was significantly higher in 1998 than in 1997, when it was 1.2 percent.

More Guideline Sources

The guideline above on cocaine dependence is only one example of the kind of material that you can find online and free of charge. The remainder of this chapter will direct you to other sources which either publish or can help you find additional guidelines on topics related to cocaine dependence. Many of the guidelines listed below address topics that may be of particular relevance to your specific situation or of special interest to only some patients with cocaine dependence. Due to space limitations these sources are listed in a concise manner. Do not hesitate to consult the following sources by either using the Internet hyperlink provided, or, in cases where the contact information is provided, contacting the publisher or author directly.

Topic Pages: MEDLINEplus

For patients wishing to go beyond guidelines published by specific Institutes of the NIH, the National Library of Medicine has created a vast and patient-oriented healthcare information portal called MEDLINEplus. Within this Internet-based system are "health topic pages." You can think of a health topic page as a guide to patient guides. To access this system, log on to **http://www.nlm.nih.gov/medlineplus/healthtopics.html**. From there you can either search using the alphabetical index or browse by broad topic areas. Recently, MEDLINEplus listed the following as being relevant to cocaine dependence:

Alcoholism
http://www.nlm.nih.gov/medlineplus/alcoholism.html

Amphetamine Abuse
http://www.nlm.nih.gov/medlineplus/amphetamineabuse.html

Club Drugs
http://www.nlm.nih.gov/medlineplus/clubdrugs.html

Marijuana Abuse
http://www.nlm.nih.gov/medlineplus/marijuanaabuse.html

Pregnancy and Substance Abuse
http://www.nlm.nih.gov/medlineplus/pregnancyandsubstanceabuse.html

Within the health topic page dedicated to cocaine dependence, the following was recently recommended to patients:

- General/Overviews

  Cocaine
  Source: Drug Enforcement Administration
  http://www.usdoj.gov/dea/concern/cocaine.html

  JAMA Patient Page: Cocaine Addiction
  Source: American Medical Association
  http://www.medem.com/medlb/article_detaillb.cfm?article_ID=ZZ
  ZW2IF4HVC&sub_cat=466

- Treatment

  Blood Pressure Medication May Improve Cocaine Treatment Results in Patients With Severe Withdrawal Symptoms
  Source: National Institute on Drug Abuse
  http://www.nida.nih.gov/NIDA_Notes/NNVol16N6/Blood.html

  Cognitive-Behavioral Approach: Treating Cocaine Addiction
  Source: National Institute on Drug Abuse
  http://www.nida.nih.gov/TXManuals/CBT/CBT4.html

  Joint Treatment of PTSD and Cocaine Abuse May Reduce Severity of Both Disorders
  Source: National Institute on Drug Abuse
  http://www.nida.nih.gov/NIDA_notes/NNVol18N1/Joint.html

  Principles of Drug Addiction Treatment: A Research-Based Guide
  Source: National Institute on Drug Abuse
  http://www.nida.nih.gov/PODAT/PODATindex.html

  Types of Treatment (Drug Addiction)
  Source: Office of National Drug Control Policy
  http://www.whitehousedrugpolicy.gov/treat/treatment.html

- Specific Conditions/Aspects

  Mind Over Matter - The Brain's Response to Stimulants
  Source: National Institute on Drug Abuse
  http://www.nida.nih.gov/MOM/STIM/MOMSTIM1.html

  Oops: How Casual Drug Use Leads to Addiction
  Source: National Institute on Drug Abuse
  http://www.nida.nih.gov/Published_Articles/Oops.html

- Children

    What You Need to Know About Drugs: Cocaine and Crack
    Source: Nemours Foundation
    http://kidshealth.org/kid/grow/drugs_alcohol/know_drugs_cocain
    e.html

- From the National Institutes of Health

    Cocaine Abuse and Addiction
    Source: National Institute on Drug Abuse
    http://www.nida.nih.gov/ResearchReports/Cocaine/Cocaine.html

    Crack and Cocaine
    Source: National Institute on Drug Abuse
    http://www.nida.nih.gov/Infofax/cocaine.html

- Latest News

    Updated Directory of Drug, Alcohol Abuse Treatment Programs Available
    Source: 04/28/2004, Substance Abuse and Mental Health Services Administration
    http://www.samhsa.gov/news/newsreleases/040427nr_directory.ht
    m

- Organizations

    American Council for Drug Education
    http://www.acde.org/

    Drug Enforcement Administration
    http://www.usdoj.gov/dea/

    National Clearinghouse for Alcohol and Drug Information
    Source: Dept. of Health and Human Services, Substance Abuse and Mental Health Services Administration
    http://www.health.org/

    National Institute on Drug Abuse
    http://www.nida.nih.gov/

    Office of National Drug Control Policy
    http://www.whitehousedrugpolicy.gov/

    Partnership for a Drug-Free America
    http://drugfreeamerica.com/

- Research

  Amphetamine or Cocaine Exposure May Limit Brain Cell Changes That Normally Occur with Life Experiences
  Source: National Institute on Drug Abuse
  http://www.nih.gov/news/pr/aug2003/nida-25.htm

  Chronic Solvent Abusers Have More Brain Abnormalities and Cognitive Impairments Than Cocaine Abusers
  Source: National Institute on Drug Abuse
  http://www.nida.nih.gov/NIDA_notes/NNVol17N4/Chronic.html

  Cocaine Abusers' Cognitive Deficits Compromise Treatment Outcomes
  Source: National Institute on Drug Abuse
  http://www.drugabuse.gov/NIDA_notes/NNvol19N1/Cocaine.html

  Cocaine May Compromise Immune System, Increase Risk of Infection
  Source: National Institute on Drug Abuse
  http://www.drugabuse.gov/NIDA_notes/NNvol18N6/Cocaine.html

  Cocaine's Effect on Blood Components May Be Linked to Heart Attack and Stroke
  Source: National Institute on Drug Abuse
  http://www.nida.nih.gov/NIDA_notes/NNVol17N6/Cocaine.html

  Combining Medications May Be Effective Treatment for "Speedball" Abuse
  Source: National Institute on Drug Abuse
  http://www.nida.nih.gov/NIDA_notes/NNVol17N3/Combining.html

  Small Study Suggests Anticonvulsant Drug Holds Promise as Therapy for Cocaine Abuse
  Source: National Institute on Drug Abuse
  http://www.nih.gov/news/pr/sep2003/nida-22.htm

  Study Finds Significant Mental Deficits in Toddlers Exposed to Cocaine Before Birth
  Source: National Institute on Drug Abuse
  http://www.nida.nih.gov/NIDA_notes/NNVol17N5/Study.html

  Study Opens Promising New Approach to Developing Medications To Prevent Relapse to Cocaine Use
  Source: National Institute on Drug Abuse
  http://www.nida.nih.gov/NIDA_notes/NNVol17N3/Promising.ht

ml

Study Sheds Light on Progression to Drug Dependence
Source: National Institute on Drug Abuse
http://www.nida.nih.gov/NIDA_notes/NNVol17N4/BBoard.html

- Statistics

  High School and Youth Trends
  Source: National Institute on Drug Abuse
  http://www.nida.nih.gov/infofax/hsyouthtrends.html

  Treatment Admissions for Injection Drug Abuse
  Source: Substance Abuse and Mental Health Services Administration
  http://www.oas.samhsa.gov/2k2/ivdrugTX/ivdrugTX.htm

  Women in Treatment for Smoked Cocaine: 2000
  Source: Substance Abuse and Mental Health Services Administration
  http://www.oas.samhsa.gov/2k3/FemCrack/FemCrack.htm

- Teenagers

  Tips for Teens: The Truth About Cocaine
  Source: Substance Abuse and Mental Health Services Administration
  http://www.health.org/govpubs/phd640/

  What's Up With Cocaine & Crack?
  Source: Drug Enforcement Administration
  http://www.usdoj.gov/dea/pubs/straight/cocaine.htm

- Women

  Cocaine Use during Pregnancy
  Source: March of Dimes Birth Defects Foundation
  http://www.marchofdimes.com/professionals/681_1169.asp

You may also choose to use the search utility provided by MEDLINEplus at the following Web address: **http://www.nlm.nih.gov/medlineplus/**. Simply type a keyword into the search box and click "Search." This utility is similar to the NIH search utility, with the exception that it only includes materials that are linked within the MEDLINEplus system (mostly patient-oriented information). It also has the disadvantage of generating unstructured results. We recommend, therefore, that you use this method only if you have a very targeted search.

The Combined Health Information Database (CHID)

CHID Online is a reference tool that maintains a database directory of thousands of journal articles and patient education guidelines on cocaine dependence and related conditions. One of the advantages of CHID over other sources is that it offers summaries that describe the guidelines available, including contact information and pricing. CHID's general Web site is **http://chid.nih.gov/**. To search this database, go to **http://chid.nih.gov/detail/detail.html**. In particular, you can use the advanced search options to look up pamphlets, reports, brochures, and information kits. The following was recently posted in this archive:

- **Cocaine: Your child and drugs**

  Source: Elk Grove Village, IL: American Academy of Pediatrics. n.d. 1 p.

  Contact: Available from Publications Department, American Academy of Pediatrics, 141 Northwest Point Boulevard, P.O. Box 927, Elk Grove Village, IL 60009-0927. Telephone: (847) 228-5005 or (800) 433-9016 / fax: (847) 228-5097 / e-mail: ksanabria@aap.org / Web site: http://www.aap.org. $15.00 for 100 copies, members; $20.00, nonmembers. Minimum order: 100 copies.

  Summary: This brochure discusses the dangers of **cocaine** and alerts parents to the warning signs of **cocaine** abuse.

- **Cocaine**

  Source: Rochester, NY: Substance and Alcohol Intervention Services for the Deaf (SAISD), Rochester Institute of Technology (RIT). 1996. 2 p.

  Contact: Available from Substance and Alcohol Intervention Services for the Deaf (SAISD). Rochester Institute of Technology (RIT), Hale-Andrews Student Life Center, 115 Lomb Memorial Drive, Rochester, NY 14623-5608. Voice/TTY (716) 475-4978; Fax (716) 475-7375; E-mail: SPCGRL@RIT.EDU. PRICE: Single copy free.

  Summary: This brochure provides basic information for deaf people about **cocaine.** The brochure describes **cocaine** and the physical effects of using it, how **cocaine** is taken into the body, some slang terms for **cocaine,** and the problem of relapses in **cocaine** use. The brochure also includes a section listing places and organizations where readers can get help, including hospitals, employee assistance programs, doctors, clergy and family counselors, the National Council on Alcoholism and Drug Dependency (NCADD), and Substance and Alcohol Intervention Services for the Deaf (SAISD). The front cover of the brochure is illustrated with the sign for **cocaine.**

- **Hey! What's Goin' Down? Well There's Crack, Heroin, Cocaine, Dilaudid, and a New Flag is Going Up! It's HIV**

  Contact: Oklahoma State Department of Health, Disease & Prevention Services, HIV/STD Service, 1000 NE 10th St, Oklahoma City, OK, 73117-1299, (405) 271-4636, http://www.health.state.ok.us/program/hivstd/index.html.

  Summary: This brochure uses comic book style lettering and illustrations to tell readers about Human immunodeficiency virus (HIV) and Acquired immunodeficiency syndrome (AIDS). It informs readers that sharing needles can be fatal because HIV is easily transmitted that way. Readers are cautioned not to share needles, or at least to clean needles and syringes with household bleach and rinse with water. They are told that having sex with anyone carrying the virus is dangerous, and the greater the number of sex partners, the greater the danger. The use of latex condoms and nonoxynol 9 is recommended. The brochure states that HIV is not transmitted by doorknobs, toilet seats, mosquitoes, drinking glasses, telephones, or swimming pools.

Healthfinder™

Healthfinder™ is an additional source sponsored by the U.S. Department of Health and Human Services which offers links to hundreds of other sites that contain healthcare information. This Web site is located at **http://www.healthfinder.gov**. Again, keyword searches can be used to find guidelines. The following was recently found in this database:

- **Cocaine Facts and Figures**

  Summary: Pure cocaine was first used in the 1880s as a local anesthetic in eye, nose, and throat surgeries because of its ability to provide anesthesia as well as to constrict blood vessels and limit bleeding.

  Source: Office of National Drug Control Policy, The White House

  http://www.healthfinder.gov/scripts/recordpass.asp?RecordType=0&RecordID=7197

The NIH Search Utility

After browsing the references listed at the beginning of this chapter, you may want to explore the NIH search utility. This allows you to search for documents on over 100 selected Web sites that comprise the NIH-WEB-SPACE. Each of these servers is "crawled" and indexed on an ongoing basis. Your search will produce a list of various documents, all of which will relate in some way to cocaine dependence. The drawbacks of this approach are that the information is not organized by theme and that the references are often a mix of information for professionals and patients. Nevertheless, a large number of the listed Web sites provide useful background information. We can only recommend this route, therefore, for relatively rare or specific disorders, or when using highly targeted searches. To use the NIH search utility, visit the following Web page: **http://search.nih.gov/index.html**.

Additional Web Sources

A number of Web sites that often link to government sites are available to the public. These can also point you in the direction of essential information. The following is a representative sample:

- AOL: **http://search.aol.com/cat.adp?id=168&layer=&from=subcats**

- Family Village: **http://www.familyvillage.wisc.edu/specific.htm**

- Google: **http://directory.google.com/Top/Health/Conditions_and_Diseases/**

- Med Help International: **http://www.medhelp.org/HealthTopics/A.html**

- Open Directory Project: **http://dmoz.org/Health/Conditions_and_Diseases/**

- Yahoo.com: **http://dir.yahoo.com/Health/Diseases_and_Conditions/**

- WebMD®Health: **http://my.webmd.com/health_topics**

Vocabulary Builder

The material in this chapter may have contained a number of unfamiliar words. The following Vocabulary Builder introduces you to terms used in this chapter that have not been covered in the previous chapter:

Alertness: A state of readiness to detect and respond to certain specified small changes occurring at random intervals in the environment. [NIH]

Cocaethylene: Hard drug formed by cocaine and alcohol. [NIH]

Ether: One of a class of organic compounds in which any two organic radicals are attached directly to a single oxygen atom. [NIH]

Fatigue: The feeling of weariness of mind and body. [NIH]

Forearm: The part between the elbow and the wrist. [NIH]

Hepatitis: Infectious disease of the liver. [NIH]

Impairment: In the context of health experience, an impairment is any loss or abnormality of psychological, physiological, or anatomical structure or function. [NIH]

Nerve: A cordlike structure of nervous tissue that connects parts of the nervous system with other tissues of the body and conveys nervous impulses to, or away from, these tissues. [NIH]

Nucleus: A body of specialized protoplasm found in nearly all cells and containing the chromosomes. [NIH]

Outpatient: A patient who is not an inmate of a hospital but receives diagnosis or treatment in a clinic or dispensary connected with the hospital. [NIH]

Patch: A piece of material used to cover or protect a wound, an injured part, etc.: a patch over the eye. [NIH]

Pediatrics: The branch of medical science concerned with children and their diseases. [NIH]

Prone: Having the front portion of the body downwards. [NIH]

Refer: To send or direct for treatment, aid, information, de decision. [NIH]

Specialist: In medicine, one who concentrates on 1 special branch of medical science. [NIH]

Stimulants: Any drug or agent which causes stimulation. [NIH]

Synapse: The region where the processes of two neurons come into close contiguity, and the nervous impulse passes from one to the other; the fibers of the two are intermeshed, but, according to the general view, there is no direct contiguity. [NIH]

Talcum: A native magnesium silicate. [NIH]

CHAPTER 2. SEEKING GUIDANCE

Overview

Some patients are comforted by the knowledge that a number of organizations dedicate their resources to helping people with cocaine dependence. These associations can become invaluable sources of information and advice. Many associations offer aftercare support, financial assistance, and other important services. Furthermore, healthcare research has shown that support groups often help people to better cope with their conditions.[10] In addition to support groups, your physician can be a valuable source of guidance and support. Therefore, finding a physician that can work with your unique situation is a very important aspect of your care.

In this chapter, we direct you to resources that can help you find patient organizations and medical specialists. We begin by describing how to find associations and peer groups that can help you better understand and cope with cocaine dependence. The chapter ends with a discussion on how to find a doctor that is right for you.

Finding Associations

There are a several Internet directories that provide lists of medical associations with information on or resources relating to cocaine dependence. By consulting all of associations listed in this chapter, you will have nearly exhausted all sources for patient associations concerned with cocaine dependence.

---

[10] Churches, synagogues, and other houses of worship might also have groups that can offer you the social support you need.

The National Health Information Center (NHIC)

The National Health Information Center (NHIC) offers a free referral service to help people find organizations that provide information about cocaine dependence. For more information, see the NHIC's Web site at **http://www.health.gov/NHIC/** or contact an information specialist by calling 1-800-336-4797.

DIRLINE

A comprehensive source of information on associations is the DIRLINE database maintained by the National Library of Medicine. The database comprises some 10,000 records of organizations, research centers, and government institutes and associations which primarily focus on health and biomedicine. DIRLINE is available via the Internet at the following Web site: **http://dirline.nlm.nih.gov/**. Simply type in "cocaine dependence" (or a synonym) or the name of a topic, and the site will list information contained in the database on all relevant organizations.

The Combined Health Information Database

Another comprehensive source of information on healthcare associations is the Combined Health Information Database. Using the "Detailed Search" option, you will need to limit your search to "Organizations" and "cocaine dependence". Type the following hyperlink into your Web browser: **http://chid.nih.gov/detail/detail.html**. To find associations, use the drop boxes at the bottom of the search page where "You may refine your search by." For publication date, select "All Years." Then, select your preferred language and the format option "Organization Resource Sheet." By making these selections and typing in "cocaine dependence" (or synonyms) into the "For these words:" box, you will only receive results on organizations dealing with cocaine dependence. You should check back periodically with this database since it is updated every 3 months.

The National Organization for Rare Disorders, Inc.

The National Organization for Rare Disorders, Inc. has prepared a Web site that provides, at no charge, lists of associations organized by specific diseases. You can access this database at the following Web site:

http://www.rarediseases.org/search/orgsearch.html.   Type   "cocaine dependence" (or a synonym) in the search box, and click "Submit Query."

Online Support Groups

In addition to support groups, commercial Internet service providers offer forums and chat rooms for people with different illnesses and conditions. WebMD®, for example, offers such a service at its Web site: **http://boards.webmd.com/roundtable**. These online self-help communities can help you connect with a network of people whose concerns are similar to yours. Online support groups are places where people can talk informally. If you read about a novel approach, consult with your doctor or other healthcare providers, as the treatments or discoveries you hear about may not be scientifically proven to be safe and effective.

Finding Drug Treatment and Alcohol Abuse Treatment Programs

To find the right drug abuse treatment program or alcohol abuse treatment program for you, two useful resources are available.

National Drug and Treatment Referral Routing Service[11]

The U.S. Department of Health and Human Services (HHS) Substance Abuse and Mental Health Services Administration's (SAMHSA) National Drug and Treatment Referral Routing Service provides a toll-free telephone number for alcohol and drug information/treatment referral assistance. The number is: **1-800-662-HELP**.

When you call the toll-free number, a recorded message gives you the following options:

1 - Printed materials on alcohol and drug information or 24-hour substance abuse treatment referral information in your area (Additional options guide you through information and referral choices, including a Spanish language message.)

2 - Location of a Substance Abuse Treatment Office in your state

---

[11] Adapted from NIAAA: **http://www.niaaa.nih.gov/other/referral.htm**.

Substance Abuse Treatment Facility Locator[12]

Sponsored by the Substance Abuse and Mental Health Services Administration (SAMHSA), this searchable directory of drug and alcohol treatment programs shows the location of facilities around the country that treat alcoholism, alcohol abuse and drug abuse problems (**http://findtreatment.samhsa.gov/**). The Locator includes more than 11,000 addiction treatment programs, including residential treatment centers, outpatient treatment programs, and hospital inpatient programs for drug addiction and alcoholism. Listings include treatment programs for marijuana, cocaine, and heroin addiction, as well as drug and alcohol treatment programs for adolescents, and adults.

SAMHSA endeavors to keep the Locator current. All information in the Locator is completely updated each year, based on facility responses to SAMHSA's National Survey of Substance Abuse Treatment Services. New facilities are added monthly. Updates to facility names, addresses, and telephone numbers are made monthly, if facilities inform SAMHSA of changes (**http://findtreatment.samhsa.gov/facilitylocatordoc.htm**).

Finding Doctors

One of the most important aspects of your treatment will be the relationship between you and your doctor or specialist. All patients with cocaine dependence must go through the process of selecting a physician. While this process will vary from person to person, the Agency for Healthcare Research and Quality makes a number of suggestions, including the following:[13]

- If you are in a managed care plan, check the plan's list of doctors first.

- Ask doctors or other health professionals who work with doctors, such as hospital nurses, for referrals.

- Call a hospital's doctor referral service, but keep in mind that these services usually refer you to doctors on staff at that particular hospital. The services do not have information on the quality of care that these doctors provide.

- Some local medical societies offer lists of member doctors. Again, these lists do not have information on the quality of care that these doctors provide.

---

[12] Adapted from SAMHSA: **http://findtreatment.samhsa.gov/**.
[13] This section has been adapted from the AHRQ:
www.ahrq.gov/consumer/qntascii/qntdr.htm.

Additional steps you can take to locate doctors include the following:

- Information on doctors in some states is available on the Internet at **http://www.docboard.org**. This Web site is run by "Administrators in Medicine," a group of state medical board directors.

- The American Board of Medical Specialties can tell you if your doctor is board certified. "Certified" means that the doctor has completed a training program in a specialty and has passed an exam, or "board," to assess his or her knowledge, skills, and experience to provide quality patient care in that specialty. Primary care doctors may also be certified as specialists. The AMBS Web site is located at **http://www.abms.org/newsearch.asp**.[14] You can also contact the ABMS by phone at 1-866-ASK-ABMS.

- You can call the American Medical Association (AMA) at 800-665-2882 for information on training, specialties, and board certification for many licensed doctors in the United States. This information also can be found in "Physician Select" at the AMA's Web site: **http://www.ama-assn.org/aps/amahg.htm**.

If the previous sources did not meet your needs, you may want to log on to the Web site of the National Organization for Rare Disorders (NORD) at **http://www.rarediseases.org/**. NORD maintains a database of doctors with expertise in various rare diseases. The Metabolic Information Network (MIN), 800-945-2188, also maintains a database of physicians with expertise in various metabolic diseases.

Selecting Your Doctor[15]

When you have compiled a list of prospective doctors, call each of their offices. First, ask if the doctor accepts your health insurance plan and if he or she is taking new patients. If the doctor is not covered by your plan, ask yourself if you are prepared to pay the extra costs. The next step is to schedule a visit with your chosen physician. During the first visit you will have the opportunity to evaluate your doctor and to find out if you feel comfortable with him or her. Ask yourself, did the doctor:

- Give me a chance to ask questions about cocaine dependence?

- Really listen to my questions?

---

[14] While board certification is a good measure of a doctor's knowledge, it is possible to receive quality care from doctors who are not board certified.

[15] This section has been adapted from the AHRQ: **www.ahrq.gov/consumer/qntascii/qntdr.htm**.

- Answer in terms I understood?

- Show respect for me?

- Ask me questions?

- Make me feel comfortable?

- Address the health problem(s) I came with?

- Ask me my preferences about different kinds of treatments for cocaine dependence?

- Spend enough time with me?

Trust your instincts when deciding if the doctor is right for you. But remember, it might take time for the relationship to develop. It takes more than one visit for you and your doctor to get to know each other.

Working with Your Doctor[16]

Research has shown that patients who have good relationships with their doctors tend to be more satisfied with their care and have better results. Here are some tips to help you and your doctor become partners:

- You know important things about your symptoms and your health history. Tell your doctor what you think he or she needs to know.

- It is important to tell your doctor personal information, even if it makes you feel embarrassed or uncomfortable.

- Bring a "health history" list with you (and keep it up to date).

- Always bring any medications you are currently taking with you to the appointment, or you can bring a list of your medications including dosage and frequency information. Talk about any allergies or reactions you have had to your medications.

- Tell your doctor about any natural or alternative medicines you are taking.

- Bring other medical information, such as x-ray films, test results, and medical records.

- Ask questions. If you don't, your doctor will assume that you understood everything that was said.

---

[16] This section has been adapted from the AHRQ:
www.ahrq.gov/consumer/qntascii/qntdr.htm.

- Write down your questions before your visit. List the most important ones first to make sure that they are addressed.

- Consider bringing a friend with you to the appointment to help you ask questions. This person can also help you understand and/or remember the answers.

- Ask your doctor to draw pictures if you think that this would help you understand.

- Take notes. Some doctors do not mind if you bring a tape recorder to help you remember things, but always ask first.

- Let your doctor know if you need more time. If there is not time that day, perhaps you can speak to a nurse or physician assistant on staff or schedule a telephone appointment.

- Take information home. Ask for written instructions. Your doctor may also have brochures and audio and videotapes that can help you.

- After leaving the doctor's office, take responsibility for your care. If you have questions, call. If your symptoms get worse or if you have problems with your medication, call. If you had tests and do not hear from your doctor, call for your test results. If your doctor recommended that you have certain tests, schedule an appointment to get them done. If your doctor said you should see an additional specialist, make an appointment.

By following these steps, you will enhance the relationship you will have with your physician.

Broader Health-Related Resources

In addition to the references above, the NIH has set up guidance Web sites that can help patients find healthcare professionals. These include:[17]

- Caregivers:
  http://www.nlm.nih.gov/medlineplus/caregivers.html

- Choosing a Doctor or Healthcare Service:
  http://www.nlm.nih.gov/medlineplus/choosingadoctororhealthcareserv ice.html

- Hospitals and Health Facilities:
  http://www.nlm.nih.gov/medlineplus/healthfacilities.html

---

[17] You can access this information at
http://www.nlm.nih.gov/medlineplus/healthsystem.html.

PART II: ADDITIONAL RESOURCES AND ADVANCED MATERIAL

ABOUT PART II

In Part II, we introduce you to additional resources and advanced research on cocaine dependence. All too often, patients who conduct their own research are overwhelmed by the difficulty in finding and organizing information. The purpose of the following chapters is to provide you an organized and structured format to help you find additional information resources on cocaine dependence. In Part II, as in Part I, our objective is not to interpret the latest advances on cocaine dependence or render an opinion. Rather, our goal is to give you access to original research and to increase your awareness of sources you may not have already considered. In this way, you will come across the advanced materials often referred to in pamphlets, books, or other general works. Once again, some of this material is technical in nature, so consultation with a professional familiar with cocaine dependence is suggested.

CHAPTER 3. STUDIES ON COCAINE DEPENDENCE

Overview

Every year, academic studies are published on cocaine dependence or related conditions. Broadly speaking, there are two types of studies. The first are peer reviewed. Generally, the content of these studies has been reviewed by scientists or physicians. Peer-reviewed studies are typically published in scientific journals and are usually available at medical libraries. The second type of studies is non-peer reviewed. These works include summary articles that do not use or report scientific results. These often appear in the popular press, newsletters, or similar periodicals.

In this chapter, we will show you how to locate peer-reviewed references and studies on cocaine dependence. We will begin by discussing research that has been summarized and is free to view by the public via the Internet. We then show you how to generate a bibliography on cocaine dependence and teach you how to keep current on new studies as they are published or undertaken by the scientific community.

The Combined Health Information Database

The Combined Health Information Database summarizes studies across numerous federal agencies. To limit your investigation to research studies and cocaine dependence, you will need to use the advanced search options. First, go to **http://chid.nih.gov/index.html**. From there, select the "Detailed Search" option (or go directly to that page with the following hyperlink: **http://chid.nih.gov/detail/detail.html**). The trick in extracting studies is found in the drop boxes at the bottom of the search page where "You may refine your search by." Select the dates and language you prefer, and the format option "Journal Article." At the top of the search form, select the number of records you would like to see (we recommend 100) and check the box to display "whole records." We recommend that you type in "cocaine dependence" (or synonyms) into the "For these words:" box. Consider using the option "anywhere in record" to make your search as broad as possible. If you want to limit the search to only a particular field, such as the title of the journal, then select this option in the "Search in these fields" drop box. The following is a sample of what you can expect from this type of search:

- **Midfacial Complications of Prolonged Cocaine Snorting**

  Source: Journal of the Canadian Dental Association. 65(4): 218-223. April 1999.

  Contact: Canadian Dental Association. 1815 Alta Vista Drive, Ottawa, ON K1G 3Y6. (613) 523-1770. E-mail: reception@cda-adc.ca. Website: www.cda-adc.ca.

  Summary: Acute and chronic ingestion of **cocaine** predisposes the abuser to a wide range of local and systemic complications. Ingesting powdered **cocaine** orally or nasally can be extremely destructive to the periodontal and midfacial anatomy. This article describes the case of a 38 year old man whose chronic **cocaine** snorting resulted in the erosion of the midfacial anatomy and recurrent sinus infections. The author presents previously published case reports specific to this problem, and discusses the oral, systemic, and behavioral effects of **cocaine** abuse. The author reminds family dentists that the injection of local anesthetic with epinephrine must be avoided for at least six hours (and preferably up to 24 hours) after **cocaine** consumption to prevent 'sympathetic overload;' this can result in a hypertensive crisis, cerebrovascular bleed, myocardial infarction, tachydysrhythmias, or cardiac arrest. The author provides tables that guide the dentist in looking for the signs and symptoms indicating an abuse problem; this can help in the crucial factor of identifying whether **cocaine** is a factor in the patient's management. Once alerted to an abuse problem, the informed dentist can educate his or her patient about the progressive consequences of continued usage and provide a referral for professional counseling. Dental treatment should be deferred to an appropriate time when life threatening complications can be avoided. 6 figures. 2 tables. 28 references.

- **Identifying Oral Lesions Associated with Crack Cocaine Use**

  Source: JADA. Journal of the American Dental Association. 125(8): 1104-1109. August 1994.

Summary: Dental patients who smoke crack **cocaine** are at higher risk for HIV infection and other medical concerns including stroke, heart failure and pulmonary hemorrhage. In this article, four cases are reported which illustrate oral ulcers caused by crack **cocaine** usage. The cases are part of an ongoing longitudinal study of oral manifestations of HIV infection, including both HIV-negative and HIV-positive patients from a cohort of intravenous drug users. The authors describe the ulcers in each patient; discuss crack **cocaine** and its use; and hypothesize how the lesions in the patients were caused. They note that although each patient's lesions had a different clinical appearance, there were two characteristics common to all of the lesions, the midpalatal location and a recent (less than 48 hours prior to examination) history of smoking crack **cocaine.** 5 figures. 1 table. 20 references. (AA-M).

- **Dental Management of a Patient with a Cocaine-Induced Maxillofacial Defect: A Case Report**

Source: SCD. Special Care in Dentistry. 20(4): 139-142. July-August 2000.

Contact: Available from Special Care Dentistry. 211 East Chicago Avenue, Chicago, IL 60611. (312) 440-2660. Fax (312) 440-2824.

Summary: There are several dental complications associated with **cocaine** abuse, including adverse reactions to dental anesthetics, postoperative bleeding, and cellulitis, which can lead to necrosis (tissue death) of orbital, nasal, and palatal bones. This article offers a report of the initial treatment rendered to a patient who had destroyed most of her hard palate over a ten year period of **cocaine** abuse. The authors describe the patient's presentation, and the dental treatment plan established by a multidisciplinary team of care providers. The authors note that drug abuse victims may present as patients in any dental office. There are no classic socioeconomic or educational profiles for abusers of **cocaine.** Though there are certain classic physiological and psychological symptoms of their condition, they may not display symptoms at all. 4 figures. 20 references.

- **Cocaine Connection: Users Imperil Their Gingiva**

Source: JADA. Journal of American Dental Association. 122(1): 85-87. January 1991.

Summary: This article describes the risks involved when **cocaine** users apply **cocaine** to the gingiva as an alternative to snorting the substance. Topics covered include the increasing use of **cocaine,** necrosis and ulceration of mucal surfaces from direct contact with **cocaine,** and the vasoconstrictive properties of **cocaine.** The authors report on a study of

181 patients with AIDS who were questioned about the duration and location of **cocaine** use by mucosal application. Nine (5 percent) of the 181 patients had focal destruction of the soft and hard tissue of the periodontium. These areas were located on the labial surfaces of the mandibular anterior teeth (7 patients) or buccal surfaces of the maxillary posterior teeth (2 patients). All 9 patients reported a minimum of several weeks of **cocaine** application to the affected areas. The authors conclude with a discussion of the implications of their findings. 18 references.

- **Crack Cocaine Use and High - Risk Behaviors Among Sexually Active Black Adolescents**

Source: Journal of Adolescent Health; Vol. 14, 1993.

Summary: This article discusses crack **cocaine** use and high-risk behaviors among sexually active African American adolescents. It observes the prevalence of five factors that promote sexually transmitted diseases (STDs), including HIV, among a sample of sexually active Black adolescent crack users and non-users in the San Francisco Bay area. The factors examined are self-reported history of STDs, more than five sexual partners per year, involvement in an exchange of sexual activity for drugs or money, a history of having sexual relations while under the influence of crack, and failure to use a condom in the most recent sexual encounter. The study concludes that risk behaviors are significantly associated with crack use and with having one or more relatives who used drugs. It suggests addressing both individual and environmental risk factors when designing intervention efforts targeted at preventing or reducing the risk of teenage drug abuse and/or STDs, including HIV.

- **How Cocaine Abuse Affects Post-Extraction Bleeding**

Source: JADA. Journal of American Dental Association. 124(12): 60-62. December 1993.

Summary: This article discusses the effects of **cocaine** and the relevance of **cocaine** abuse to clinical dentistry. The authors present a case report in which severe bleeding occurred after an extraction. The authors describe the physiological effects of **cocaine** and discuss the difficulties of ascertaining its use in patients because of its illegality and the stigma associated with **cocaine** abuse. They stress that surgical dental treatment is not appropriate on a patient with acute **cocaine** abuse. 19 references. (AA-M).

- **Palate Perforation from Cocaine Abuse**

  Source: Otolaryngology-Head and Neck Surgery. 116(4): 565-566. April 1997.

  Summary: This article presents a case report of a palate perforation from cocaine abuse. A 37 year old Hispanic woman had a longstanding history of cocaine use at presentation. She had a nasal septal perforation for several years and now reported a palatal defect of 6 months' duration. She noted crusting in her nose that was relieved by thorough and vigorous rubbing of her nasal cavity with cotton swabs, pencils, and pens. The patient subsequently underwent a thorough evaluation for nasal malignancies and infections, results of which were negative. The patient had continued snorting cocaine and cleaning her nose, and the defect slowly enlarged during the previous 6 months. The authors discuss how chronic inhalation of cocaine can cause nasal and mucoperichondrial ischemia, which can lead to atrophic changes in the mucosal lining. In addition, recurrent mucosal irritation of nasally applied chemicals leads to the formation of a nasal septal defect. As the ischemic process continues to hinder healing, the area becomes necrotic and the existing defect enlarges. 1 figure. 3 references.

- **Researchers Study Impact of Prenatal Cocaine Exposure on Communication**

  Source: ADVANCE for Speech-Language Pathologists and Audiologists. 5(36): 8-9. September 11, 1995.

  Contact: Available from Merion Publishers, Inc. 659 Park Avenue, Box 61556, King of Prussia, PA 19406-0956. (800) 355-1088 or (610) 265-7812.

  Summary: This article, from a professional newsletter for speech-language pathologists and audiologists, discusses research investigating the impact of prenatal cocaine exposure on communication. Topics covered include the use of semantic relationships in language to study the potential effect of prenatal cocaine exposure; determining drug exposure; monitoring and evaluating these children in order to determine if and when intervention will be required; testing and attention difficulties in children who had been exposed to drugs; utilizing natural language sample data collected during free play periods; attention deficit problems in this population; the maturation of the brainstem and how prenatal cocaine exposure can affect the auditory pathway; the role of the child's environment on speech and language delays; and problems with a lack of funding for research in this area. The article concludes with the addresses and telephone numbers of the primary researchers interviewed in the article.

Federally Funded Research on Cocaine Dependence

The U.S. Government supports a variety of research studies relating to cocaine dependence and associated conditions. These studies are tracked by the Office of Extramural Research at the National Institutes of Health.[18] CRISP (Computerized Retrieval of Information on Scientific Projects) is a searchable database of federally funded biomedical research projects conducted at universities, hospitals, and other institutions. Visit CRISP at **http://crisp.cit.nih.gov/crisp/crisp_query.generate_screen**. You can perform targeted searches by various criteria including geography, date, as well as topics related to cocaine dependence and related conditions.

For most of the studies, the agencies reporting into CRISP provide summaries or abstracts. As opposed to clinical trial research using patients, many federally funded studies use animals or simulated models to explore cocaine dependence and related conditions. In some cases, therefore, it may be difficult to understand how some basic or fundamental research could eventually translate into medical practice. The following sample is typical of the type of information found when searching the CRISP database for cocaine dependence:

- **Project Title: A THERAPEUTIC WORKPLACE FOR HOMELESS ALCOHOLICS**

  Principal Investigator & Institution: Silverman, Kenneth; Associate Provessor; Psychiatry and Behavioral Scis; Johns Hopkins University 3400 N Charles St Baltimore, Md 21218

  Timing: Fiscal Year 2002; Project Start 01-MAY-2000; Project End 30-APR-2005

  Summary: APPLICANT'S ABSTRACT: Few populations are beset with the constellation of economic, social and health problems that afflict homeless individuals. Alcoholism is one of their most common and serious problems. Given the nature and severity of their problems, the Institute of Medicine has suggested that the homeless need specialized substance abuse interventions. We propose to examine the efficacy of a novel treatment for chronically unemployed substance abusers, the Therapeutic Workplace, in homeless, alcohol-dependent adults. Prior research has shown that this intervention is effective in the treatment of

---

[18] Healthcare projects are funded by the National Institutes of Health (NIH), Substance Abuse and Mental Health Services (SAMHSA), Health Resources and Services Administration (HRSA), Food and Drug Administration (FDA), Centers for Disease Control and Prevention (CDCP), Agency for Healthcare Research and Quality (AHRQ), and Office of Assistant Secretary of Health (OASH).

heroin and **cocaine** dependence. The intervention integrates abstinence reinforcement contingencies of proven efficacy into a model supported work program. Patients are paid to perform data entry jobs in the Therapeutic Workplace. Those lacking needed skills are given intensive training. To reinforce abstinence from alcohol, patients can work and earn salary only when they remain abstinent from alcohol as assessed in weekday morning and random daily breath-alcohol tests. Patients are paid in vouchers instead of cash to reduce the chance they will use their earnings to Purchase alcohol or drugs. A randomized trial is planned over 5 years to evaluate the efficacy of this intervention and to assess the contribution of the abstinence reinforcement component in homeless, alcohol-dependent adults who complete an inpatient alcohol detoxification. After the detoxification, 156 participants will be invited to attend the workplace for 6 months and randomly assigned to one of three groups that will differ in the requirements for voucher reinforcement. One group will receive the full therapeutic workplace intervention in which vouchers are contingent on both abstinence and work. A second group will be paid for work, but will not have to provide an alcohol-free breath sample to gain access to the workplace (vouchers contingent on work only). A third group will receive vouchers on a noncontingent basis. This group will control for the increases in wealth associated with voucher reinforcement. Critical measures of alcohol use, other drug use, HIV risk behaviors, employment and housing will be assessed. We expect the most abstinence when both abstinence and work are required to earn vouchers. This study will allow for the rigorous evaluation of a novel approach to the treatment of alcohol dependence, the Therapeutic Workplace, in a group of homeless, alcohol-dependent individuals who desperately need effective interventions to control their alcohol use, and to improve their chronic conditions of unemployment and homelessness.

Website: http://crisp.cit.nih.gov/crisp/Crisp_Query.Generate_Screen

- **Project Title: ADOLESCENCE: A SENSITIVE PERIOD FOR NICOTINE ADDICTION**

Principal Investigator & Institution: Levin, Edward D.; Associate Professor; Psychiatry; Duke University Durham, Nc 27710

Timing: Fiscal Year 2004; Project Start 01-APR-2004; Project End 31-MAR-2009

Summary: (provided by applicant): The great majority of tobacco addiction begins during adolescence, but very little is known about the neurobehavioral effects of nicotine in adolescents compared to adults. Adolescents are still undergoing important neurodevelopmental changes on the path to adulthood. Nicotine exposure in adolescence may have lasting impacts on this late neurodevelopment. There are suggestions in the clinical literature that more heavily addicted smokers begin smoking earlier in adolescence, but the impact of nicotine self-administration during adolescence versus self-selection bias whereby people more prone to heavy addiction also begin earlier, cannot be ethically unconfounded in humans. This project is based on our hypothesis beginning nicotine self-administration during adolescence leads to greater nicotine intake and dependence than beginning in adulthood. Our preliminary data demonstrated in the rat model of nicotine self-administration that rats with adolescent-onset nicotine self-administration self-administer substantially higher total doses of nicotine than adult-onset rats, This higher rate of nicotine self-administration continues into adulthood with an approximate doubling of nicotine self-administration. The proposed experiments will determine the causal relationship between adolescent-onset nicotine self-administration and enhanced long-term nicotine self-administration with these Specific Aims. 1. Determine the pharmacokinetics and dose-effect functions of nicotine in adolescents and adult rats. 2. Determine the impact of nicotine replacement and nicotinic antagonist therapy on nicotine self-administration in adolescent-onset and adult-onset nicotine self-administration. 3. Determine the age threshold for the adult-like nicotine self-administration. 4. Determine if adolescent-onset nicotine self-administration enhances **cocaine** dependence. 5. Determine sex differences in adolescent-onset nicotine self-administration. Nicotine pharmacokinetic measurements in adolescent and adult rats will be used to determine the effect of altered distribution and metabolism versus pharmacodynamic factors in accounting for age-related differences in nicotine self-administration. Benefits of this research include a more relevant animal model of adolescent-onset smoking, improved understanding of how adolescent-onset nicotine use potentiates nicotine intake, a cause and effect determination of the gateway hypothesis of adolescent nicotine use leading to harder drugs and the development of better treatments for adolescent-onset nicotine dependence.

Website: http://crisp.cit.nih.gov/crisp/Crisp_Query.Generate_Screen

- **Project Title: AFTERCARE FOR SUBSTANCE ABUSERS**

Principal Investigator & Institution: Mckay, James R.; Associate Professor; Psychiatry; University of Pennsylvania 3451 Walnut Street Philadelphia, Pa 19104

Timing: Fiscal Year 2002; Project Start 01-APR-1998; Project End 31-MAR-2004

Summary: Applicant's Abstract An Independent Scientist Award (K02) is requested to allow the candidate to continue to focus on and to expand his research programs on the impact of aftercare for substance abusers and the assessment of factors in relapse. The award would also make it possible for the candidate to pursue additional training in longitudinal data analytic techniques, cost-effective research, and assessment instrument development. These training experiences will be accomplished through a combination of formal course work and directed readings with acknowledged experts in these areas. The candidate's long-term career goal is to integrate findings from studies of various approaches to continuing care, or "aftercare," and studies of factors in relapse to generate more effective and cost-effective approaches to relapse prevention in substance abusers. As described in the research plan, during the term of support from this proposed Independent Scientist Award the candidate will serve as Principal Investigator on two RO1 grants that evaluate the effectiveness and cost-effectiveness of aftercare of **cocaine** and alcohol dependent individuals who have completed a primary treatment program. As these projects are similar, only the **cocaine** study is described in detail. In this project, entitled "Aftercare for **Cocaine** Patients: Effectiveness and Costs," **cocaine** dependent patients who complete intensive outpatient rehabilitation (IOP) will be randomly assigned to one of the following interventions: (1) Minimal aftercare (MIN), a combination of referral to self-help groups and brief telephone case-management; (2) Standard disease model aftercare counseling (STND), provided through two group therapy sessions per week; and (3) Individual aftercare (IND), provided through one individual cognitive-behavioral, relapse prevention session and one group therapy session per week. The effectiveness analysis will include the testing of main effect and patient by treatment "matching" hypotheses generated by prior work by the candidate and other investigators. The cost-effectiveness analysis, which will be done in collaboration with Dr. Donald Shepard of Brandeis University, will focus on the identification of the types of patients who are treated most cost effectively in each aftercare condition. Based on prior research, it is anticipated that the IND condition will be particularly effective, relative to the other conditions, for poor prognosis patients, such as those who did not achieve remission from **cocaine** dependence during IOP and those with greater psychiatric severity. Outcome measures in this study will include measures of **cocaine** and alcohol use and frequency of behaviors that place patients at high risk for contracting or spreading AIDS. The funding provided by the KO2 award also will allow the candidate to further the development and refinement of the **Cocaine** Relapse Interview, an assessment instrument that was initially developed with a First Award.

Website: http://crisp.cit.nih.gov/crisp/Crisp_Query.Generate_Screen

- **Project Title: BEHAVIORAL FACTORS IN DRUG TOLERANCE**

Principal Investigator & Institution: Branch, Marc N.; Professor; Psychology; University of Florida Gainesville, Fl 32611

Timing: Fiscal Year 2002; Project Start 01-SEP-2002; Project End 31-JUL-2007

Summary: (provided by applicant): The general significance of the proposed research is that it may have relevance to the development of dependence on **cocaine. Cocaine** use and dependence remain significant health issues in the United States. For example, recent surveys indicated that more than 5.6 million Americans had used **cocaine** within the past year, and that more than 23 million have taken the drug at some time in their lifetimes. Interestingly, estimates indicate that only about 5 to 10% of those who use **cocaine** eventually become dependent on it. It appears, therefore, that **cocaine** tends not to be immediately addictive. The factors that lead to dependence have not been identified, but clinical evidence suggests that a prolonged period of intermittent use of the drug often precedes the development of dependence. The proposed research is aimed at furthering our knowledge concerning behavioral effects of relatively long-term intermittent exposure to **cocaine.** Laboratory study of effects of long-term intermittent exposure to **cocaine** has yielded a puzzling array of results. Sometimes tolerance is observed, sometimes sensitization. Previous investigations, however, have indicated that experiential/behavioral factors can determine whether or not tolerance or sensitization occurs to cocaine's effects. The proposed research is aimed at adding to our knowledge of how experiential factors interact with repeated **cocaine** exposure. The specific research aims of this application are to: 1.) Expand our analyses of the interaction between explicitly conditioned operant behavior (as a model of purposive behavior) and general activity during repeated exposure to **cocaine.** Our recent finding that presence of an operant contingency prevented the observation of sensitization to the drug's effects on general activity has set the basis for this aim. 2.) Continue to examine the role of alterations in rate of reinforcement as a predictor of tolerance to effects of **cocaine.** 3) Continue analyses of reinforcement-schedule-parameter dependent tolerance. We plan to determine if such tolerance is "contingent," if and how it is related to behavioral economic factors, and how rate of reinforcement and ratio contingencies interact. This application is to provide support for the PI so that he may devote at least 75% of his time to research on the foregoing issues. The study of long-term, intermittent exposure to **cocaine** has potential relevance to the genesis of **cocaine** dependence. Understanding of the processes that occur under long-term, intermittent exposure should facilitate the development of effective treatment and, especially, prevention programs.

Website: http://crisp.cit.nih.gov/crisp/Crisp_Query.Generate_Screen

- **Project Title: BEHAVIORAL STRATEGIES TO MAXIMIXE PHARMACOTHERAPY EFFICACY FOR COCAINE DEPENDENCE**

Principal Investigator & Institution: Schmitz, Joy M.; Professor; University of Texas Hlth Sci Ctr Houston Box 20036 Houston, Tx 77225

Timing: Fiscal Year 2002; Project Start 01-SEP-2002; Project End 31-AUG-2003

Summary: Treatments to reduce **cocaine** use have been both pharmacological based on hypothesized biological mechanisms action, and psychological, based on behavioral and cognitive-behavioral theory. Most pharmacotherapies for **cocaine** dependence are still in need of confirmation. During the original funding period of this grant, our research at the SAMDRC has been pivotal in identifying the role of agonist medication treatments for **cocaine** dependence. We have demonstrated that levodopa (L-dopa) along with carbidopa can be safely administered and has discernable efficacy over placebo in the ambulatory treatment of **cocaine** dependence. The optimal use of this pharmacotherapy, however, is not likely to depend on the behavioral/environment context in which the medication is administered. Cognitive-behavioral approaches and contingency management procedures are two behaviorally based therapies for **cocaine** addiction that have been empirically evaluated. The purpose of this research is to determine whether these two popular behavioral approaches, independently or combined, serve to enhance a promising new pharmacologic strategy. Two studies will be conducted concurrently. Study 1 will employ a randomized, between groups, additive research design, to test the hypothesis that the combination of RP and Contingency Management Procedures (CMP) can potentiate the efficacy of L- dopa/carbidopa. Three therapy conditions of varying intensity will be compared: (1) clinical management (CM) only; (2) CM+RP, and (3) CM +CMP. The incremental efficacy of these therapy conditions will be examined under active and placebo medication conditions. A total sample of 120 **cocaine** dependent individuals will be randomly assigned to one of the six treatment conditions. Study 2 will parametrically assess which type of contingent incentive, when compared with RP, facilities the efficacy of agonist pharmacotherapy. Participants will receive RP therapy in combination with a CMP that targets clinic attendance, medication compliance, or **cocaine** abstinence. A total sample of 120 **cocaine** dependent individuals will be randomly assigned to one of the six treatment conditions. Both studies will be conducted concurrently, using nearly identical recruitment, intake, and assessment procedures. Assignment to treatment group will be random, using an urn randomizing technique to assure balanced distribution of baseline characteristics that may influence outcome. Standard outcome variables related to **cocaine** (urine toxicology screens and patient self report), addiction problem severity, medication compliance, and clinic visit attendance will be collected during twelve weeks of treatment and one year follow up. Assessment of potential prognostic dimensions, including severity of **cocaine** dependence, concurrent alcohol use, motivation for treatment and level of readiness to change, will be used to identify patient characteristics associated with optimal outcome in these well-defined treatments. These studies are direct, logical extensions of our research on the integration of behavior therapy with promising pharmacotherapy for the treatment of **cocaine** dependence.

Website: http://crisp.cit.nih.gov/crisp/Crisp_Query.Generate_Screen

- **Project Title: BEHAVIORAL TREATMENT OF ADOLESCENT MARIJUANA ABUSE**

Principal Investigator & Institution: Budney, Alan J.; Associate Professor; Psychiatry; University of Vermont & St Agric College 340 Waterman Building Burlington, Vt 05405

Timing: Fiscal Year 2002; Project Start 01-MAY-2002; Project End 30-APR-2006

Summary: Treatment seeking marijuana abuse among adolescents increased dramatically during the 1990s, yet not consensus exists on how to best treat this clinical population. Well-controlled clinical trials are lacking, and most treatments examined have had difficulty documenting initial periods of marijuana abstinence. The primary aim of this proposal is to extend our prior contingency-management treatment development research on adult marijuana and **cocaine** dependence by creating an effective, developmentally appropriate intervention for adolescent marijuana abuse/dependence. Specific Aim 1 is to develop, manualize, and pilot a contingency management intervention that includes two components. First, a voucher program will enhance the adolescent's engagement in the treatment process and engender initial marijuana abstinence by providing immediate positive reinforcement for documented abstinence. Second, a parent training program will enhance and maintain the positive effects of the vouchers by teaching parents how to effectively use contingency management in the home environment A randomized trial will determine whether the contingency- management intervention enhances outcomes when added to a standard cognitive-behavioral therapy. Specific Aim 3 is to determine if this intervention effectively changes specific parental and adolescent behavior deemed important risk factors for ongoing substance abuse. Systematic Assessment of parenting behavior, peer associations, family cohesion, and delinquent behavior will provide an initial evaluation of the mechanisms by which this intervention affects outcome. The proposed treatment model holds much promise for success. The voucher program has demonstrated efficacy with different types of drug- dependent adults. The home-based contingency management program is effective with conduct problems and delinquency, i.e., problems that co- occur in the majority of adolescent substance abusers. If successful, future studies will examine the relative contribution of specific components of the CM intervention.

Website: http://crisp.cit.nih.gov/crisp/Crisp_Query.Generate_Screen

- **Project Title: BIOBEHAVIORAL HETEROGENEITY OF CRACK COCAINE DEPENDENCE**

Principal Investigator & Institution: Pricheps, Leslie S.; Psychiatry; New York University School of Medicine 550 1St Ave New York, Ny 10016

Timing: Fiscal Year 2002; Project Start 01-APR-1993; Project End 30-JUN-2004

Summary: (provided by applicant) During the period of our ongoing study we have published results demonstrating the existence of a characteristic replicable and persistent profile of quantitative EEG (QEEG) abnormalities associated with long-term **cocaine** dependence. Electrophysiological heterogeneity (QEEG subtypes) existed at baseline, independent of length of exposure to **cocaine,** but significantly related to length of stay in treatment (continued abstinence). Significant interactions between subtype membership, comorbidity and gender were found to exist. An electrophysiological database has been constructed containing EEG, EP, neuropsychological, demographic and clinical data, collected from 452 evaluations from 149 subjects, at baseline and follow-up intervals of up to 18 months sustained abstinence. Preliminary study has revealed that some QEEG features persist while others move toward normal with sustained abstinence. Normalization, when it occurred, was at different rates for different QEEG features and significantly interacted with gender. This renewal application has been designed to examine the implications and significance of the results of the previous years of study, and will allow us to: [11 identify the specific features of the QEEG profile which remain abnormal in the chronic **cocaine** users during prolonged abstinence, and to study the incidence of such features in order to determine whether these are 'traits present prior to initiation of **cocaine** use or develop with chronic exposure. We hypothesize that the delta deficit in frontal cortex found in all subtypes may be such a 'trait, reflecting decreased activity of delta generating neurons in lower cortical layers as a consequence of decreased dopaminergic thalamo-cortical drive and predict that it will appear with high incidence in non-drug using siblings; [2] identify the specific features of the QEEG profile which reflect an abnormal 'state', becoming more normal with prolonged abstinence, and predict that it will not display higher incidence in non-using siblings. We hypothesize that the global alpha excess is such a feature, probably reflecting decreased ascending reticular activation of thalamo-cortical interactions, as a consequence of either deficient serotonergic transmission or striatal-nigral inhibition, and that it will gradually normalize during prolonged abstinence; [3] determine whether gender significantly interacts with change of abnormal features with sustained abstinence; [4] determine if additional features become more normal with confirmed abstinence extending to 24 months. Application of new mathematical algorithms will permit identification of the most probable neuroanatomical sources generating the QEEG, which may improve understanding of underlying mechanisms and help target new medications.

Website: http://crisp.cit.nih.gov/crisp/Crisp_Query.Generate_Screen

- **Project Title: BRAIN RECOVERY FOLLOWING ABSTINENCE FROM COCAINE**

Principal Investigator & Institution: Nierenberg, Jay;; Nathan S. Kline Institute for Psych Res Psychiatric Research Orangeburg, Ny 10962

Timing: Fiscal Year 2002; Project Start 01-SEP-2002; Project End 31-AUG-2004

Summary: (provided by applicant): Evidence from neuroimaging studies suggests that chronic **cocaine** use leads to white matter (WM) injury in frontal brain regions. Cocaine-induced damage to cortical WM can result in cognitive and behavioral deficits that may impact recovery and ongoing abstinence. There has been little in vivo study of the duration of cocaine's effect on WM microstructure, following abstinence; nor has the relationship between WM microstructure and cognitive function in active **cocaine** dependence (CD) or during recovery been addressed. Whether cocaine-induced changes in brain structure and function can partly or fully recover following the cessation of drug use has significant implications for the ongoing medical management of patients with CD, including their psychiatric treatment. Diffusion Tensor Imaging (DTI) is a magnetic resonance imaging (MRI) technique that can be applied to the study of WM integrity in vivo. DTI can be used to assess WM integrity by quantifying the magnitude and direction of tissue water mobility. Because water diffusion in WM is anisotropic (i.e., it is greater along the longitudinal extent of a nerve fiber when compared to diffusion along the short axis), this anisotropy can be quantified and used to assess the microstructural organization of WM using scalar measures such as fractional anisotropy (FA). Recent data have demonstrated decreased FA in the frontal WM in patients with active CD. This proposal intends to use DTI to study the persistence of cocaine's effect on WM integrity following cessation of **cocaine** use. We propose a cross-sectional design to study patients with a history of CD using MRI and neurocognitive assessments. Subjects will be recruited from a therapeutic community (Daytop) and compared with a group of healthy control subjects. Using DTI offers a significant opportunity to begin elucidating the relationship between WM integrity and recovery of neuropsychological function following **cocaine** abstinence. These data will help assess the feasibility of a longitudinal study of WM changes related to CD and potentially inform future treatment options.

Website: http://crisp.cit.nih.gov/crisp/Crisp_Query.Generate_Screen

- **Project Title: BRAIN SUBSTRATES OF SELF-CONTROL IN ADDICTION**

Principal Investigator & Institution: Monterosso, John R.; Assistant Professor; Psychiatry; University of Pennsylvania 3451 Walnut Street Philadelphia, Pa 19104

Timing: Fiscal Year 2002; Project Start 01-SEP-2001; Project End 30-JUN-2002

Summary: (Provided by Applicant) The goal of this K01 proposal is to provide John Monterosso, Ph.D., with the training and support to become an independent investigator in the field of clinical substance abuse research. The research plan builds on the candidate's expertise in animal models of impulsivity; its basic aim is to measure analogous constructs in **cocaine** dependent patients and to use these measurements in conjunction with cue reactivity to better characterize patients and to better predict treatment outcomes. The training plan provides extensive clinical exposure, individual mentoring in areas related to the research, and structured didactics. Both the research and training plans are opportunistic, utilizing readily-available patient populations from ongoing research, and seasoned investigators in the University of Pennsylvania research community. Dr. Anna Rose Childress will provide primary mentorship and daily supervision in the proposed research; her expertise lies in the phenomenology of **cocaine** dependence, cue-induced craving, and its brain substrates. Dr. Ronald Ehrman will provide expertise in the laboratory measurement of cue reactivity, and in statistical modeling. Dr. Charles O'Brien will provide expertise on the neurobiology of addiction, will ensure support for successful execution of the project, and will chair an Advisory Board of selected investigators who will be a resource to the candidate and monitor his development. Relapse is a cardinal feature of the addictions, and the one which exacts the greatest human and economic costs. Understanding its mechanisms is critical to reducing these costs. Though cue-induced craving and arousal have been offered by us, and by others, as one possible mechanism, craving has been an imperfect predictor of drug use: not every craving episode eventuates in relapse, and patients vary in their ability to manage these episodes. Host variables may help explain this variability. Since the reward of drug is immediate and the benefits of abstinence are delayed, individual differences in sensitivity to future consequences may be an important variable. Tasks have recently been developed for assessing this dimension: one derived from an animal model of impulsivity, and two others from neuropsychological research with orbitofrontal patients, who show extreme behavioral "myopia" (Damasio, 1994). We have combined these methods into a "Myopia Battery (MB)" for use in the proposed studies. We have conducted a large pilot study with encouraging results. Differences in myopia may be particularly useful for understanding the disconnect between reported craving and drug use/relapse. In Study 1, cocaine-dependent patients participating in a large-scale treatment outcome study (n= 120) will be assessed on cue reactivity/craving, ASP, Impulsivity, I.Q. and will be administered the MB. The MB will also be administered to a group of matched controls (n=80). In Study 2, the MB will be administered to **cocaine** patients (n=60) participating in ongoing PET studies that directly assess orbitofrontal activity. Our primary hypotheses are: 1) cocaine-dependent patients will perform worse on the MB than controls; 2) performance on the MB will be especially poor in cocaine-dependent patients with ASP; 3) performance on the MB will be related to the variability of patients' ability to manage craving states without relapsing, and 4) MB performance will be correlated with orbitofrontal functioning. The link between severe myopia and orbitofrontal impairment is particularly exciting given emerging evidence (including that collected recently in our own lab) of orbitofrontal deficits in **cocaine** addicts relative to controls. Whether the dysfunction is a predisposing factor for, or a consequence of, stimulant use - or both - it could undermine an important psychological resource for recovery.

Website: http://crisp.cit.nih.gov/crisp/Crisp_Query.Generate_Screen

- **Project Title: CBT AND MODAFINIL FOR COCAINE ADDICTION**

Principal Investigator & Institution: Malcolm, Robert J.; Professor; Psychiatry and Behavioral Scis; Medical University of South Carolina P O Box 250854 Charleston, Sc 29425

Timing: Fiscal Year 2003; Project Start 30-SEP-2003; Project End 30-JUN-2007

Summary: (provided by applicant): Thus far, an effective pharmacologic treatment for **cocaine** dependence has not been discovered. The present trial proposes cognitive behavior therapy (CBT) as the psychosocial platform to compare two doses of modafinil with placebo for the treatment of **cocaine** addiction. Modafinil is a marketed, atypical stimulant which has been approved by the FDA for the treatment of nacrolepsy. Modafinil acts intracellularly in several nuclei in the anterior hypothalamus to promote cortical activation, but does not alter dopamine systems. Controlled trials with modafinil indicate that it decreases hypersomnolence, elevates mood, enhances attention/concentration, and decreases appetite. Several preclinical human trials indicate that abuse potential of modafinil is low. Side effect profile for modafinil is modest and modafinil does not have pharmacokinetic interactions with **cocaine,** amphetamines, or methylphenidate. In a human laboratory study (n=12) from our group, Modafinil 400 and 800 mg suppressed subjective "high," "drug effect," and "amount willing to pay for high" to both low doses (20 mg) and high doses (40 mg) of IV **cocaine.** We postulate that modafinil serves as an atypical agonist replacement therapy for **cocaine.** Modafinil should ameliorate the symptoms of **cocaine** abstinence, blunt multiple dimensions of the **cocaine** "high" and enhance benefits of the CBT. To test these hypotheses and the safety of modafinil, we propose a two week screening baseline period followed by an eight week randomized parallel study of modafinil 200 mg, 400 mg and placebo daily. Follow up will occur four and eight weeks after all therapies cease. Outcome measures will include the number of **cocaine** non-use days and consecutive non-use days as assessed by self-report that will be confirmed by urine assays for quantitative benzoylecgonine three times a week. Secondary assessments will include measures of mood, daytime sleepiness, and subjective aspects of **cocaine** withdrawal and **cocaine** "high." Compliance with placebo and study medications will be assessed by quantitative urine riboflavin levels and serum modafinil levels. Safety will be assessed by a combination of self-report and repeated physical examinations, laboratory studies, ECGs, and monitoring by an independent data safety monitoring board.

Website: http://crisp.cit.nih.gov/crisp/Crisp_Query.Generate_Screen

- **Project Title: COCAETHYLENE COCAINE AGONIST THERAPY/TOLERANCE INDUCTION**

  Principal Investigator & Institution: Mccance-Katz, Elinore F.; Associate Professor; Psychiatry and Behavioral Scis; Yeshiva University 500 W 185Th St New York, Ny 10033

  Timing: Fiscal Year 2002; Project Start 15-APR-2001; Project End 31-MAR-2003

  Summary: The search for an effective pharmacotherapy for the treatment of **cocaine** dependence has been elusive, but the serious medical and psychological morbidity and social costs of **cocaine** abuse underscore the need to continue research in the area of **cocaine** medications development. In this application, we propose studies to determine whether **cocaine** agonist (substitution) therapy with C2 substituted benzoyloxytropane analogs of **cocaine** might be safe and efficacious as pharmacotherapy treatments for **cocaine** dependence. The C2 substituted **cocaine** analogs, while sharing some pharmacological properties with **cocaine,** have other dissimilar properties that potentially make them useful as pharmacotherapeutic agents to treat **cocaine** dependence. We propose to use cocaethylene, the C2 ethyl ester of benzoylecgonine, as a prototype drug to test the concept that agonist treatment may block and/or produce tolerance to the acute effects of **cocaine.** This proposal will examine the question of the safety of cocaethylene administered to volunteers by examination of cocaethylene pharmacokinetics, physiological, and behavioral responses following infusion of the drug. A paradigm has also been developed based on preclinical studies showing induction of tolerance to acute **cocaine** responses in rodents which will be undertaken in human subjects. This protocol will determine whether tolerance to cardiovascular and subjective responses to **cocaine** can be induced following cocaethylene infusion. Positive findings from these studies could be followed in future studies with clinical trials to assess the efficacy of this class of drugs in the treatment of **cocaine** dependence.

  Website: http://crisp.cit.nih.gov/crisp/Crisp_Query.Generate_Screen

- **Project Title: COCAINE & CHEST PAIN IN THE ED: SERVICE & OUTCOMES**

  Principal Investigator & Institution: Booth, Brenda M.; Professor of Psychiatry; Psychiatry and Behavioral Scis; University of Arkansas Med Scis Ltl Rock Little Rock, Ar 72205

  Timing: Fiscal Year 2002; Project Start 30-SEP-2001; Project End 31-AUG-2005

Summary: (provided by applicant) Little is known about the clinical picture of **cocaine** users presenting with chest pain in the ED from the substance abuse or health services perspective. Almost all of the research on **cocaine** users presenting to the ED with chest pain has been conducted from the perspective of the ED physician and hence has focused on cardiac outcomes and mortality. Before we can develop interventions for this high-risk group of **cocaine** users, we need to understand who is at greatest risk for poor outcome and who is least likely to enter treatment in order to target interventions for those most in need. Likewise, we need to know where and when high-risk individuals intersect with the health care system to determine the optimal timing and setting for interventions. We propose a prospective observational study to provide the foundation for subsequent intervention research. We propose to study a consecutive cohort (N=300) of individuals presenting to the Hurley Medical Center ED, Flint, MI with chest pain and recent **cocaine** use and to follow them longitudinally for a year after their ED presentation with interviews at 3, 6, and 12 months. The specific aims of the study are: (1) To develop a comprehensive portrait of a consecutive cohort of **cocaine** users presenting to the ED with chest pain; (2) To identify specific locations where study participants interact with the health service system in the year following their ED visit and to identify the key patient characteristics associated with types of service use; (3) To identify access barriers to engaging in treatment and use of other services including primary care; (4) To measure one-year outcomes for this Cohort and to identify key socio-demographic and clinical characteristics of cocaine-using individuals with poor or good outcomes in the year after their ED visit for chest pain; and (5) To identify the timing and service setting for future interventions, based on findings from Specific Aims 1-4. The proposed study will study barriers to obtaining treatment, including access (multi-dimensional measures including accessibility, availability, acceptability, and affordability of treatment services), motivation (readiness to change), and need for treatment, including severity of **cocaine** dependence, comorbid conditions including other substance dependence, and comorbid medical conditions. Therefore, this proposed longitudinal observational study will identify key observational data and directions for future work to develop interventions in the ED or elsewhere to enhance treatment engagement, linkages to primary care, and changes in drug use for this understudied population already experiencing potentially harmful medical consequences of their drug use.

Website: http://crisp.cit.nih.gov/crisp/Crisp_Query.Generate_Screen

- **Project Title: COCAINE ADDICTION:MEDICATION STRATEGIES AND EVALUTION**

Principal Investigator & Institution: Bergman, Jack; Associate Professor; Mc Lean Hospital (Belmont, Ma) Belmont, Ma 02478

Timing: Fiscal Year 2002; Project Start 30-SEP-1996; Project End 30-JUN-2007

Summary: (provided by applicant): Drug addiction arising from abuse of **cocaine** and other psychomotor stimulants continues to be a critical public health concern. Currently, effective pharmacotherapies are not available to combat the addictive power of **cocaine.** Consequently, medication strategies and candidate medications that reduce cocaine's reinforcing strength need to be identified. The proposed research is designed to address these problems with innovative self-administration procedures in which dose-effect functions for the relative reinforcing strength of **cocaine** can be rapidly determined. Self-administration procedures in nonhuman primates have been integral to previous studies of abuse liability and drug dependence; however, procedures that are suitably modified to identify medications that alter reinforcing strength, particularly in chronic studies and under varying behavioral conditions, have not yet been advanced. In our novel procedure, rhesus monkeys learn to distribute their behavior throughout the session on the basis of the relative reinforcing strengths of an i.v. solution that is available for self-injection and an alternative reinforcer (food). This procedure is especially designed to divorce the reinforcing strength of drugs from their other behavioral effects. In proposed studies, the distribution of behavior will be determined under varying conditions of response cost and response suppression to establish the full range of cocaine's relative reinforcing strength. Next, the acute and chronic effects of drugs that represent different agonist-based medication strategies will be fully evaluated. Strategies will be based upon indirect and direct monoaminergic mechanisms that may be associated with the reinforcing or other subjective effects of stimulant drugs. It is expected that some strategies may more effectively combat the reinforcing strength of **cocaine** when it is low whereas other strategies may be useful over a wider range of conditions. The effects of selected drugs in combination also will be evaluated to explore the possibility that mechanistic synergism may expand the effectiveness or increase the potency of medications. Finally, the effects of candidate medications on cocaine's overt behavioral effects (visual scanning/checking) also will be evaluated during chronic exposure. These effects may be related to behavioral toxicity, and will provide important information with which to evaluate the therapeutic advantage of different agonist-based medication strategies. Overall, our proposed studies in monkeys will provide significant advances for evaluating the reinforcing strength of **cocaine** and for assessing the effectiveness with which different agonist-based medications may combat the addictive power of stimulant drugs.

Website: http://crisp.cit.nih.gov/crisp/Crisp_Query.Generate_Screen

- **Project Title: COCAINE AND BRAIN EXTRACELLULAR MATRIX**

Principal Investigator & Institution: Sorg, Barbara A.; Associate Professor; Vet & Comp Anat/Pharm/Physiol; Washington State University 423 Neill Hall Pullman, Wa 99164

Timing: Fiscal Year 2002; Project Start 30-SEP-2001; Project End 31-AUG-2004

Summary: (provided by the applicant) Repeated **cocaine** exposure induces neural plasticity as implied by the development of dependence and sensitization. An under explored but critical aspect of cocaine-dependent plasticity is the impact of **cocaine** on proteins involved in synaptic remodeling during drug-seeking behaviors. This proposal focuses on the proteins that regulate the extracellular matrix (ECM). These proteins are critical for dynamic processes involved in synaptic reorganization during learning. We envision that the ECM acts as a scaffold to optimally align pre- and postsynaptic elements, which must be transiently degraded during synaptic remodeling. Since drug abuse is believed to involve a learning process, molecules involved in remodeling should be altered in brain areas implicated in drug abuse. This notion is supported by recent studies reporting morphological changes in brain regions critical for drug-taking behavior. We hypothesize that these morphological changes require shifts in the expression of ECM proteins, which are dependent on the regulators, matrix metalloproteinases (MMPs) and tissue inhibitors of MMPs (TIMPs). Recent work in our laboratories has demonstrated that activity of the enzyme MMP-9 in the hippocampus is correlated with active learning of a water maze spatial learning task. In addition, acute **cocaine** treatment increases MMP-9 activity in the nucleus accumbens and medial prefrontal cortex, with a concomitant decrease in the ventral tegmental area. In contrast, only small changes were found in the substantia nigra and striatum, suggesting a specificity of cocaine's effects on plasticity of mesocorticolimbic pathways. The proposed studies will assess the level of expression of MMPs and TIMPs critical for remodeling processes believed to occur during learning and extinction of a **cocaine** conditioned place preference (CPP) task. These studies will determine which brain regions exhibit plastic changes associated with the pairing of contextual information with **cocaine,** whether or not the same brain sites are involved in the extinction of **cocaine** CPP behavior, and if these molecules can be further altered once initial learning of the CPP task has taken place. We postulate that repeated **cocaine** initially produces synaptic rearrangement in specific brain regions linked to drug craving and addiction, and that changes in MMPs/TIMPs are indicators of this rearrangement. Moreover, subsequent to repeated **cocaine** treatment, there may be an attenuation or loss of neural plasticity in these brain sites that contributes to the long-lasting nature of addiction.

Website: http://crisp.cit.nih.gov/crisp/Crisp_Query.Generate_Screen

- **Project Title: COCAINE AND POLYDRUG ABUSE: NEW MEDICATION STRATEGIES**

Principal Investigator & Institution: Mello, Nancy K.; Professor of Psychology; Mc Lean Hospital (Belmont, Ma) Belmont, Ma 02478

Timing: Fiscal Year 2002; Project Start 15-MAR-2002; Project End 28-FEB-2007

Summary: This is a new application for a NIDA Program Project (P-01) entitled **Cocaine** and Polydrug Abuse: New Medication Strategies. **Cocaine** abuse remains one of the nation's most serious drug abuse problems, and as yet, there are no effective anti-cocaine medications. **Cocaine** is often abused in combination with heroin, and dual dependence on **cocaine** and opioids further complicates medication based treatment. Four inter- related clinical and pre-clinical research projects are proposed to develop novel medications for the treatment of **cocaine** abuse and polydrug abuse. These multi-disciplinary collaborative projects involve behavioral science, endocrinology, neurobiology and pharmacology. An innovative new preclinical model of speedball (cocaine+heroin) abuse will be used to evaluate novel medication strategies, and to test the hypothesis that medication combinations targeted at both the **cocaine** and the opioid components of the speedball will be more effective than treatment with either anti-cocaine or anti-opioid medications alone. Acute and chronic treatment with potential anti-cocaine medications (endocrine modulators, dopamine reuptake inhibitors; dopamine agonists and antagonists) and anti-opioid medications (high and intermediate efficacy mu agonists and a new long-acting mu antagonist) will be evaluated. In addition to pharmacological approaches, we propose to evaluate novel biologic approaches to reduce **cocaine** abuse that are based on our recent discoveries of cocaine-neuroendocrine interactions. We hypothesize that the acute neuroendocrine effects of **cocaine** may contribute to its abuse- related effects and that analysis of cocaine-endocrine interactions will guide new strategies for medications development. The temporal covariance between **cocaine** stimulation of anterior pituitary, gonadal and adrenal hormones will be examined in both clinical and preclinical studies. The behavioral relevance of cocaine's acute endocrine effects will be evaluated both in clinical studies and preclinical studies of biologic approaches to **cocaine** abuse treatment. The pharmacological mechanisms underlying cocaine's acute endocrine effects will be evaluated with selective monoamine agonists and antagonists in preclinical studies. In addition, we propose to systematically examine changes in the acute endocrine profile of **cocaine** produced by (a) repeated **cocaine** dosing in a binge pattern, (b) the addition of heroin to **cocaine** to simulate milieu on the efficacy of medications for **cocaine** abuse treatment will e examined. These studies should clarify the ways in which **cocaine** abuse influences and is influenced by neuroendocrine factors. Advances in understanding the neurobiological determinants of the abuse-related effects of drugs should facilitate the development of more effective treatment medications.

Website: http://crisp.cit.nih.gov/crisp/Crisp_Query.Generate_Screen

- **Project Title: COCAINE DEPENDENCE AND COGNITIVE CONTROL OF BEHAVIOR**

Principal Investigator & Institution: Kilts, Clinton D.; Professor and Vice-Chair of Research; Psychiatry and Behavioral Scis; Emory University 1784 North Decatur Road Atlanta, Ga 30322

Timing: Fiscal Year 2003; Project Start 15-AUG-2003; Project End 30-APR-2007

Summary: (provided by applicant): **Cocaine** dependence (CD) is defined by the loss of control over drug seeking and use behavior despite clear adverse consequences of drug use. The conceptual framework of the proposed project asserts that **cocaine** addiction represents a disorder of cognitive control of behavior with definable neural correlates. The objective of this proposal is to use event-related fMRI to test hypotheses related to a neural model of the effect of CD on context-modulated cognitive control. Aim 1 of the project would use a Go-NoGo task involving human faces to assess the behavioral and neural correlates of the effect of CD on response inhibition. Aims 2 and 3 would assess the specific impact of conditioned **cocaine** cues on cognitive control. Studies would assess the effect of CD on the behavioral, neural, psychophysiological and cognitive correlates of attempts to volitionally regulate the drug craving response to mental imagery of **cocaine** cues (Aim 2). Comparisons at early (7-21 days) vs. prolonged (60-75 days) periods of **cocaine** abstinence would test further the neural model. Additional studies would use a **cocaine** counting word Stroop task (cocStroop) to define the behavioral and neural correlates of cognitive interference by **cocaine** cues (Aim 3). Aim 4 would use a Prisoners Dilemma game variation as a naturalistic social model to define the neural substrates of a CD-related abnormality in the expression and regulation of social aggression. Aim 5 would determine whether impairments in cognitive control of behavior represent vulnerability factors for **cocaine** addiction. The behavioral and neural correlates of response inhibition, cognitive interference and social aggression would be assessed in an "at risk" sample of cocaine-naive, same-sex siblings of CD probands. The long-term goal of these studies is to develop a novel understanding of the processes related to the acquisition, maintenance and social consequences of **cocaine** addiction.

Website: http://crisp.cit.nih.gov/crisp/Crisp_Query.Generate_Screen

- **Project Title: COCAINE DEPENDENCE: EEG SLEEP AND CYTOKINES**

Principal Investigator & Institution: Irwin, Michael R.; Professor; Psychiatry & Biobehav Sciences; University of California Los Angeles 10920 Wilshire Blvd., Suite 1200 Los Angeles, Ca 90024

Timing: Fiscal Year 2002; Project Start 30-SEP-2002; Project End 31-MAY-2006

Summary: (provided by applicant): Sleep disturbance is a prominent complaint of **cocaine** dependent patients during usage, and also following withdrawal and abstinence. However, the high frequency of disordered sleep stands in sharp contrast with limited effort to fully evaluate sleep or to identify the mechanisms that account for sleep abnormalities associated with chronic **cocaine** abuse. Given evidence that **cocaine** addiction also leads to a striking increase in the risk of infectious disease, we hypothesize that the complex cytokine network is one physiological system that mediates both sleep and immune abnormalities in **cocaine** dependence. Basic observations demonstrate that cytokines play a key role in the regulation of sleep. Translation of cytokine-sleep mechanisms into the clinic show that sleep loss and disturbances of sleep architecture are coincident with alterations in pro-inflammatory and helper T cell type 1/type 2 (Th1/Th2) cytokines, and that cytokine abnormalities predict disordered sleep in **cocaine** dependent patients. Thus, the over-arching objective of this study is to evaluate sleep and the reciprocal relationships between sleep and cytokine expression in **cocaine** dependent patients during acute and protracted abstinence as compared to controls. Acute administration of **cocaine** will serve as a pharmacologic probe of cytokine-sleep regulatory processes. The specific aims of this study are to: 1) evaluate whether **cocaine** and **cocaine** dependence are associated with disturbances of sleep including loss of delta sleep and increases of REM sleep; 2) determine the predictive validity of proteomic measures of nocturnal pro-inflammatory-, Th1, and Th2 cytokines on sleep depth in **cocaine** dependent subjects during acute- and protracted abstinence and following acute **cocaine** administration; 3) examine the consequences of disordered sleep on the expression of pro-inflammatory, Th1, and Th2 cytokines and daytime sleepiness during acute- and protracted abstinence and following acute **cocaine** administration. Given the prominence of sleep disturbance in **cocaine** dependent subjects and evidence of sleep architecture abnormalities into recovery, understanding the bi-directional relationships between cytokines and sleep in **cocaine** dependence has implications for answering why sleep is disordered in **cocaine** dependent patients and for the development of novel treatments for sleep disturbance in **cocaine** dependence.

Website: http://crisp.cit.nih.gov/crisp/Crisp_Query.Generate_Screen

- **Project Title: COCAINE SELF ADMINISTRATION IN DOPAMINE KNOCKOUT MICE**

Principal Investigator & Institution: Caine, Simon B.;; Mc Lean Hospital (Belmont, Ma) Belmont, Ma 02478

Timing: Fiscal Year 2002; Project Start 12-MAR-1999; Project End 29-FEB-2004

Summary: Studies are proposed to use gene-targeted "knockout" mice to analyze the roles of different dopaminergic systems in the reinforcing effects of **cocaine.** Compelling pharmacological and neurobiologic evidence suggests that the abuse-related effects of **cocaine** are mediated by dopaminergic systems, and dopamine-based strategies provide promising avenues for development of new medications to treat **cocaine** abuse and dependence. The more specific identification of molecular targets for design and synthesis of dopamine-related medications may be greatly assisted by systematic analyses of mechanisms mediating cocaine's reinforcing effects in knockout mice. Although drugs acting at the dopamine transporter or at D1-like or D2- like receptors can modify some abuse-related effects of **cocaine,** the roles of these proteins in cocaine's effects are not fully understood. Genetic technology in mice that permits the deletion of a single protein by "knockout" of its functional gene provides a highly specific tool that may help to elucidate the roles pharmacologically. For example, the modification of **cocaine** self-administration by mixed D2/D3 compounds may be due to D2 or D3 actions alone or in combination. Studies in mice that lack the D2 receptor will permit a clearer analysis of the role of the D3 receptor in such effects. The proposed self-administration will: (1) examine the reinforcing effects of **cocaine** in mice lacking the dopamine transporter or to the D1 or D2 receptor, and (2) use these mice to specify more precisely the receptor mechanisms involved in the modification of **cocaine** self-administration by non-selective dopaminergic compounds. An important feature of this proposal is that self-administration studies in parental inbred strains and studies of responding maintained by a non-drug reinforcer will be conducted to provide a comprehensive basis for interpreting results of self-administration studies in knockout mice. In addition, studies in male and female mice will allow assessment of gender differences in genetic and pharmacological influences on **cocaine** self-administration. Overall, this research will increase our understanding of the roles of specific dopaminergic proteins in cocaine's abuse-related effects and help to identify the most appropriate targets for medications development. Moreover, integrating gene-targeting strategies with pharmacological and drug self-administration techniques will provide a framework for future studies using yet more advanced genetic technology to identify molecular mechanisms of cocaine's abuse-related effects.

Website: http://crisp.cit.nih.gov/crisp/Crisp_Query.Generate_Screen

- **Project Title: COCAINE, DISULFIRAM & DBH: A PHARMACOMECHANISTIC STUDY**

Principal Investigator & Institution: Malison, Robert T.; Professor; Psychiatry; Yale University 47 College Street, Suite 203 New Haven, Ct 065208047

Timing: Fiscal Year 2002; Project Start 30-SEP-2002; Project End 30-JUN-2005

Summary: (provided by applicant): A broadly effective pharmacotherapy for **cocaine** dependence remains an unrealized national priority. Of the multiple medications tested to date, only disulfiram has shown consistent, albeit modest, efficacy in clinical trials. While its efficacy is well demonstrated, it s therapeutic mechanism of action is largely unknown. Initial rationales for disulfiram s use in **cocaine** dependence derived from observations of high rates of co-morbid alcohol intake. However, recent studies indicate comparably improved outcomes in non-alcohol abusing cohorts. The latter observation has shifted attention away from peripheral targets of the drug (i.e., alcohol dehydrogenase) to neurobiologically more relevant candidates. One possible mediator is dopamine beta-hydroxylase (DbetaH), the enzyme that converts dopamine to norepinephrine. However, the direct relevance of DbetaH to **cocaine** reward remains to be established. The current R01 application will test the hypothesis that DbetaH is an important mediator of cocaine-induced euphoria in human **cocaine** abusers. Specifically, we will examine the effects of 1) allelic variation in the gene encoding DbetaH (DBH), 2) pharmacologic antagonism (disulfiram) of DbetaH function, and 3) gene-drug interactions on cocaine-induced euphoria in chronically dependent subjects. To do so, we have developed and validated a novel laboratory paradigm of "binge" **cocaine** self-administration based on patient-controlled analgesia techniques. Preliminary results in 12 subjects provide direct support for Aim #1 and suggest that "low activity" alleles at DBH are associated with a normal dose-responsively to cocaine-induced euphoria (p = 0.007), while individuals homozygous for the wild type allele have a flat, anhedonic curve). Direct demonstration of DbetaH s relevance to **cocaine** reward by convergent genetic, pharmacological, and pharmacogenetic data would provide powerful neurobiological support for DbetaH as a prime medication development target for **cocaine** dependence.

Website: http://crisp.cit.nih.gov/crisp/Crisp_Query.Generate_Screen

- **Project Title: COCAINE/SEX HORMONE/5HT--MOLECULAR & BEHAVIORAL ANALYSES**

Principal Investigator & Institution: Thomas, Mary L.; Pharmacology and Toxicology; University of Texas Medical Br Galveston 301 University Blvd Galveston, Tx 77555

Timing: Fiscal Year 2002; Project Start 01-AUG-1998; Project End 30-JUN-2004

Summary: (Applicant's Abstract) The acute and chronic effects of psychostimulants, such as **cocaine** and amphetamine derivatives, are more pronounced in females than males. There is evidence to suggest that these gender differences are hormonally, rather than developmentally, based. The long-term goal of this project is to determine the cellular and molecular substrates that underlie the modulation of stimulant-induced behaviors by the female sex hormones estrogen (E) and progesterone (P). In the present proposal, we will test the hypothesis that the interaction of sex hormones with serotonin (5-HT) function lays the foundation for the behavioral response to **cocaine;** the actions of **cocaine** to inhibit 5-HT reuptake contribute to its behavioral effects while inhibition of dopamine (DA) reuptake is defined as a primary mediator. Hormone levels will be controlled experimentally using groups of female rats that have undergone ovariectomy (OVX), with or without replacement with E and P. In Specific Aim 1, molecular biology approaches will be used to assess the impact of ovarian steroids on steady-state levels of the 5-HT transporter mRNA in midbrain and 5-HT1A, 5-HT1B, and 5-HT2c receptor mRNA in reward-relevant brain areas. The concomitant effects of these treatments on levels of mRNA for DA transporter, DA1 and DA2 receptors, and E and P receptors will also be determined. Behavioral and pharmacological tools will be used to assess the relative contribution of 5-HT1A, 5-HT1B, and 5-HT2C receptors to the locomotor stimulation (Specific Aim 2) and sensitization (Specific Aim 3) induced by **cocaine** in the face of given hormone environments. In Specific Aim 4, the functional significance of sex hormone and 5-HT interactions will be assessed in the drug discrimination paradigm to provide an animal model of the "subjective" effects of **cocaine.** Intact or OVX female rats will be trained to discriminate **cocaine** from saline and the neuropharmacological profile will be investigated using specific 5-HT and DA agonists and antagonists in the absence and presence of ovarian hormones. A comparative study of the locomotor stimulatory, sensitization and discriminative stimulus effects of the abused amphetamine derivative (+/-)-3,4-methylenedioxymethamphetamine (MDMA) will be conducted in parallel groups of rats to assess the generality of hormonal regulation to another psychostimulant, one whose behavioral effects are thought to be mediated in large part by 5-HT mechanisms. The results of these studies will provide important information concerning the fundamental mechanisms underlying both steroid-5-HT interactions and gender differences in the responsivity to psychostimulants. As a consequence, new insight into potential therapeutic strategies for drug dependence in women as well as the enhanced vulnerability of women to mood and anxiety disorders will be obtained.

Website: http://crisp.cit.nih.gov/crisp/Crisp_Query.Generate_Screen

- **Project Title: COGNITION IN COCAINE DEPENDENCE: ASSESSMENT & THERAPY**

Principal Investigator & Institution: Aharonovich, Efrat; Psychiatry; Columbia University Health Sciences Po Box 49 New York, Ny 10032

Timing: Fiscal Year 2003; Project Start 10-SEP-2003; Project End 30-APR-2008

Summary: (provided by applicant): Cognitive impairment, commonly found among substance abusers, may reduce the effectiveness of manualized psychosocial treatments. If so, tailoring such treatments to the patients' needs should improve effectiveness. The goal of this mentored clinical scientist award is to enhance the developing clinical research skills of Efrat Aharonovich, Ph.D. through research on cognitive deficits and manualized psychosocial treatments for substance abuse patients. In 2001, Dr. Aharonovich joined the faculty in the Division as Assistant Professor of Clinical Psychology in Psychiatry. Her pilot studies on cognitive functioning and treatment outcome in substance abuse patients provide preliminary support for her hypothesis that cognitive functioning affects treatment outcome. Dr. Aharonovich is co-PI on a NIDA-funded study of depressed heroin addicts, and she will shortly receive NIDA funds for an exploratory study of cognitive deficits and treatment outcome in non-depressed **cocaine** abusing patients. However, to become an independent clinical researcher, Dr. Aharonovich will need formal course work, mentoring, and release of time from her extensive clinical and administrative responsibilities so that she can concentrate on developing her own research. In the next several years, Dr. Aharonovich plans to conduct mentored formative research and clinical treatment trials of behavioral interventions modified for cognitively impaired substance abusers. This research and additional training will prepare Dr. Aharonovich well to meet her long-term research career goal of improving the effectiveness of behavioral interventions for substance abuse patients. Under the sponsorship and guidance of Dr. Edward Nunes, together with other Columbia University faculty, Dr. Aharonovich's training plan combines formal course work with clinical research experience. She will work closely with several preceptors to receive training in the following areas: methods of conducting clinical treatment trials, neuropsychological assessment batteries for substance abusers, instrument development, study design and interpretation, and biostatistics. Her research plan includes a study of the effects of cognitive deficits on the outcome of Cognitive Behavioral Therapy (CBT) in substance abuse patients, the use of this information to tailor CBT for cognitively impaired substance abuse patients, and a randomized clinical trial of the effectiveness of the modified CBT. The combined mentoring, training and research plan will provide Dr. Aharonovich with unique training, and will afford her the opportunity to develop an independent clinical research career focused on the development of new behavioral approaches to the treatment of substance abuse disorders.

Website: http://crisp.cit.nih.gov/crisp/Crisp_Query.Generate_Screen

- **Project Title: COMMUNITY-FRIENDLY MANUAL GUIDED DRUG COUNSELING**

Principal Investigator & Institution: Crits-Christoph, Paul F.; Associate Professor; Psychiatry; University of Pennsylvania 3451 Walnut Street Philadelphia, Pa 19104

Timing: Fiscal Year 2002; Project Start 30-SEP-2002; Project End 30-JUN-2005

Summary: (provided by applicant): We propose here treatment development work to create and test a "community-friendly" manual-based individual plus group drug counseling package. The NIDA Collaborative **Cocaine** Treatment Study (Crits-Christoph et at., 1999) recently reported that manual-based individual drug counseling (IDC) plus group drug counseling (GDC) has superior drug use outcomes compared to cognitive-behavior therapy plus GDC, psychodynamic therapy plus GDC, and GDC alone. Proposed changes to IDC and GDC to make them more "community-friendly" include changes to both the duration and content of the treatment models. The proposed treatment development work will include (1) obtaining feedback on the new treatment manuals by a sample of 15 community-based drug counselors, (2) evaluating whether a group of drug counselors can successfully learn to implement the new manuals, (3) evaluating counselors' experiences in learning and conducting the new treatments, (4) conducting a pilot randomized evaluation of the outcomes of the new package of individual plus group drug counseling compared to group drug counseling alone, (5) obtaining ratings of treatment fidelity to assess whether the new individual and group drug counseling approaches can be differentiated from the original therapies, (6) assessing patient reactions to the new treatment, and (7) conducting a preliminary investigation of potential mediators of change of the new treatments. The pilot randomized trial will involve assignment of 40 patients meeting DSM-IV criteria for **cocaine** dependence to either new versions of individual plus group drug counseling or group drug counseling alone. Assessments will be done at time of intake and weekly (for urines and self-report of **cocaine** use) or monthly (for other outcome measures) during a 3-month treatment phase. The primary efficacy measures will be the ASI Drug Use Composite scale and a composite **cocaine** use measure that incorporates urine data, Addiction Severity Index Interview data, and weekly self-report of **cocaine** use. Mediation of drug use change will be examined by assessing beliefs about substance use, endorsement of 12-step behaviors and beliefs, and attendance/ participation in 12-step meetings at baseline, weekly for the first month and monthly thereafter. The data gathered from this treatment development project will inform the design of a subsequent larger study.

Website: http://crisp.cit.nih.gov/crisp/Crisp_Query.Generate_Screen

- **Project Title: COMORBID DISORDERS IN TREATMENT OF OPIATE DEPENDENCE**

Principal Investigator & Institution: Gonzalez-Haddad, Gerardo; Psychiatry; Yale University 47 College Street, Suite 203 New Haven, Ct 065208047

Timing: Fiscal Year 2002; Project Start 01-JUL-2001; Project End 30-JUN-2006

Summary: (Provided by Applicant) This application is to study comorbid disorders that affect the treatment of opiate dependence. The specific aims of the proposed program of research are as follows: Study 1 will examine comorbid depression as a predictive factor in treatment with desipramine and contingency management of **cocaine** abusing opiate dependent subjects maintained on buprenorphine by secondary data analysis of a completed randomized clinical trial. Study 2 will evaluate the efficacy of sertraline in the treatment of **cocaine** dependent patients with comorbid depression in a recently started double-blind randomized clinical trial. Study 3 will determine changes of health care cost after treatment of opiate dependence in the Veterans Affairs health delivery system using existing administrative databases. It will determine whether confounding factors, especially comorbid depression and **cocaine** dependence, may affect changes in costs. The overall aim of the proposal is to provide me with a supervised patient oriented research and educational experience that will enable me to become an independent investigator in substance abuse. My specific career development goals are to: (1) Acquire in-depth knowledge of the neuropharmacology of **cocaine** and opiate dependence, and of substance induced mood disorders. (2) Develop expertise in clinical research and management of **cocaine** and opiate dependence, and current pharmacotherapies. (3) Develop skills in Mental Health Service research related to substance abuse. The proposed career development plan utilizes the collaboration of Thomas Kosten, MD in developing expertise executing randomized clinical trials, Robert Rosenheck, MD in developing skills in mental health services research and Kevin Sevarino, MD, PhD in clinical management of opiate dependence. The educational experience includes a four year period of formal coursework at the Interdepartmental Neuroscience Program at the Yale School of Medicine and at the Yale School of Epidemiology and Public Health. This K23 research career award will enable me to start an academic career focusing on research in **cocaine** and opiate dependence and to develop a bridge between clinical trials and services research.

Website: http://crisp.cit.nih.gov/crisp/Crisp_Query.Generate_Screen

- **Project Title: COMORBIDITY IN COCAINE AND OPIOID PHARMACOTHERAPY**

Principal Investigator & Institution: Kosten, Thomas R.; Professor of Psychiatry; Psychiatry; Yale University 47 College Street, Suite 203 New Haven, Ct 065208047

Timing: Fiscal Year 2002; Project Start 01-APR-2000; Project End 31-AUG-2005

Summary: (Applicant's Abstract) This application requests a Research Scientist Award to enable the candidate to pursue full time research and research training aimed at improving the pharmacotherapy of **cocaine** and opioid dependence. During the award period, the applicant will conduct pharmacotherapy trials of two types: a) combinations of novel pharmacotherapies with behavioral interventions targeted at **cocaine** dependent patients with comorbidities such as depression and opioid dependence, b) treatments for **cocaine** associated cerebral perfusion defects assessed using SPECT neuroimaging. The Research Plan uses behavioral contingencies to move forward our 10 years of work showing the efficacy of desipramine (DMI) and its combination with buprenorphine (BUP) for reducing **cocaine** abuse. The plan provides a detailed description of our 24 week, randomized placebo-controlled, double blind clinical trial using DMI in combination with contingency management for 160 patients who are maintained on buprenorphine for comorbid opioid and **cocaine** dependence. The contingency group will get a voucher worth a set monetary value that increases for consecutively drug-free urines (weeks 1-19) or a voucher with a fixed value under an increasing ratio of number of consecutive drug free urines per voucher (weeks 13-24). Subjects not in the contingency group get monetary vouchers independent of their illicit **cocaine** use.

Website: http://crisp.cit.nih.gov/crisp/Crisp_Query.Generate_Screen

- **Project Title: CORTICOTROPIN RELEASING FACTOR MECHANISMS AND COCAINE**

Principal Investigator & Institution: Gallagher, Joel P.; Pharmacology and Toxicology; University of Texas Medical Br Galveston 301 University Blvd Galveston, Tx 77555

Timing: Fiscal Year 2002; Project Start 25-APR-1999; Project End 31-MAR-2004

Summary: (applicant's abstract): Accumulating evidence suggests that the corticotropin releasing factor (CRF) neurotransmitter system may play a prominent role in the mediation of motivational aspects of drug dependence and that CRF receptors participate in the arousal-enhancing properties of psychostimulants and in behavioral sensitization. The objective of the proposed research is to define the membrane mechanism of action of the CRF neuro- transmitter system in control and after chronic **cocaine** administration in two limbic areas, the septum and the amygdala. This project will test the hypothesis that the effects of CRF agonists and antagonists in control neurons are mediated through different receptors in the septum and amygdala and that the altered effects of CRF after chronic **cocaine** are due to modulation of specific CRF receptors. In these studies, CRF, urocortin - an endogenous CRF-like peptide, CRF (9-33) - a CRF binding protein inhibitor, and peptide and non-peptide CRF receptor antagonists will be analyzed using whole patch and intracellular sharp electrode recording. Electrophysiological data will be compared in naive control, saline control, and chronic **cocaine** animals. The following specific aims will be addressed: 1. Define the effect of CRF, urocortin, the CRF binding protein inhibitor, and CRF receptor antagonists on synaptic transmission and on membrane conductance in septal and amygdala neurons, 2. Determine receptors mediating CRF actions by analyzing the effect of the specific CRF-R1 receptor and non-specific antagonists on the agonists' responses, 3. Analyze effects of CRF, urocortin, the CRF binding protein inhibitor, and CRF receptor antagonists, on synaptic transmission and membrane conductance in the septum and amygdala in saline control and chronic **cocaine** treated animals, and 4. Determine the time course of the development of CRF receptor-mediated changes and the persistence of these changes. The proposed studies will contribute valuable insight into the mechanisms of CRF actions in chronic **cocaine** addiction and its possible motivational role in drug dependence. These results may also provide critical information regarding non-peptide and peptide antagonists of CRF as potentially effective pharmacotherapies in the treatment of chronic **cocaine** dependence.

Website: http://crisp.cit.nih.gov/crisp/Crisp_Query.Generate_Screen

- **Project Title: DISCOVERY OF NOVEL PHARMACOTHERAPIES: COCAINE DEPENDENCE**

Principal Investigator & Institution: Meltzer, Peter C.; President; Organix, Inc. Woburn, Ma 01801

Timing: Fiscal Year 2004; Project Start 30-SEP-1997; Project End 28-FEB-2009

Summary: (provided by applicant): **Cocaine** dependence is a problem of national significance. In the past decade there has been a considerable advance in the understanding of the chemistry and pharmacology of **cocaine** dependence. Notwithstanding, no **cocaine** pharmacotherapy has yet been approved by the FDA. A number of lead compounds are undergoing pharmacological evaluation as potential therapeutic agents. Cocaine's reinforcing properties and stimulant effects are associated with its propensity to bind to monoamine transporters. The goal of this project is to design potential pharmacotherapies for **cocaine** dependence. We will focus on the development of an understanding of the interaction between ligand and monoamine neurotransmitter uptake systems. We propose to expand our search for compounds that bind to DAT and SERT mechanisms but disturb dopamine (DA) uptake minimally, for compounds with slow onset and long duration of action, and for mechanism-based inhibitors of **cocaine** binding. We will focus on three classes: 8-oxabicyclo[3,2,1]octanes (oxatropanes), 8-azabicyclo[3,2,1]octanes (tropanes) and pyrovalerone analogues. The Specific Aims are: Synthesis and evaluation of (i) non-nitrogen tropane analogs, (ii) 6- and 7 hydroxylated 8-azatropane prodrugs, (iii) 6- and 7-hydroxylated 8-oxatropan(en)es, (iv) dopamine sparing **cocaine** antagonists that bind irreversibly to the **cocaine** site, (v) 3-heterobiaryltropanes. (vi) analogues of pyrovalerone.

Website: http://crisp.cit.nih.gov/crisp/Crisp_Query.Generate_Screen

- **Project Title: DISULFIRAM FOR COCAINE ABUSE IN BUPRENORPHINE TREATMENT**

Principal Investigator & Institution: Schottenfeld, Richard S.; Professor; Psychiatry; Yale University 47 College Street, Suite 203 New Haven, Ct 065208047

Timing: Fiscal Year 2002; Project Start 10-APR-2000; Project End 29-FEB-2004

Summary: Applicant's Abstract We are proposing a placebo-controlled clinical trial to evaluate the efficacy and potential mechanisms of action of disulfiram (vs. placebo) for treating **cocaine** abuse in buprenorphine maintained subjects (N=180) with concurrent opiate dependence and **cocaine** abuse or dependence. Because of its safety in overdose situations and decreased abuse liability, buprenorphine may be widely used outside of narcotic treatment programs (e.g., in primary care or office settings). Thus it is of considerable importance to evaluate adjunctive pharmacologic treatments that may improve its efficacy for treating concurrent opioid and **cocaine** dependence. Convergent findings from epidemiologic, laboratory and clinical trials, including the results of a preliminary study conducted in preparation for this application, support the potential efficacy of disulfiram; a medication used to treat alcohol dependence, for the treatment of **cocaine** abuse. Disulfiram's efficacy for **cocaine** may result from preventing concurrent alcohol use, which can precipitate **cocaine** relapse, or from its inhibition of dopamine-beta-hydroxylase, the enzyme that converts dopamine to norepinephrine, which may reduce craving and increase the anxiogenic or dysphoric effects of **cocaine** administration. Accordingly, to explore whether disulfiram efficacy for **cocaine** dependence is mediated by its effects on alcohol consumption or on central DBH and dopamine activity, baseline alcohol severity, and DBH genotypes which are associated with high or low DBH activity will be evaluated as predictors of differential treatment response. Subjects meeting DSM-IV criteria for opioid dependence and **cocaine** abuse or dependence will be stabilized on buprenorphine (24 mg daily, sublingual tablets) for 2 weeks before being randomly assigned to 12 weeks of treatment with disulfiram 250 mg daily or placebo, provided under double-blind conditions. An urn randomization procedure will be used to balance the treatment groups on gender, depressive symptoms, baseline alcohol use and **cocaine** use severity. Manual-guided group drug counseling will be the platform psychotherapy provided weekly for all subjects. Primary outcome measures include reductions in **cocaine** use assessed by three times weekly urines and self-report. Secondary outcomes measures include reductions in illicit opioid use and HIV risk behaviors. Primary data analyses will focus on an intention-to-treat sample and will utilize mixed models analysis of variance and a factorial analysis of variance. The effects of baseline predictors and their interactions with treatment condition on these outcomes will also be evaluated.

Website: http://crisp.cit.nih.gov/crisp/Crisp_Query.Generate_Screen

- **Project Title: DISULFIRAM FOR COCAINE ABUSE IN METHADONE- PATIENTS**

Principal Investigator & Institution: Oliveto Beaudoin, Alison; Psychiatry; Yale University 47 College Street, Suite 203 New Haven, Ct 065208047

Timing: Fiscal Year 2002; Project Start 01-MAY-2001; Project End 31-MAR-2006

Summary: (Applicant's Abstract) Because **cocaine** use remains epidemic among most opioid maintenance programs and pharmacological therapeutic strategies specifically aimed at cocaine's dopaminergic actions have shown little efficacy in unselected populations, this proposal will examine a novel pharmacological strategy for treating **cocaine** abuse in opioid-maintained **cocaine** abusers; i.e., treatment with disulfiram. Specifically, the aim of this proposal is to examine the effects of disulfiram (0, 62.5, 125, or 250mg /day) on treatment outcome in methadone-maintained **cocaine** abusers. This 14-wk, double blind, randomized clinical trial will provide treatment for 160 opioid- and cocaine-dependent individuals (18-65 years). Participants will be placed on methadone maintenance during weeks 1-2, at which time level of **cocaine** use is assessed. Then participants will continue on methadone maintenance and be randomly assigned to receive one of the following doses of disulfiram: 0, 62.5, 125, or 250 mg/day. During stabilization on methadone (wks 1-2), participants typically are administered increasing doses of methadone on a daily basis until maintenance doses are attained. Then during the treatment phase (weeks 5-14), participants continue to receive their daily maintenance doses of methadone. In addition, they receive disulfiram/placebo on a daily basis. At the end the study, participants will undergo detoxification from methadone over a 4-week period. In order to enhance outcome, all participants receive weekly 1-hour psychotherapy (Cognitive Behavioral Treatment) with experienced clinicians specifically trained to deliver the therapy and who will receive ongoing supervision. The primary outcomes will be retention and reduction in opioid and **cocaine** use, as assessed by self-report and confirmed by thrice-weekly urinalyses. Secondary outcomes will include reductions in other illicit drug and alcohol use, as well as improvements in psychosocial functioning. The prognostic relevance of genotype at the dopamine beta-hydroxylase locus, dopamine beta-hydroxylase enzyme activity, and severity of **cocaine** dependence will also be examined.

Website: http://crisp.cit.nih.gov/crisp/Crisp_Query.Generate_Screen

• Project Title: DOPAMINE TRANSPORTER AGENTS AGAINST COCAINE DEPENDENCE

Principal Investigator & Institution: Dutta, Aloke K.; Associate Professor of Medicinal Chemist; Pharmaceutical Sciences; Wayne State University 656 W. Kirby Detroit, Mi 48202

Timing: Fiscal Year 2002; Project Start 30-SEP-1999; Project End 31-AUG-2004

Summary: Cocaine is a strong reinforcer which led to its wide-spread use as a major drug of abuse in U.S.A in the last two decades. The development of a medication to treat this addiction is an urgent requirement. The central mechanism of the action of **cocaine** is attributed to its binding to the dopamine (DA) transporter system in the brain. Many structurally diverse compounds that bind selectively to the DAT, have been developed with an aim to block **cocaine** dependence in the central nervous system (CNS), but they met with only limited success. Recently, a high affinity DAT- specific compound GBR 12909 was found to have longer duration of action, was self-administered less potently than **cocaine,** and could antagonize some of the **cocaine** action. In our structure- activity relationship (SAR) study, we have shown the development of novel piperidine analogs of GBR 12909-related potent DAT- specific compounds. Our follow-up SAR study led to the development of a second generation of compounds in this class with far more selectivity for the DAT than conventional GBR molecules. In one of our recent studies, replacement of the benzhydrylic O-atom by an N-atom is these DAT-specific compounds, led to the development of potent and more polar, new-generation N-analog molecules. Furthermore, some of our analogs showed remarkable selectivity for binding to the **cocaine** binding site compared to the dopamine reuptake site in the cloned human transporters binding assay. The values of their uptake to binding ratio were far greater than values of any other existing compounds. In our initial in-vivo motor action studies in mice, two of these analogs were less stimulatnt than **cocaine** and GBR 12909 at similar doses. In combination studies with **cocaine,** these compounds attenuated the locomotor stimulatory effect of **cocaine** efficiently. We now propose to follow up on the SAR studies of our lead compounds to develop potent and selective compounds for the DAT with high dopamine uptake to binding ratio. Selected compounds will be tested for their effects on locomotor action and drug discrimination studies to observe their ability to block **cocaine** action. Our goal is to develop an effective medication against **cocaine** addiction.

Website: http://crisp.cit.nih.gov/crisp/Crisp_Query.Generate_Screen

- **Project Title: EFFECTS OF COCAINE ON SIV AIDS & CNS DISEASE**

Principal Investigator & Institution: Zink, M Christine.; Professor; Comparative Medicine; Johns Hopkins University 3400 N Charles St Baltimore, Md 21218

Timing: Fiscal Year 2002; Project Start 30-SEP-1999; Project End 31-JUL-2004

Summary: Cocaine use is associated with behaviors that increase exposure to HIV. However, it is not known whether **cocaine** use accelerates the progression to AIDS, increases the incidence or severity of AIDS dementia, or increases the likelihood that an individual exposed to HIV will become infected. Some of the confusion over these possible interactions between **cocaine** and HIV lies in the inherent difficulties of studying human populations of drug users, including problems establishing the duration of **cocaine** use, the amount and formulation of **cocaine** consumed, the route of administration, and the concurrent use of the drugs and/or alcohol. SIV infection in macaques is an excellent model for studies of the neurological events in HIV-infected people because it causes clinical and pathological changes similar to HIV and alterations in cognitive/behavioral function similar to those seen in AIDS dementia. The SIV/macaque model has several strengths: macaques can be inoculated with molecularly cloned, biologically characterized viruses, they can be euthanized at different stages of infection to study tissue changes and virus gene expression, and macaque studies do not have the confounding effects of antiviral treatment. Further, macaques can be administered drugs such as **cocaine** on a known schedule to determine the effects of those drugs on cognitive/behavioral function and on the pathogenesis of SIV infection. The SIV/macaque model is currently an untapped resource for studies of the cognitive/behavioral consequences of injection drug use in the context of HIV infection. Our hypothesis is that **cocaine** accelerates the progression to AIDS and the development of CNS lesions and dementia, and thus augments or accelerates the production of cognitive/behavioral deficits. Further, we hypothesize that **cocaine** increases the susceptibility to infection in macaques exposed to SIV by the mucosal route. The proposed research will employ the SIV/macaque model of HIV/AIDS to determine whether acute or chronic **cocaine** use alters 1) the progression to AIDS, 2) the incidence or severity of CNS lesions, 3) cognitive/behavioral function during different stages of SIV infection, and 4) the susceptibility to infection after exposure to SIV. **Cocaine** is proposed as the prototypic drug of abuse in these studies due to its widespread use, its known immunosuppressive effects, its association with HIV in humans, and the absence of physical dependence following its long-term use (e.g., as contrasted with opiates).

Website: http://crisp.cit.nih.gov/crisp/Crisp_Query.Generate_Screen

- **Project Title: EFFECTS OF DRUG INDUCED BRAIN INJURY ON COGNITION**

Principal Investigator & Institution: Lim, Kelvin O.; Professor; Psychiatry; University of Minnesota Twin Cities 200 Oak Street Se Minneapolis, Mn 554552070

Timing: Fiscal Year 2002; Project Start 05-OCT-2001; Project End 31-MAY-2004

Summary: (Adapted from applicant's abstract): There is increasing evidence that white matter is injured in **cocaine** dependence (CD). **Cocaine** and its metabolites have potent vasoconstrictive and neurotoxic properties. White matter lesions in CD subjects have been observed with magnetic resonance imaging (MRI). Brain perfusion defects are present even after several months of abstinence. Chronic hypoperfusion in animal models has been shown to result in white matter injury and learning impairment. White matter injury can impair cortical communication resulting in cognitive and behavioral alterations. Although white matter provides the physical foundation for cortical connectivity, there has been iime in vivo study of white matter, perhaps because of a lack of appropriate tools. Diffusion Tensor Imaging (DTI) is an MRI method which is uniquely suited to the study of white matter because it can be used to quantify the magnitude and directionality of tissue water mobility (ie., self-diffusion) in three dimensions. Structures in white matter (WM), such as myelin sheaths, axon membranes, cytoskeletal elements and white matter tracts, can act as barriers to water mobility, causing the water molecules to move farther along paths that are parallel to fibers rather than those mat are perpendicular to these fibers. When there is a directional dependence of water mobility, the diffusion is described as being anisotropic. This anisotropy can be quantified in a scalar value, fractional anisotropy (FA) and used to assess the microstructural organization of white matter fibers. Highly regular, organized fibers will have high anisotropy; less well-organized fibers will have lower anisotropy measures. We have used DTJ in a series of clinical research studies and have demonstrated differences in white matter anisotropy due to normal aging, schizophrenia, and alcoholism. In addition, we have demonstrated significant correlations between white matter anisotropy and cognitive measures in schizophrenia and alcoholism. In this application, we propose to study **cocaine** dependent patients and normal controls with DTI and neurocognitive assessments. Our Specific Aims are to: 1) Determine if there are abnormalities in WM FA in **cocaine** dependent (CD) subjects compared with controls (NC) 2) Determine if there is a relationship between WM FA and cognitive impairment in CD subjects.

Website: http://crisp.cit.nih.gov/crisp/Crisp_Query.Generate_Screen

- **Project Title: EFFECTS OF DRUG USE AND CESSATION ON MONKEY BRAIN**

Principal Investigator & Institution: Ronen, Itamar; Radiology; University of Minnesota Twin Cities 200 Oak Street Se Minneapolis, Mn 554552070

Timing: Fiscal Year 2002; Project Start 30-SEP-2002; Project End 31-AUG-2004

Summary: (provided by applicant): Human studies show that **cocaine** dependence affects the microstructure of white matter, probably as a result of vasoconstrictive effects of the drug. Little is known, however, about the temporal development of the white matter injury and the changes in cerebral vasculature during the dependence period, or about the recovery of both with cessation of the drug use. Magnetic resonance imaging (MRI) provides tools that are highly suitable for investigating in a non-invasive manner the anatomical, structural and functional and chemical characteristics of the brain. In this application we propose to implement a set of MRI techniques for investigating the effects of the use of **cocaine** on monkey brain, in particular its effects on white matter microstructure on gray/white matter volumes, on the vascularity and perfusion of gray and white matter and on the neurochemical profile of the monkey brain. These techniques will be used to perform a preliminary study on a small and well-controlled population of monkeys. Aim 1. To develop a robust methodology for investigating structural, anatomical and functional measures in monkey brains. Aim 2. To collect preliminary data on the effects of drug use and its cessation on monkey brain. We hypothesize that: 1. Long term **cocaine** self-administration will result in brain changes in the monkeys similar to those seen in human studies. 2. Cessation of drug use will result in a normalization of brain measures. This will address the important issue of whether or not there is significant brain recovery following cessation of drug use.

Website: http://crisp.cit.nih.gov/crisp/Crisp_Query.Generate_Screen

- **Project Title: ESCALATING COCAINE SELF-ADMINISTRATION: NMDA MECHANISMS**

Principal Investigator & Institution: Allen, Richard M.; Psychology; University of Colorado at Denver P.O. Box 173364 Denver, Co 802173364

Timing: Fiscal Year 2002; Project Start 01-AUG-2002; Project End 31-JUL-2004

Summary: (provided by applicant): **Cocaine** abuse represents a serious threat to personal and public health. The increased consumption of **cocaine** in heavy users of the drug is thought to drive demand for **cocaine** in the United States and lead to greater threats to personal and public health. Indeed, four of the seven DSM-IV criteria for Substance Dependence relate to the amount of drug consumed by a user. Although animal models (such as the drug self-administration procedure) have contributed greatly to our understanding of the behavioral and neurobiological mechanisms that underlie drug use, this critical aspect of drug dependence (increased consumption) has not been extensively modeled or explored. Recently, however, an animal model has been described in which rats given 6-hour access to **cocaine** in daily self-administration sessions increase their drug consumption over time. This behavioral adaptation (increased consumption) is not observed with standard short-access (1 or 2 hr) self-administration procedures. Based on the changes in rats' responding for a range of doses of **cocaine** that follow extended-access **cocaine** self-administration sessions, this behavioral adaptation has been described as an example of drug sensitization. Unfortunately, there is virtually no information available that describes the neurobiological correlates associated with increased **cocaine** consumption under these conditions. There is evidence, however, that the reinforcing and behavioral effects of **cocaine** involve glutamatergic activity. Further, sensitization to the locomotor stimulating effects of **cocaine** involves activation of N-methyl-D-aspartate (NMDA) glutamate receptors, and is prevented when rats are treated with NMDA receptor antagonists. It is possible, therefore, that the neurobiological mechanisms that underlie increased **cocaine** consumption are similar to those that underlie other forms of **cocaine** sensitization. The purpose of this proposal is to determine the nature of the changes that underlie the increases in **cocaine** consumption that occur when rats are permitted long access to **cocaine.** The experiments proposed in this application test the hypothesis that the mechanisms that underlie this behavioral adaptation (increased consumption) are similar to those that underlie other forms of adaptation to repeated drug exposure, such as tolerance and sensitization. Specifically, this proposal critically tests the hypothesis that the transition from stable **cocaine** intake to increased **cocaine** consumption involves activation of NMDA receptors, and that this behavioral adaptation is preventable when rats receive chronically an NMDA receptor antagonist throughout extended-access **cocaine** self-administration sessions.

Website: http://crisp.cit.nih.gov/crisp/Crisp_Query.Generate_Screen

- **Project Title: FACTORS IN DRUG DEPENDENCE**

Principal Investigator & Institution: Walsh, Sharon L.; Professor; Psychiatry and Behavioral Scis; Johns Hopkins University 3400 N Charles St Baltimore, Md 21218

Timing: Fiscal Year 2002; Project Start 01-MAY-2002; Project End 30-APR-2007

Summary: The broad objective of this RFA is to increase our understanding of the factors involved in the transition from drug use to drug dependence (the "switch"). Few clinical studies have sought to examine directly factors in humans that may differentiate individuals who intensify their use to a state of dependence compared to those who sustain regular, but controlled, patterns of use. **Cocaine** dependence is an excellent model system for examination of factors underlying drug dependence as **cocaine** is highly reinforcing, is used in binges- indicative of a loss of control, and its abuse is a persistent public health problem. The present application will employ an array of psychiatric, behavioral, pharmacological and pharmacokinetic technologies to examine differences between carefully-matched **cocaine** users with and without **cocaine** dependence under controlled inpatient laboratory conditions. These studies capitalize upon preclinical paradigms designed to assess drug-seeking behavior including self-administration and priming procedures. Experiment I will compare cocaine-dependent users to sporadic users (n=12/group) on measures of impulsivity and sensation seeking, direct pharmacodynamic and pharmacokinetic response to intravenous **cocaine,** and on indices of cocaine-seeking in both a relapse choice self-administration procedure and a progressive ratio self-administration procedure with **cocaine.** Outcome measures for the behavioral paradigms will include the rate of drug-taking, break-point, and estimates of relative reinforcing value in the presence of alternative reinforcers. In addition, novel measures of loss of control, which contrast the subjects' intent about drug use and their actual drug-seeking behavior, will be examined. Experiment II will compare separate groups of cocaine- dependent individuals to carefully-matched, sporadic **cocaine** using individuals (n=12/group) on their relative susceptibility or resilience to priming-induced cocaine-seeking. The priming effects of **cocaine,** alcohol and heroin on cocaine-seeking will be examined in a relapse choice procedure. In addition to this primary outcome, measures of impulsivity and sensation-seeking will be used to examine group differences and as correlates for behavioral outcomes as in Experiment I, and group comparisons will be made for pharmacodynamic and pharmacokinetic differences to **cocaine,** alcohol and heroin. These studies will provide novel information about differences between cocaine-dependent individuals who demonstrate a loss of control over drug use (i.e., those for whom the "switch" is on) to individuals who are able to maintain a regular and controlled pattern of **cocaine** use (i.e., those for whom the "switch" is off). Overall, these projects may identify factors that are predictive of the loss of control in **cocaine** use and may identify fundamental pharmacological or behavioral factors that differentiate individuals who do from those who do not transition to **cocaine** dependence.

Website: http://crisp.cit.nih.gov/crisp/Crisp_Query.Generate_Screen

- **Project Title: FAMILY STUDY OF COCAINE DEPENDENCE**

Principal Investigator & Institution: Bierut, Laura J.; Director; Psychiatry; Washington University Lindell and Skinker Blvd St. Louis, Mo 63130

Timing: Fiscal Year 2002; Project Start 01-SEP-2000; Project End 30-JUN-2005

Summary: (Applicant's abstract): This 5-year case control family study of **cocaine** dependence will examine familial and non-familial antecedents and consequences associated with **cocaine** dependence. The specific aims of this study are: (i) to examine familial transmission of **cocaine** dependence and related psychopathology; (ii) to study interrelationships between individual 'and familial factors that are associated with **cocaine** use, abuse, and dependence; (iii) to specify predisposing factors and outcomes of **cocaine** use, abuse, and dependence, and their relationship to family factors; and (iv) to compare results of this study with data from a large multi- site family study of alcoholism, the Collaborative Study on the Genetics of Alcoholism (COGA). To accomplish these goals, 500 **cocaine** dependent subjects in treatment, 500 community-based subjects, and their nearest aged full siblings will be recruited (total of 2000 subjects). Personal interviews will be performed to determine the rates of **cocaine** use, abuse, and dependence along with alcohol, nicotine, and other substance dependence. In addition, lifetime psychiatric histories will be obtained for major depressive disorder, anxiety disorders, post-traumatic stress disorder, conduct disorder, attention deficit, and hyperactivity. Adverse circumstances including school difficulties, high-risk sexual behaviors, IV drug use violence, and legal difficulties will be assessed. Histories of all first-degree relatives will be obtained from all the subjects. This information will permit analyses of individual and familial factors that are involved in the development of **cocaine** use, abuse, and dependence, and familial patterns of psychopathology related to **cocaine** dependence. By surveying groups of high and low risk individuals for the development of **cocaine** use, abuse, and dependence, the proposed study will generate a unique understanding of the natural history, etiology, and consequences of **cocaine** dependence in our communities.

Website: http://crisp.cit.nih.gov/crisp/Crisp_Query.Generate_Screen

- **Project Title: FUNCTIONAL BRAIN MAPPING OF COCAINE ACTION**

Principal Investigator & Institution: Rosen, Bruce R.; Professor of Radiology; Massachusetts General Hospital 55 Fruit St Boston, Ma 02114

Timing: Fiscal Year 2002; Project Start 30-SEP-1994; Project End 30-JUN-2004

Summary: A major unmet goal of drug abuse research is to understand the neural substrates of reinforcement of drugs of abuse in humans and the role that these mechanisms may play in initiating and sustaining drug dependence. This proposal for a Program Project is a renewal of our currently funded PO1 from the National Institute on Drug Abuse, "fMRI of **Cocaine** Action". The overall goal of this program continues to be the utilization and refinement of state of the art techniques to produce interpretable brain maps, functional anatomy of human subjective states that occur in response to c0caine, with particular emphasis during the funding cycle on the braid reward circuitry mediating **cocaine** response in humans, using functional magnetic resonance imaging (fMRI) as the principal tool. To effectively perform the experiments to test these hypotheses, three Projects and three Cores. As in our current funding cycle, Project 1 is an fMRI study of regional brain activation by **cocaine** in cocaine-dependent human subjects. The objective of Project 1 is to investigate of brain reward circuitry in mediating the **cocaine** response in humans, and to distinguish euphoria-like brain activation from craving-like brain activation. Project 2 has evolved to begin the important work of developing rodent models to more completely understand pharmacologically mediated MRI signal changes observed after administration of dopamine ligands. The studies proposed in Project 2 are of fundamental importance for understanding and interpreting functional imaging data following **cocaine** administration in animals and humans. Project 3 utilizes rodent models, including both drug-naive and cocaine- dependent rats and, new to this funding cycle, knockout mice, to address specific pharmacological and drug dependence issues which cannot be readily addressed in humans. We anticipate that results from these experiments, will identify the role of particular neurotransmitter mechanisms (namely, dopaminergic and serotonergic) that underlie the pattern of cocaine-induced brain activation. The hypothesis driven experiments using state of the art functional imaging techniques that we proposed in Project 1, in concert with experiments proposed in Project 2 focused on identifying mechanisms coupling psychostimulant administration to cerebrovascular response, are designed to provide a deeper understanding of the mechanism of **cocaine** action. The Program Project mechanism is ideal for a multi-disciplinary project with these goals in mind. We anticipate that the experiments in rodents will advance our understanding of acute and chronic effects of **cocaine** on brain function, facilitating interpretation of data from Project 1, thereby providing a crucial effects of **cocaine** on brain function, facilitating interpretation of data from Project, thereby providing a crucial link in understanding the fMRI correlates and neurobiology consequences of **cocaine** addiction in humans.

Website: http://crisp.cit.nih.gov/crisp/Crisp_Query.Generate_Screen

- **Project Title: GABA B AGONISTS IN HUMAN COCAINE DEPENDENCE**

Principal Investigator & Institution: Childress, Anna R.; Research Associate Professor; Psychiatry; University of Pennsylvania 3451 Walnut Street Philadelphia, Pa 19104

Timing: Fiscal Year 2002; Project Start 01-SEP-1999; Project End 30-JUN-2004

Summary: After more than a decade of intensive efforts, researchers have yet to find a medication effective in human **cocaine** craving and dependence. Though brain dopamine (DA) systems have regularly been implicated both in **cocaine** reward and **cocaine** craving, direct manipulation of these systems with available agonists or antagonists has provided underwhelming clinical results: dopamimetics often seem to worsen craving (perhaps by acting as an internal cue reminiscent of cocaine), and neuroleptics have side-effects which make them unappealing as treatment agents. Recently, Roberts et al. discovered that GABA B agonists have, by far, the most selective effect on **cocaine** reward and incentive motivation of any compound (among dozens) systematically tested by their laboratory. Other evidence suggests GABA B agonists can inhibit DA release, offering a possible mechanism for their potential to blunt both the direct, and conditioned, effects of **cocaine.** Inspired by Dr. Roberts' preclinical findings, our clinical site initiated pilot work with baclofen, a prototypic GABA B agonist used safely in humans for decades as an anti-spastic. This research determined a dose-range of baclofen well-tolerated by **cocaine** patients, and additionally suggested that it may block cue-induced **cocaine** craving and "high". The long-term objective of the application is to provide coordinated and cost-effective development and testing of the GABA B agonist baclofen in **cocaine** dependence, making use of the considerable clinical expertise of Dr. Childress' team in **cocaine** treatment, **cocaine** cue reactivity, medication trials, and safety trials employing **cocaine** administration. As any candidate medication for **cocaine** treatment will eventually be used in conjunction with **cocaine,** examining the interaction of the agent with **cocaine** under protected, controlled conditions is an important safety step in medication development. In drug development, medications are usually first tested for safety, then for efficacy (effect under optimal, controlled conditions), and finally for "real-world" effectiveness. This sequence often entails several independent experiments over a very extended period of time. In contrast, Study 1 in the current application offers an innovative inpatient safety trial which will obtain several distinct efficacy measures, all within the same experiment. Specifically, Study 1 will determine 1) the safety of baclofen in combination with **cocaine,** 2) the efficacy of baclofen in blocking cocaine's subjective (particularly rewarding) effects, 3) the efficacy of baclofen in reducing the craving and arousal induced by cocaine-related cues, and 4) the efficacy of baclofen in blocking cocaine-triggered craving. Though this information could be collected in several independent experiments, the proposed design results in considerable savings in the total number of patients to be studied, and greatly increases the speed with which findings in these critical domains can be acquired. Three groups of **cocaine** inpatients (n=20 per group) will be studied in a double-blind, between-groups 10mg b.i.d., 10mg b.i.d., 20mg b.i.d.), random-assignment design. An additional placebo group will examine the effect of expecting **cocaine** on cue reactivity, an issue of direct relevance for use of cue methodologies in medications development. Study 2 will subsequently examine the effectiveness of baclofen vs. placebo (n=30 per group) in the treatment of **cocaine** outpatients, using a double-blind, random-assignment, controlled 12-week trial with subsequent medication and treatment taper. Dependent variables in Study 2 will include drug use as measured by frequent urine toxicologies, ambient and cue-elicited craving. treatment retention, and standard measures of clinical function.

Website: http://crisp.cit.nih.gov/crisp/Crisp_Query.Generate_Screen

- **Project Title: GENDER DIFFERENCE IN RESPONSE TO CUES IN COCAINE DEPENDENCE**

  Principal Investigator & Institution: Brady, Kathleen T.;; Medical University of South Carolina P O Box 250854 Charleston, Sc 29425

  Timing: Fiscal Year 2002; Project Start 01-SEP-2002; Project End 31-AUG-2007

  Summary: (provided by applicant): A critical area in the investigation of gender differences in **cocaine** dependence is differences in factors influencing initiation, maintenance and relapse to drug use. Human laboratory studies indicate that both cocaine-related cues and negative emotional stimuli can elicit craving in cocaine-dependent individuals. There is some evidence to suggest that this effect may be more robust in women as compared to men. Animal studies have clearly demonstrated that exposure to stress facilitates both the initiation and reinstatement of substance use in previously dependent animals. The hypothalamic-pituitary-adrenal (HPA) axis, one of the most important hormonal systems involved in the stress response, is likely to be an important mediator of stress-facilitated drug self-ad ministration. Of particular relevance to this proposal, there are important gender differences in the response of the HPA axis to stress. Preliminary data from our group suggest gender differences in the biologic and subjective response to these different types of stressors. In this proposed study, we plan to build upon these intriguing findings. Specifically HPA axis (e.g., ACTH, cortisol), physiologic (e.g., HR, GSR) and subjective response to the presentation of cocaine-related cues and negative affect-inducing cues will be compared in cocainedependent men, women and matched control groups without **cocaine** dependence. A CRH stimulation test will also be performed. Following the test procedures, individuals will return for a follow-up visit at one week and one month to assess the amount and subjective attributions of drug use. In summary, this project is designed to build upon our ongoing research in the area of stress reactivity and substance use disorders. Specifically, this study will complement Project 1, which focuses on gender differences in animal models of reinstatement and will focus on gender differences in response to differing stimuli associated with relapse. Exploration of potential neurobiologic underpinnings of gender differences in precipitants relapse to drug use can have important implications for prevention and treatment.

Website: http://crisp.cit.nih.gov/crisp/Crisp_Query.Generate_Screen

- **Project Title: GENETICS OF COCAINE DEPENDENCE**

Principal Investigator & Institution: Gelernter, Joel E.; Professor; Psychiatry; Yale University 47 College Street, Suite 203 New Haven, Ct 065208047

Timing: Fiscal Year 2002; Project Start 30-SEP-1999; Project End 31-AUG-2004

Summary: This is an RO1 proposal to study the genetics of **cocaine** dependence using a collection of small nuclear families, each including (at least) an affected sibling pair (ASP). The clinical work will take place at four university-based programs in CT (Univ. CT and Yale), MA (McLean Hospital), and SC (Med. Univ. of South Carolina), and the laboratory and statistical work at Yale and Boston University School of Medicine. This project will provide information that will, eventually, substantially increase understanding of the mechanisms of **cocaine** dependence, and lead to new ways to attack this pervasive societal problem therapeutically. The purpose of this proposal is to identify chromosomal regions containing genes predisposing to **cocaine** dependence (CD). The aims are to collect a set of 500 small nuclear families, primarily ASPs, and (whenever possible) additional siblings and parents; and to complete a 10 cM genome scan using STR markers and an automated sequencer. Affection will be defined according to DSM-IV diagnostic criteria, ascertained using the Semi-Structured Assessment for the Genetics of Alcoholism (SSAGA) as the primary instrument. The principal method of analysis will be sibling pair linkage; this will be augmented by linkage disequilibrium methods. An important genetic contribution to risk for CD is strongly supported by clinical genetic data. This sample will have sufficient power to detect linkage under reasonable assumptions of heterogeneity. As for any complex trait, while the proposed sample size cannot be proven a priori to be sufficient to complete gene mapping, it is necessary, and the cell lines prepared as part of this study may be a component of any future mapping efforts. These data, combined with mapping data from other substance dependence (SD) disorders, will ultimately help to resolve basic questions about the extent of unique, vs. shared, genetic contribution to various SD phenotypes. This will be the first large-scale linkage study of CD. Given that CD is a complex trait, a large ASP study that will allow genetic analysis without assumptions about trait transmission will provide the best chance to map genes related to this dangerous, prevalent disorder.

Website: http://crisp.cit.nih.gov/crisp/Crisp_Query.Generate_Screen

- **Project Title: HIV AND COCAINE USE--CARDIOVASCULAR EFFECTS AND THERAPY**

Principal Investigator & Institution: Margolin, Arthur; Research Scientist; Psychiatry; Yale University 47 College Street, Suite 203 New Haven, Ct 065208047

Timing: Fiscal Year 2002; Project Start 15-JUN-1999; Project End 31-MAY-2004

Summary: The proposed study was formulated in response to RFA HL-98-012 requesting applications to investigate cardiovascular complications from **cocaine** abuse in HIV infection, with a focus on the call for clinical studies to identify effective treatment protocols. **Cocaine** use by HIV-positive individuals represents a primary vector of infection to non-infected individuals, and may also adversely affect disease progression, including increasing risk for cardiovascular dysfunction. A treatment approach targeting both **cocaine** use and cardiovascular disorders simultaneously would therefore be extremely beneficial in an HIV- positive, cocaine-abusing patient population. The proposed study capitalizes on the multiple effects of the angiotensin converting enzyme (ACE) inhibitor, fosinopril, in numerous tissue systems, and will investigate its ability to reduce **cocaine** use through activity in the brain, and to reverse or prevent the cardiotoxic effects of **cocaine** and HIV disease by actions upon the heart and cardiovascular system, including platelet aggregation factors. In the proposed five-year study, one hundred and twenty-four HIV- positive cocaine-dependent methadone-maintained patients will be randomly assigned to receive either fosinopril (20 mg/day) or placebo for six months. The specific aims of this study are: (a) to investigate the efficacy of fosinopril for the treatment of **cocaine** dependence in HIV-positive methadone-maintained patients, based on twice weekly urine toxicology screens; (b) to determine the ability of fosinopril to improve cardiac functioning by comparing pre- and post-treatment two-dimensional and Doppler echocardiograms, and (c) to investigate the ability of fosinopril to decrease platelet reactivity to physiological agonists. Biological and psychosocial risk factors for cardiovascular disorders (including CD4 count, viral load, antiretroviral medications, family history of cardiovascular disease, severity of addiction, depression, and subjective cardiovascular distress during **cocaine** use) will also be examined.

Website: http://crisp.cit.nih.gov/crisp/Crisp_Query.Generate_Screen

- **Project Title: HUMAN BEHAVIORAL PHARMACOLOGY OF DRUG ABUSE**

Principal Investigator & Institution: Bigelow, George E.; Professor and Director; Psychiatry and Behavioral Scis; Johns Hopkins University 3400 N Charles St Baltimore, Md 21218

Timing: Fiscal Year 2002; Project Start 01-JAN-1993; Project End 31-DEC-2003

Summary: (Applicant's Abstract) This is an application for competitive renewal of K-series career award support for years 21-25. The focus of the applicant's research career is on the human behavioral pharmacology of drug abuse. The applicant directs a large and multi faceted clinical research program that includes two major components: (1) residential human laboratory studies related to the clinical pharmacology of opioids, of **cocaine,** and of potential pharmacotherapies for opioid or **cocaine** dependence; and (2) outpatient controlled clinical trials of behavioral and pharmacological treatments for opioid or **cocaine** dependence. The research program is also the site of a postdoctoral research training program, which has a history of training productive new scientists as drug abuse researchers, and of which the applicant is director. The applicant proposes to continue as research program director, and as training program director, and to conduct during this renewal period an inter-related series of human laboratory studies and outpatient clinical trials directed toward the behavioral pharmacological understanding and treatment of opioid and **cocaine** abuse. The opioid clinical pharmacology studies will evaluate the effects of opioids with kappa-receptor agonist activity in comparison to mu-receptor agonists, and will assess and characterize the effects of an opioid antagonist combination product (buprenorphine plus naloxone) that is being developed as an opioid dependence pharmacotherapy. The **cocaine** clinical pharmacology studies will test potential anti-cocaine pharmacotherapies by assessing whether response to **cocaine** challenge is altered by pretreatment with various agents (chronic oral **cocaine,** the opioid kappa agonist enadoline, the serotonergic agent tryptophan). The opioid dependence clinical trials will compare the efficacy and patient acceptability of three opioid agonist substitution pharmacotherapies (methadone, LAAM, buprenorphine). The **cocaine** dependence clinical trials will evaluate the efficacy of the serotonergic agents tryptophan and fluoxetine in the context of an incentive-based behavior therapy program.

Website: http://crisp.cit.nih.gov/crisp/Crisp_Query.Generate_Screen

- **Project Title: HUMAN GENETICS OF DRUG-ABUSE RELATED PHENOTYPES**

Principal Investigator & Institution: Cubells, Joseph F.; Associate Professor and Director; Psychiatry; Yale University 47 College Street, Suite 203 New Haven, Ct 065208047

Timing: Fiscal Year 2003; Project Start 01-JUL-2003; Project End 30-JUN-2008

Summary: (provided by applicant): K02 Independent Scientist Career Development Award for Joseph F. Cubells,MD, PhD This proposal seeks support for the candidate's continued development as a research psychiatrist specializing in human genetics of drug-abuse-related phenotypes. The overarching hypothesis organizing both the Research Plan and the Career Plan is that sequence variation at specific loci will exert measurable effects on specific drug-abuse-related phenotypes. This hypothesis is predicated on the importance of identifying and characterizing appropriate phenotypes, which will reflect the effects of one or a few genes with high penetrance. Three projects are proposed in the Research Plan. Project 1, which is well under way, is the candidate's R01-funded research on the human genetics of cocaine-induced psychosis (DA 12422). The project seeks to collect DNA samples from unrelated individuals with **cocaine** dependence, and from family trios containing cocaine-dependent probands; these probands are carefully characterized for cocaine-induced psychotic symptoms, and for axis-1 substance-abuse and psychiatric diagnoses, as well as for plasma levels of the catecholamine-synthetic enzyme dopamine beta-hydroxylase. Project 2 will build on work accomplished in Project 1, to examine how linkage disequilbrium among nearby polymorphisms influences phenotypic variation in quantitative traits. Project 3 will elucidate genetic influences on nicotine-dependence-related phenotypes by examining the influence of functional variation at the COMT locus on human neurocognitive function and acoustic startle responses in smoking and nonsmoking subjects, with and without schizophrenia. The Career Development Plan will entail collaboration with colleagues at Yale University and the University of Connecticut, whose expertises range from evaluation of complex phenotypes, to molecular genetics, to statistical genetics. In addition, the candidate plans specific coursework, both at Yale, and at off-campus sites, to strengthen his expertise in a both molecular, statistical and clinical genetics. The latter goal will be accomplished by the candidate directing the newly-established Yale Human Behavioral Genetics Clinic, which offers psychiatric and substance-abuse services to patients with genetic illnesses.

Website: http://crisp.cit.nih.gov/crisp/Crisp_Query.Generate_Screen

- **Project Title: IMAGING DOPAMINE/SEROTONIN MECHANISMS IN COCAINE CRAVING**

Principal Investigator & Institution: Wong, Dean F.; Vice Chair for Research; Radiology; Johns Hopkins University 3400 N Charles St Baltimore, Md 21218

Timing: Fiscal Year 2003; Project Start 01-SEP-1997; Project End 31-AUG-2004

Summary: Craving has been implicated as a major contributor both to relapse and maintenance of addiction following abstinence in **cocaine** abusers. Although a mechanistic understanding of the biological basis of **cocaine** craving could identify therapeutic approaches to reduce **cocaine** dependence, information on the involvement of specific neurochemical systems in this phenomenon is scarce. Ongoing and previous studies in human volunteers have shown that environmental stimuli related to drug taking selectively increase cerebral glucose metabolism (Grant, 1995) and perfusion (Childress et all 1996) in cortical and limbic areas of brain and that activation in the dorsolateral prefrontal cortex and amygdala is correlated with self-reports of craving (London, 1996). We propose to elucidate the role of dopaminergic and serotonergic systems in spontaneous and cue-elicited **cocaine** craving, in an integrated approach utilizing positron emission tomOgraphy (PET) scanning and selective radioligands for dopamine(DA) and serotonin (5-HT) receptors and transporters. Neurochemical markers, assayed by PET, will be related to self-reports of craving in **cocaine** abusers, and will be compared to measures in control subjects who have no significant history of illicit dmg abuse. Our premise is that, not only is there considerable evidence in the literature for the role of dopamine and serotonin in craving, but that the activated areas, previously seen in the amygdala and dorsal lateral prefrontal cortex can be examined further by examination of these neurotransmitter systems. We hypothesize that in our experimental paradigm following withdrawal, extracellular dopamine and to a lesser extent serntonin will be decreased. It is then predicted that both intrasynaptic DA (InsDA) and intrasynaptic 5HT (Ins5HT) will increase following the pharmacologic challenge and that cue-elicited craving will correlate significantly with this increase. It is predicted that spontaneous craving however, will correlate negatively with D1 D2 and 5HT 2a receptors. Finally, it is predicted that both when cue-elicited craving is induced during PET imaging, increased InsDA and 5HT will be measurable and will correlate significantly with the craving score. Testing of these hypotheses will provide novel and fundamental answers to craving mechanisms.

Website: http://crisp.cit.nih.gov/crisp/Crisp_Query.Generate_Screen

- **Project Title: IMAGING VENTROSTRIATAL DOPAMINE SYSTEM IN COCAINE ABUSE**

Principal Investigator & Institution: Laruelle, Marc A.; Associate Professor; New York State Psychiatric Institute 1051 Riverside Dr New York, Ny 100321098

Timing: Fiscal Year 2002; Project Start 10-MAY-1997; Project End 30-APR-2005

Summary: (provided by applicant): Preclinical studies suggest that the mesolimbic dopamine (DA) system to the nucleus accumbens is critically involved in **cocaine** addiction. Yet alterations of DA transmission in the ventral striatum of **cocaine** abusers are still poorly understood. Recent progress in positron emission tomograph (PET) camera resolution permits direct evaluation of the mesolimbic DA function in human **cocaine** users. In preliminary data, we probed the responsivity of DA neurons to an amphetamine challenge, by measuring the decrease in [11C]raclopride binding potential resulting from the increase in synaptic DA induced by amphetamine. In healthy subjects, amphetamine-induced DA release is higher in ventral compared to dorsal striatum. In contrast, studies in detoxified subjects with a long history (15 years) of heavy **cocaine** dependence revealed a dramatic blunting of amphetamine-induced DA release in the ventral striatum. This finding suggests that years of **cocaine** abuse might be associated with a severe pathology of mesolimbic DA neurons. The general aim of this proposal is to confirm this observation in a larger group of subjects (specific aim 1), and to combine this measurement with determination of dopamine transporters (DAT) availability with the selective DAT PET radiotracer [11C]PE21 (specific aim 2). As the DAT is exclusively located on DA terminals, this evaluation will provide a comprehensive picture of presynaptic DA function in the ventral striatum in cocine abusers. Alteration in presynaptic DA function might be associated with development of tolerance to **cocaine.** This hypothesis will be investigated by correlating the imaging results with the subjective effects of **cocaine** self administration (specific aim 3). If confirmed, such a result would support the general hypothesis that years of **cocaine** exposure result in pathological adaptation of mesolimbic DA function. Given the role of this system in incentive learning, it is predicted that such a pathology would result in inability to learn and encode new "natural" rewarding behaviors and would contribute to the maintenance of the addictive behavior. Understanding the neurochemical abnormalities associated with the development and maintenance of **cocaine** addiction is critical to guide future treatment interventions.

Website: http://crisp.cit.nih.gov/crisp/Crisp_Query.Generate_Screen

- **Project Title: INPATIENT STABILIZATION IN TREATMENT OF COCAINE DEPENDENCE**

Principal Investigator & Institution: Dackis, Charles A.; Assistant Professor of Psychaitry and Ch; University of Pennsylvania 3451 Walnut Street Philadelphia, Pa 19104

Timing: Fiscal Year 2002; Project Start 30-SEP-1992; Project End 30-JUN-2007

Summary: (provided by applicant) Previous comparison studies of inpatient and outpatient forms of treatment for substance dependence have made direct comparisons of the outcomes and costs of these two forms of care under the assumption that both were designed to perform the same rehabilitation function. The present project proposes to compare two groups of 125 **cocaine** dependent patients randomly assigned to receive either Direct Admission to Intensive Outpatient treatment or to Brief (6-day) Inpatient Stabilization prior to Day Hospital rehabilitation. This study is unlike prior cost effectiveness comparisons because it specifically assumes that inpatient and outpatient treatments should not be evaluated on common outcome criteria. Instead, the study assumes that the appropriate function of inpatient care is to remove the barriers to and prepare the patient for outpatient care. Thus, the outcomes to be compared between the two groups include, engagement, retention and performance in Intensive Outpatient care, post-treatment outcomes as well as the total costs of each type of care. Patients will be evaluated at the start of the study, throughout the course of inpatient and Intensive Outpatient treatment and at six-month follow-up using validated instruments and procedures. All patient and treatment costs in both groups will be measured for comparative analyses. Specific hypotheses are that patients who receive brief stabilization first, will be more likely to engage in outpatient treatment, to complete that treatment and to have better outcomes at follow-up, than those randomly assigned directly to the Intensive Outpatient program. We believe the study is particularly pertinent to contemporary questions of cost, outcome and value in substance abuse treatment.

Website: http://crisp.cit.nih.gov/crisp/Crisp_Query.Generate_Screen

- **Project Title: INTRAVENOUS COCAINE DISCRIMINATION IN HUMANS**

Principal Investigator & Institution: Johanson, Chris-Ellyn; Professor; Psychiatry & Behav Neuroscis; Wayne State University 656 W. Kirby Detroit, Mi 48202

Timing: Fiscal Year 2002; Project Start 15-JUL-2002; Project End 31-MAY-2005

Summary: (provided by applicant): **Cocaine** abuse/dependence remains a major social and public health problem. There are a significant number of **cocaine** dependent individuals for whom current behavioral treatment interventions are ineffective. Finding a successful pharmacological treatment for **cocaine** abuse/dependence continues to be an important yet elusive goal. Several compounds have been shown in pre-clinical studies to attenuate the discriminative stimulus and reinforcing effects of intravenous **cocaine** but when these medications have been tested in clinical trials, none have proven effective. It is not clear whether the lack of concordance is a function of the behavioral procedures that are used in these models or to a species difference. One strategy to answer this question is to conduct similar studies in humans to assess the validity of the animal models. Although there are established methods for studying the subjective, physiological, and reinforcing effects of intravenous **cocaine** in humans, drug discrimination methods with intravenous **cocaine** have not been developed. The potential advantage of studying the discriminative stimulus effects of drugs is that this procedure is particularly well suited for studying mechanisms underlying the dependence-related effects of drugs and has the potential to be relatively efficient, allowing several candidate medications to be evaluated over a relatively short period of time. The goal of this application is to establish the validity of an intravenous **cocaine** discrimination paradigm in humans. In the first study, human participants will be trained to discriminate the effects of intravenous **cocaine** injections. Dose-response functions will then be generated with **cocaine** doses higher and lower than the training dose and generalization tests will be conducted with doses of a drug similar pharmacologically to **cocaine** (d-amphetamine) and a drug different from **cocaine** (pentobarbital) to determine the specificity of the paradigm. The second study will determine whether oral **cocaine** can attenuate the subjective, physiological, and discriminative stimulus effects of intravenous **cocaine** injections. Although oral **cocaine** would be an unlikely medication for **cocaine** dependence, studies of the reinforcing effects of **cocaine** have demonstrated that they are blocked following the administration of oral **cocaine** and that this approach functions as a proof of concept in the absence of established blocking agents. These studies as a whole will investigate a promising new strategy for developing treatment medications for **cocaine** abuse/dependence. If successful, this will be an efficient paradigm for examining the ability of compounds to attenuate the effects of **cocaine** in humans and may lead to a successful pharmacological treatment for **cocaine** abuse/dependence.

Website: http://crisp.cit.nih.gov/crisp/Crisp_Query.Generate_Screen

- **Project Title: KAPPA RECEPTOR SELECTIVE PET LIGANDS**

Principal Investigator & Institution: Hwang, Dah-Ren;; New York State Psychiatric Institute 1051 Riverside Dr New York, Ny 100321098

Timing: Fiscal Year 2002; Project Start 30-SEP-2002; Project End 31-JUL-2007

Summary: (provided by applicant): Neuroreceptor imaging techniques using positron emission tomography allow the in vivo investigation of the neurotransmitter systems in psychiatric disease. As a result, radioligand imaging can provide direction for targeted treatment strategies. This is of critical importance in developing future pharmacotherapy for substance abuse. Both preclinical and clinical studies indicate that the "direct pathway" plays a critical role in relapse. The direct pathway consists of the GABAergic neurons of the striatum that project back to the substantial nigra/VTA, and which contain the D1 receptor and dynorphin. We have currently begun studies in **cocaine** dependence with a D1radioligand. Therefore the goal oft his application is the development of a radioligand for the kappa receptor, which can be employed in future studies of substance dependence. In the R21 portion of this application, we propose to develop both an agonist (GR103545) and antagonist (JDTic) radiotracer, as well as their analogs, for the kappa receptor. The development of these radiotracers will begin with the optimization of their synthesis, in order to ensure the most effective and reliable chemistry. These compounds will be evaluated in vitro in order to measure their affinity for the receptor and to establish their selectivity for the kappa receptor. Those ligands shown to have a high affinity and selectivity will then be evaluated in vivo in biodistribtuion studies in rodents, followed by studies in non-human primates. The studies in baboons will be used to establish the selectivity for the kappa receptor in vivo, the susceptibility of the radioligand to endogenous dynorphin, and to develop the imaging analysis of the radioligands. The candidate radioligands that meet the criteria outlined in the milestones will be chosen for the R33 portion of this application, which includes toxicology studies and test/retest studies in healthy human volunteers. The studies in human subjects will be performed in order to establish the selectivity for the kappa receptor in humans and to determine optimal scanning protocol. At the end of the award period, we expect to have developed both a kappa agonist and antagonist, which will be available for a wide range of research centers.

Website: http://crisp.cit.nih.gov/crisp/Crisp_Query.Generate_Screen

- **Project Title: LAB TRIALS TO DEVELOP MEDICATIONS FOR COCAINE DEPENDENCE**

Principal Investigator & Institution: Johnson, Bankole A.; Wurzbach Distinguished Professor and Dep; Psychiatry; University of Texas Hlth Sci Ctr San Ant 7703 Floyd Curl Dr San Antonio, Tx 78229

Timing: Fiscal Year 2002; Project Start 30-SEP-1999; Project End 31-AUG-2003

Summary: L-type calcium channel antagonists are promising agents for the treatment of **cocaine** dependence, presumably because they reduce cocaine's rewarding effects associated with abuse liability. We propose two experiments using state-of-the-art human abuse liability assessment techniques to examine the subjective, behavioral, and physiological effects of **cocaine** both alone and in combination with the L-type calcium channel antagonist, isradipine. Both studies will be double-blind and placebo-controlled using balanced (for sequence and ordinal position) cross-over designs in male and female non treatment seeking **cocaine** abusers (total n = 42). The first experiment, which is a logical and systematic extension of pre-clinical work and our own preliminary studies, will test the hypothesis that acute isradipine significantly reduces acute cocaine-mediated changes in subjective mood and other abuse liability assessments. As a secondary objective of this experiment, we will characterize the effects of **cocaine** on cognitive function and physiological response in non-fatigued subjects during drug-taking, and determine if, and by how much, these effects are altered by isradipine. The second experiment will test the hypothesis that repeated isradipine administration will antagonize the rewarding effects of acute **cocaine.** In addition, as a secondary objective, we will determine if repeated isradipine administration will be well tolerated, produce no adverse effects on cognitive or psychomotor function, and reduce cocaine's pressor effects. In essence, Exp. number I provides a proof-of-concept analysis of isradipine's ability to reduce cocaine's abuse potential. Exp. number 2 directly assesses issues of potential clinical effectiveness and tolerability with which to guide clinical trials. Confirmation that isradipine is well tolerated and effective in the human laboratory would provide a solid rationale to begin clinical trials using this agent for the treatment of **cocaine** dependent populations. Whereas no pharmacological treatment is yet known or expected to be entirely sufficient in preventing **cocaine** abuse and dependence, studies such as these should improve our knowledge of mechanistic pharmacological and behavioral processes associated with **cocaine** use, and may contribute to the development of an effective treatment agent. This project supports NIDA's mission to understand the bio-behavioral effects of **cocaine** dependence, and to develop effective medications for its treatment.

Website: http://crisp.cit.nih.gov/crisp/Crisp_Query.Generate_Screen

- ## Project Title: LIMBIC SENSITIVITY IN COCAINE ADDICTION

Principal Investigator & Institution: Adinoff, Bryon H.; Professor of Psychiatry; Psychiatry; University of Texas Sw Med Ctr/Dallas Dallas, Tx 753909105

Timing: Fiscal Year 2003; Project Start 10-AUG-1998; Project End 31-AUG-2006

Summary: (provided by applicant): The limbic system is an integrated brain area involved in the regulation of reward, motivation, emotional expression, and memory. These regions are considered critical to the development and persistence of addiction. In our currently-funded proposal, the regional cerebral blood flow (rCBF) response to the limbicstimulant procaine was assessed relative to saline in cocaine-addicted subjects (n=38) and healthy controls (n=37). Our findings revealed that cocaine-addicted men and women exhibit a blunted limbic rCBF response to procaine compared to age and gender matched controls. Procaine, unlike **cocaine,** has minimal interaction with the monoamine transporters, but has potent affinity with both cholinergic and 5HT3 receptors. Preclinical studies indicate that these latter receptor systems are altered following the acute and chronic administration of **cocaine,** and disruptions in these systems may modulate subsequent drug reinforcement. Our competitive renewal is designed to further elucidate the putative neurobiologic differences in the cholinergic and 5HT3 systems revealed by procaine. Hypotheses: We hypothesize that cocaine-addicted subjects will demonstrate impairment of the cholinergic and 5HT3 receptor systems. Preliminary Studies: To explore cholinergic and 5HT3 receptor functioning, healthy controls (n=3) and cocaine-addicted subjects (n=3) were administered (1) the cholinergic agonist physostigmine, (2) the muscarinic cholinergic antagonist scopolamine, (3) the 5HT3 antagonist ondansetron, and (4) saline. Preliminary analyses suggest that the limbic rCBF response (relative to saline) following all three probes is blunted in cocaine-addicted subjects compared to controls. Methods: Male (n=12) and female (n=12) cocaine-addicted subjects between two and six weeks abstinence will be compared to age and gender matched controls (12 male and 12 female). All subjects will receive physostigmine, scopolamine, ondansetron, and saline. Single photon emission computed tomography (SPECT) and SPM analytic techniques will be used to assess rCBF and differences within and between groups. Significance: The cholinergic and 5HT3 receptor systems have not previously been studied in cocaine-addicted subjects using neuroimaging techniques. Our competing renewal will be used to identify specific changes in these neuroreceptor systems, providing avenues for new pharmacologic investigations in the treatment of **cocaine** dependence.

Website: http://crisp.cit.nih.gov/crisp/Crisp_Query.Generate_Screen

- **Project Title: MAGNETIC RESONANCE, EEG AND BEHAVIOR AFTER COCAINE**

Principal Investigator & Institution: Renshaw, Perry F.; Director; Mc Lean Hospital (Belmont, Ma) Belmont, Ma 02478

Timing: Fiscal Year 2002; Project Start 30-SEP-1994; Project End 31-MAR-2004

Summary: During the first three years of funding, we used proton and phosphorus magnetic resonance spectroscopy (MRS) and functional magnetic resonance imaging (fMRI) techniques, to document important changes in brain chemistry and hemodynamics following acute **cocaine** administration. We have also used fMRI methods to demonstrate changes in cerebral metabolism associated with **cocaine** cue-induced craving. Studies which merge electroencephalography (EEG) with fMRI to evaluate task- and drug-induced effects on cortical electrical activity are also underway. Important accomplishments include the documentation of cocaine-induced vasospasm and decreased cerebral blood volume following acute **cocaine** administration, the demonstration that exposure to **cocaine** cues leads to changes in cerebral metabolism which can be detected using blood oxygen level dependent (BOLD) fMRI, and the identification of a novel treatment strategy for **cocaine** dependent individuals. This competing continuation requests five years of funding to pursue a series of studies on the acute and chronic effects of **cocaine** on the human brain. In this application, we will continue to study the effects of acute **cocaine** administration, taking advantage both of insights derived from our prior work as well as advances in magnetic resonance methods. As an important new direction for this research effort, based on findings obtained during the current funding period, we also propose investigations on the effects of chronic **cocaine** use and early abstinence on the brain. Relatively few studies to date have focused on changes in brain chemistry or metabolism associated with recovery from **cocaine** dependence, despite their importance for efforts to develop more effective therapies. We propose a total of eight separate studies, involving 392 subjects who will complete 524 magnetic resonance examinations. These studies are designed to investigate the neuroanatomic bases of cocaine-induced euphoria and cue-induced craving, processes which contribute to chronic **cocaine** use and dependence. As pharmacologic strategies for the treatment of **cocaine** abuse and dependence include the use of dopaminergic and GABAergic agents, we will assess changes in retinal dopamine metabolism and brain GABA concentrations in cocaine-dependent subjects. This research will also evaluate whether acute **cocaine** administration is associated with transient cerebral ischemia and whether chronic **cocaine** use leads to neuronal death and/or diminished cerebrovascular reserve.

Website: http://crisp.cit.nih.gov/crisp/Crisp_Query.Generate_Screen

- **Project Title: MEDICATION DEVELOPMENT FOR COCAINE ABUSE--CDP CHOLINE**

Principal Investigator & Institution: Lukas, Scott E.; Professor of Psychiatry (Pharmacology) a; Mc Lean Hospital (Belmont, Ma) Belmont, Ma 02478

Timing: Fiscal Year 2003; Project Start 10-APR-1999; Project End 31-MAR-2004

Summary: (Applicant's Abstract) This is a revised application that focuses on the development of a novel medication for **cocaine** dependence--CDP-choline. This naturally occurring nucleotide is a major component in phospholipid metabolism and is an integral ingredient in membrane synthesis. It is approved for use in Europe to treat head trauma and a variety of neurological degenerative disorders. Interestingly, it also enhances dopamine activity. Thus, CDP-choline's efficacy as a treatment for **cocaine** dependence may be high because it repairs two putative consequences of chronic **cocaine** abuse: 1) membrane damage, and 2) depleted dopamine levels. Two experiments are proposed in this three year study. The first is a challenge study designed to assess the acute effects of **cocaine** administration in CDP-choline treated non-dependent, casual **cocaine** users. A multidisciplinary assessment battery including EEG, physiologic, subjective responses and plasma **cocaine** and metabolite levels will be conducted after **cocaine** or placebo challenge. This experiment will be conducted in the first six months of the project and will provide basic information on how cocaine's effects are altered by this medication. Study 2 is a 6-week placebo-controlled clinical trial of CDP-choline in **cocaine** dependent men and women. Follow-up assessments will be made at 8, 12 and 26 weeks. In an attempt to gain insight into the possible mechanism of CDP- choline's effects, two different assessments of CNS function will be conducted at baseline, after 6 weeks of treatment and at the 12 week follow-up visit. The first is a cue reactivity challenge using subjective reports of craving, physiologic and EEG activity after neutral, emotionally laden and cocaine-related stimuli. The second assessment is Magnetic Resonance Spectroscopy (MRS), which will be used to measure changes in brain chemistry that reflect neuronal damage. One of the major appeals of CDP-choline is its low inherent toxicity. Large doses have been given for relatively long periods of time with no adverse effects. The implication of this is that CDP-choline may be safe enough to treat **cocaine** dependence in pregnant women and adolescents and may even be useful for treating infants who are born to cocaine-dependent mothers. Although we have collected very encouraging preliminary data on CDP-choline's effects in cocaine-dependent male and female subjects, we recognize that it is not a "magic bullet" and that CDP-choline may serve as an important adjunct to other psychotherapy or pharmacotherapy programs.

Website: http://crisp.cit.nih.gov/crisp/Crisp_Query.Generate_Screen

- **Project Title: MEDICATIONS FOR COMORBID COCAINE AND ALCOHOL DEPENDENCE**

Principal Investigator & Institution: Johnson, Rolley E.; Associate Professor; Psychiatry and Behavioral Scis; Johns Hopkins University 3400 N Charles St Baltimore, Md 21218

Timing: Fiscal Year 2002; Project Start 30-SEP-2002; Project End 31-MAR-2003

Summary: (provided by applicant): **Cocaine** abuse and dependence continues to be a major public health problem with up to 3 million people in need of treatment. Over the past decade, medications including dopamine agonists, antagonists, tricyclic antidepressants, selective serotonin reuptake inhibitors, opiate mixed agonist-antagonists, and opioid antagonist have been studied for thetreatment of this disorder. No efficacious medication has been found to treat **cocaine** abusing or dependent patients. The lack of a efficacious medication for **cocaine** dependence has led to the proposal to treat co-morbid disorders found with high frequency in **cocaine** abusing patients, especially when these disorders are thought to enhance or perpetuate the use of **cocaine.** Alcohol abuse/dependence is the most common co-morbid condition found in **cocaine** abusing patients; as many as 85% of patients with **cocaine** dependence also have a diagnosis of alcohol abuse or dependence. Since alcohol use is common among **cocaine** abusers, it is possible that treatment of co-morbid alcohol use could lead to decreases in **cocaine** use. Disulfiram is approved for the treatment of alcohol abuse. Thus, it is possible to test the hypothesis that treatment of alcoholism in **cocaine** abusing patients will lead to improvements in **cocaine** use, as well as alcohol use. Disulfiram inhibits the enzyme that breaks down acetaldehyde (the first metabolite of alcohol) thus causing an increase in acetaldehyde which produces unpleasant aversive effects. It also inhibits opamine P-hydroxylase causing an increase in dopamine and decrease in norepinephrine that may result in attenuation of **cocaine** craving and euphoria and thus decrease the desire to use **cocaine.** This may explain the reported reduction in **cocaine** use in opioid dependent patients treated with disulfiram. Thus, disulfiram appears to have potential for impacting significantly on the treatment of **cocaine** addicts. This study assesses the efficacy of disulfiram at two different doses levels (62.5 mg and 250 mg) to treat **cocaine** dependent patients with a dual diagnosis of **cocaine** dependence and alcohol abuse or dependence. A randomized, placebo controlled, parallel 3-group design is utilized in conjunction with manual-guided Cognitive-Behavioral Therapy (CBT). Primary outcome measures include: 1) continuous **cocaine** (qualitative and quantitative) and alcohol abstinence, 2) retention time in treatment, and 3) frequency and quantity of **cocaine** and alcohol use. Secondary measures include: 1) use of other illicit drugs, 2) side effects data, 3) safety data, 4) self- and observer global reports and 5) other subjective measures (e.g., psychosocial adjustment, time spent in use, reduction in time spent in use, severity of withdrawal, etc.). This study will utilize rigorous clinical trials methodology to provide critical scientific and safety data for assessing disulfiram as a treatment for primary **cocaine** dependence and associated alcohol abuse and dependence.

Website: http://crisp.cit.nih.gov/crisp/Crisp_Query.Generate_Screen

- **Project Title: NATIONAL DRUG ABUSE TREATMENT CLINICAL TRIALS NETWORK**

Principal Investigator & Institution: Hubbard, Robert L.; Director; Psychiatry; Duke University Durham, Nc 27710

Timing: Fiscal Year 2002; Project Start 10-JAN-2001; Project End 31-DEC-2005

Summary: (Applicant's Abstract) This is the first resubmission of a proposal to establish a Southeastern Duke Node in the NIDA National Drug Abuse Clinical Trials Network. We will partner with at least 10 real world community-based treatment programs (CTPs). The CTPs reflect diverse demographics; several are in rural or small town settings. CTPs will not only implement existing research protocols but will collaborate with Node scientists to develop new research concepts. The coordination of the CTPs and the interface with other Nodes and NIDA will be directed by a Regional Research and Training Center (RRTC) that represents a confederation of investigators, trainers and research monitors from Duke University Medical Center (DUMC) Department of Psychiatry, the Duke Clinical Research Institute (DCRI), and the National Development and Research Institutes (NDRI) each with their own strengths and a history of collaborating with each other. The RRTC will maintain the clinical infrastructure and the research infrastructure and will be responsible for all aspects of conducting clinical trials. Concept research proposals that can utilize the unique scope of the CTN are delineated: 1) Multi-modal CBT for adolescent substance abusers with internalizing disorders and 2) Selegiline/CBT for **cocaine** dependence. To enhance our contribution to the CTN's focus on multi-center, effectiveness research designs, we have designated Dr. Robert Hubbard as PI and added a cadre of DUMC-DCRI experts on effectiveness research who will broaden the inclusiveness, generalizability and usefulness of our studies.

Website: http://crisp.cit.nih.gov/crisp/Crisp_Query.Generate_Screen

- **Project Title: NEURAL FUNCTION IN COCAINE DEPENDENCE AND RELAPSE**

Principal Investigator & Institution: Clark, Vincent P.; Assistant Professor; Psychology; University of New Mexico Albuquerque Controller's Office Albuquerque, Nm 87131

Timing: Fiscal Year 2002; Project Start 30-SEP-2001; Project End 30-JUN-2005

Summary: (provided by applicant) Our long term goal is to apply functional magnetic resonance imaging (fMRl), event-related potentials (ERPs), structured interviews and neuropsychological testing for the prediction of relapse to **cocaine** use in abstinent **cocaine** dependent patients. The objectives of this application are to study the effects of **cocaine** dependence on brain activity and cognition, and test which measures, or combination of measures, best predicts relapse. The rationale behind this research is that the amplitude of the frontal P300 ERP component has been found to be a reliable predictor of relapse to **cocaine** abuse in abstinent cocaine-dependent patients in treatment. However, the specific neural and cognitive factors that underlie this finding are unknown. FMRI has a spatial resolution that is ideal for imaging the neural architecture of the human brain, and could provide an improved measure of relapse potential. Newly developed methods for performing event-related fMRI will be used to obtain the anatomical locations of neural fields that respond to the same stimuli that generate the P300 ERP component. Recently abstinent **cocaine** dependent patients will be recruited from local treatment programs after two weeks of abstinence. Abstinence will be verified over a six-month period. Healthy non-drug-dependent volunteers will also be studied. Neuropsychological testing will examine the behavioral consequences of neurophysiological differences found between groups. The combination of ERP, fMRI and neuropsychological methods will provide a precise analysis of changes in brain activity, and their consequences for cognitive task performance, during **cocaine** withdrawal in humans. It is anticipated that information obtained in the present series of experiments will be useful in understanding the mechanisms of **cocaine** dependence and relapse, and in improving treatments for this disorder.

Website: http://crisp.cit.nih.gov/crisp/Crisp_Query.Generate_Screen

- **Project Title: NEURAL MECHANISMS OF DRUG SEEKING BEHAVIOR**

Principal Investigator & Institution: Neisewander, Janet L.; Associate Professor; Psychology; Arizona State University P.O. Box 873503 Tempe, Az 852873503

Timing: Fiscal Year 2002; Project Start 10-JUN-1997; Project End 30-APR-2006

Summary: Cocaine dependence is viewed as a chronic condition because of the high incidence of relapse that occurs even after prolonged periods of abstinence. Thus, successful treatment of **cocaine** dependence must include prevention of relapse. Factors contributing to relapse include incentive motivational effects (e.g., craving) produced by **cocaine** itself or by exposure to cocaine-associated cues (e.g., paraphernalia, cocaine-taking environment, etc). Recent evidence suggests that different neural mechanisms underlie incentive motivational effects of **cocaine** versus **cocaine** cues. Leading theories suggest that these mechanisms likely involve changes in monoamine systems, yet little research has been done to test this hypothesis in regard to the involvement of the monoamine, serotonin (5-HT). The objective of this proposal is to examine the role of 5-HT systems in incentive motivation for **cocaine.** The hypotheses are that increasing 5-HT brain levels or 5-HT1A stimulation will decrease incentive motivation for **cocaine,** whereas decreasing stimulation of 5-HT2 receptors will decrease incentive motivation for **cocaine.** These hypotheses will be tested by examining cocaine-seeking behavior (i.e., operant responding in the absence of **cocaine** reinforcement that is thought to reflect motivation for cocaine) after administration of drugs that either alter serotonin release or stimulation of 5-HT1A or 5-HT2 receptors. The effects of these drugs on extinction of cocaine-seeking behavior and reinstatement by presentations of cocaine-paired cues will be examined in animals in a drug-free state. Next, effects of these drugs with and without **cocaine** co-administration on reinstatement of cocaine-seeking behavior will be examined. Finally, behavioral specificity of observed effects will be examined by comparing them to the effects of the drugs on sucrose-seeking behavior. These experiments will help to elucidate 5-HT mechanisms involved in incentive motivation for **cocaine** and will likely have important implications for developing treatments for **cocaine** dependence.

Website: http://crisp.cit.nih.gov/crisp/Crisp_Query.Generate_Screen

- **Project Title: NEURAL SUBSTRATES OF HUMAN COCAINE SELF-ADMINISTRATION**

Principal Investigator & Institution: Risinger, Robert C.; Assistant Professor; Psychiatry and Behavioral Med; Medical College of Wisconsin Po Box26509 Milwaukee, Wi 532260509

Timing: Fiscal Year 2002; Project Start 01-SEP-2001; Project End 30-JUN-2004

Summary: It is widely believed that cocaine's ability to reinforce its own administration leads to the sustained, repeated, and heavy use of **cocaine.** Interventions to treat human **cocaine** abuse attempt to alter the reward or motivation associated with compulsive use. As models of drug-induced reinforcement, self-administration (SA) paradigms are felt to best approximate naturalistic **cocaine** abuse. These and other models of dependence have demonstrated that **cocaine** activates the dopaminergic mesocorticolimbic (MCL) system. At the same time, there is emerging evidence from first preclinical and now human models to suggest that, the hedonic euphoriant effect response to drugs of abuse, although related to activation in striatal, limbic, and paralimbic structures may not be essential to the reinforcing effects of drugs of abuse. Indeed, a number of neuroimaging studies have confirmed that passive **cocaine** administration in humans activates mesolimbic structures and that this activation is related to behavioral effects. On the other hand, the neurobiological consequences of passive **cocaine** injections are substantially different from self-administered **cocaine.** While several animal models of compulsive drug seeking behavior exist, little is known about the neural substrates for the motivation and reinforcement of human **cocaine** use. This proposal seeks to determine the neuroanatomical sites and neurocognitive mechanisms associated with the reinforcement and reward of **cocaine** SA in human **cocaine** dependent individuals using fMRI. Pharmacological and behavioral models will be applied to identify and characterize those neural regions associated with **cocaine** dose-response, the anticipation of reward associated with SA, as well as determine those regions related to the reinforcement and reward of self-injection in contrast with passive investigator administered **cocaine.** The characterization of human neural substrates of **cocaine** reinforcement will lead to a better understanding of the neurobiological pathways underpinning the drive to use **cocaine** and may help to explain vulnerability to drug abuse. It is expected that such information will be essential to developing more effective clinical treatment strategies by providing insight into the compulsion to abuse this addicting drug.

Website: http://crisp.cit.nih.gov/crisp/Crisp_Query.Generate_Screen

- **Project Title: NEUROBIOLOGICAL PARAMETERS OF COCAINE REINFORCEMENT**

Principal Investigator & Institution: Smith, James E.; Professor and Chairman; Physiology and Pharmacology; Wake Forest University Health Sciences Winston-Salem, Nc 27157

Timing: Fiscal Year 2004; Project Start 01-JAN-1988; Project End 28-FEB-2009

Summary: (provided by applicant): The search for the neurobiological processes that underlie chemical dependence has entered the fourth decade of heightened investigation. The proliferation of neurotransmitter receptor subtypes has initiated a renaissance in potential new, more selective therapies for a number of neurological disorders. Hopefully, the definition of the subclasses of neurotransmitter receptors underlying **cocaine** self-administration will lead to new pharmacotherapeutic adjuncts for the treatment of these debilitating disorders. The overall goal of the research outlined in this competitive renewal application is to investigate the role of cholinergic neurons in intravenous **cocaine** self-administration. Recently completed acetylcholine (ACh) turnover rate studies implicate cholinergic innervations of several brain regions in **cocaine** self-administration. Cholinergic neurotoxin induced lesions that effect three of these regions [nucleus accumbens (NAcc), ventral pallidum (VP) and medial septum- (MS) vertical limb of the diagonal band (vlDA)] resulted in a shift to the left in the dose-intake relationship for self-administered **cocaine.** Experiments proposed in this next funding period will concentrate on the characterization of the role of cholinergic neurons in the NAcc, VP, vlDA and MS in **cocaine** self-administration using intracranial administration of receptor sub-type selective agonists, a selective cholinergic neurotoxin, in vivo microdialysis, targeted gene expression and immunohistochemistry. The overall research strategy will be first to administer muscarinic and nicotinic receptor agonists directly into the NAcc and assess effects upon the threshold for **cocaine** self-administration and extracellular fluid levels of dopamine, glutamate and gamma-aminobutyric acid. Agonists selective for the M4 muscarinic and alpha7 nicotinic receptors wilt be administered into the NAcc of **cocaine** self-administering rats to assess effects upon the threshold for **cocaine** self-administration and extracellular fluid levels of dopamine, glutamate and gamma-aminobutyric acid.This will be followed by similar experiments in the ventral pallidum. A transgenic mouse strain developed in Japan that utilizes immunotoxin mediated cell targeting to selectively remove cholinergic cells will be used to determine if NAcc cholinergic neuronal systems are also involved in mouse **cocaine** self-administration. This will be followed by experiments using a selective cholinergic neurotoxin, 192 IgG-saporin, to selectively remove cholinergic neurons in the vlDB and the MS and assess effects upon thresholds for intravenous **cocaine** self-administration. Targeted gene expression with real time reverse transcriptase polymerase chain reaction followed by Western blot analysis will then be used to identify the up or down regulation of cholinergic receptor subtypes potentially involved. This approach should result in the characterization of the specific cholinergic neuronal systems and receptors responsible for the shift to the left in the dose intake relationship and further define the importance of cholinergic cell systems in drug self-administration.

Website: http://crisp.cit.nih.gov/crisp/Crisp_Query.Generate_Screen

• Project Title: NEUROIMAGING OG NOVELTY DETECTION IN COCAINE DEPENDENCE

Principal Investigator & Institution: Berns, Gregory S.; Associate Professor; Psychiatry and Behavioral Scis; Emory University 1784 North Decatur Road Atlanta, Ga 30322

Timing: Fiscal Year 2002; Project Start 05-SEP-1999; Project End 31-AUG-2004

Summary: This revised proposal for a Mentored Clinical Scientist Development Award (MCSDA) provides the applicant with an optimal scientific environment for training in the functional neuroimaging of **cocaine** dependence. The career development and research plans are designed to enhance the applicant's scientific skills in both positron emission tomography (PET) and functional magnetic resonance imaging (fMRI), with the long term goals of linking changes in behavior with changes in neuronal function. In conjunction with the proposed research, the career development plan will foster the applicant's growth as an independent investigator in the cognitive neuroscience of addiction. A large body of evidence has implicated mesoaccumbal and mesolimbic circuits in **cocaine** dependence, yet elucidating the relationship between the function of these regions and the addiction syndrome has been hampered by the lack of knowledge about the role of these structures in human cognition. One impediment has been the absence of a functional, nonpharmacologic probe specific to the mesoaccumbal/limbic system. Targeted functional imaging paradigms, such as using working memory tasks to probe the frontal lobes, have made important advancements in the understanding of other psychiatric disorders. Based on computational models of cellular reward and information transmission, we have developed an innovative behavioral task anatomically targeted to the mesoaccumbal/limbic system. Preliminary PET data demonstrates that striatal activity normally increases in response to novel contextual information, but **cocaine** addicts display a decreased striatal response. The central hypothesis of this proposal is that monitoring for novelty is a normal function of the mesoaccumbal/limbic circuit, and this function becomes altered through chronic **cocaine** use. The preliminary findings further suggest that **cocaine** addicts have a different response to reinforcement, generating the secondary hypothesis that the neural substrates that code for reward will show a different response to monetary incentive. To test these hypotheses, three specific aims are identified: 1) Using PET, compare the striatal/accumbal response to novel information in a cohort of **cocaine** addicts and matched controls. 2) Simultaneously compare the striatal response to monetary reward in these cohorts. 3) Test the hypothesis that the striatum responds to novel information on a single-event basis by using fMRI to examine the time course of these responses. Taken together with a series of courses, seminars, and mentoring activities, this will yield important new insights into the cognitive neuroscience of human addiction and the specific roles that the mesoaccumbal and mesolimbic circuits play in **cocaine** dependence.

Website: http://crisp.cit.nih.gov/crisp/Crisp_Query.Generate_Screen

- **Project Title: NEUROPSYCHOPHARMACOL INTERACTIONS - COCAINE & SEROTONIN**

Principal Investigator & Institution: Cunningham, Kathryn; Associate Professor; Pharmacology and Toxicology; University of Texas Medical Br Galveston 301 University Blvd Galveston, Tx 77555

Timing: Fiscal Year 2002; Project Start 01-MAY-1996; Project End 30-APR-2005

Summary: (provided by applicant) **Cocaine** abuse continues to impose serious medical, psychological and criminal challenges for society. A thorough understanding of the neural basis underlying the effects of **cocaine** is critical to the development of science-based treatment protocols for **cocaine** dependence. Serotonin (5-hydroxytryptamine, 5-HT) is involved in the etiology of psychotic (e.g., schizophrenia) and affective disorders (e.g., anxiety, depression) which are often experienced by **cocaine** abusers. The innervation and localization of 5-HT1B receptors (5-HT1BR) and 5-HT2CR in mesocorticolimbic circuits and our preliminary data support differential roles of each receptor in modulating basal and cocaine-stimulated behavior. In the present proposal, the role of 5-HT1BR and 5-HT2CR in the acute locomotor stimulant and discriminative stimulus effects of **cocaine** will be investigated using novel 5-HT1BR and 5-HT2CR ligands and after knockdown or overexpression of 5-HT1BR or 5-HT2CR. The pattern of immediate early gene expression in the presence vs. absence of 5-HT1BR or 5-HT2CR ligands will be employed to guide studies to localize the site of action of 5-HT1BR and 5-HT2CR, respectively. Based upon this map, microinfusions of 5-HT1BR or 5-HT2CR ligands, antisense oligonucleotides or viral vectors encoding the 5-HT1BR or 5-HT2CR will be targeted to specific mesocorticolimbic nuclei to clarify the role of brain 5-HT1BR and 5-HT2CR in basal and cocaine-evoked behaviors. Modifications in 5-HT1BR and 5-HT2CR during withdrawal from chronic **cocaine** will also be established via analysis of hyperactivity induced by 5-HT1BR and 5-HT2CR agonists and levels of 5-HT1BR and 5-HT2CR mRNA and protein expression, respectively. The research goal of this K02 is to pursue the development of new methodologies based on molecular biology, genomics and proteomics and the application of these methodologies to elucidate the neural mechanisms that underlie the in vivo effects of **cocaine.** I propose to gain further training in measures of gene expression, including DNA microarrays and "real-time" PCR, in order to establish the impact of **cocaine** on the steady state levels of mRNA for monoamine transporters and receptors. In addition, we will develop the skills required to conduct virally-mediated gene transfers for the overexpression of receptor proteins in specific brain circuits. The teaching goal is to expand my efforts in drug dependence education in both the academic and community arenas. These educational endeavors, exemplified by my directorship of a NIDA Training Grant in the pharmacology of abused drugs and the mentoring of junior scientists in the laboratory will be enhanced by the development of a curriculum for the training of health care professionals in the science-based treatment of drug dependence. The research administrative goal of the K02 is to continue my involvement in research initiatives in drug abuse on the campus and nationally. Thus, the release time and salary support provided by this K02 would continue to enhance the development of my career in the science of drug dependence.

Website: http://crisp.cit.nih.gov/crisp/Crisp_Query.Generate_Screen

- **Project Title: NOVEL APPROACHES TO ALCOHOLISM PHARMACOTHERAPY AND RISK**

Principal Investigator & Institution: Kranzler, Henry R.; Professor of Psychiatry; Psychiatry; University of Connecticut Sch of Med/Dnt Bb20, Mc 2806 Farmington, Ct 060302806

Timing: Fiscal Year 2002; Project Start 01-AUG-2002; Project End 31-JUL-2007

Summary: (provided by applicant): This Mid-Career Investigator Award (K24) will provide the candidate with an opportunity to continue his career development, to continue to mentor beginning clinical investigators and to continue research in the pharmacotherapy of alcoholism and the genetics of alcohol and drug dependence. The research plan includes five projects, three of which have been funded and are ongoing; the others are being considered for funding or under scientific review. The ultimate research goal of proposal is the synthesis of findings from neuropsychopharmacology and genetics to yield a coherent pharmacogenetic approach to the etiology and treatment of alcoholism. The specific research aims of the proposal are 1) to complete data analysis and report preparation for a study of targeted naltrexone for early problem drinkers (data collection for which was recently completed), 2) to complete ongoing studies of the genetics of **cocaine** dependence (CD) and opioid dependence (OD), 3) to conduct a study of the genetics of alcohol dependence (AD) using the method of linkage disequilibrium and 4) to conduct a study examining the safety, efficacy, mechanism of action and duration of effects of sertraline in alcoholics who are subtyped by age of alcoholism onset. The mentoring plan will focus on training psychiatric residents, postdoctoral fellows in addiction psychiatry, postdoctoral fellows in alcohol research, and junior faculty in psychiatry and medicine to conduct patient-oriented research. That training will focus on clinical research methods, data interpretation, manuscript and grant preparation, research ethics and human subjects protections. Mentoring will occur through trainees' participation in the research projects and through lectures and seminars that are offered through the Alcohol Research Center, Department of Psychiatry, and the General Clinical Research Center at the University of Connecticut School of Medicine. This range of research and educational activities offers a rich matrix of opportunities for trainees and junior investigators in patient-oriented research. In addition, the K24 will enable the candidate to take coursework in areas that are important to his continued development as an investigator and mentor. Over the next five years, the candidate seeks to: 1) maintain full-time effort in research and research mentoring, 2) increase the depth and breadth of his own skills through specific training in molecular genetics, biostatistics and bioinformaties and through continued collaboration with established experts in these areas, 3) continue the dissemination of research findings through presentation at scientific meetings and publication in the scientific literature and 4) help to train the next generation of investigators who will advance the field of patient-oriented research in alcoholism and drug dependence.

Website: http://crisp.cit.nih.gov/crisp/Crisp_Query.Generate_Screen

- **Project Title: NOVEL COCAINE PHARMACOTHERAPIES: LAB STUDIES**

Principal Investigator & Institution: Haney, Margaret; Assistant Professor; Psychiatry; Columbia University Health Sciences Po Box 49 New York, Ny 10032

Timing: Fiscal Year 2002; Project Start 30-SEP-1996; Project End 30-JUN-2004

Summary: (Applicant's Abstract) There is no effective pharmacotherapy for **cocaine** abuse and dependence despite extensive testing of potential medications. The clinical data suggest that the search for direct-acting dopaminergic agents effective in treating **cocaine** abuse is unlikely to be productive, and investigations of other agents which perturb the noradrenergic and serotonergic systems have been equally disappointing. Recent data suggest that both NMDA and GABA may provide new avenues for pharmacological intervention in the treatment of **cocaine** abuse. We propose to continue our laboratory investigation into novel potential medications for the treatment of **cocaine** abusers by evaluating the NMDA antagonist, dextromethorphan, and the GABAergic agents, vigabatrin and gabapentin. We will include measures of **cocaine** self-administration under a modified progressive ratio procedure, a **cocaine** discrimination procedure and measures of subjective effects, including **cocaine** craving. This expanded profile of the ways in which these potential treatment medications interact with **cocaine** use and the consequences of that use, will allow us to make more informed decisions in designing specific pharmacological interventions to treat **cocaine** abusers. All participants will be tested under double blind conditions with placebo and active medication maintenance and with multiple doses of smoked **cocaine.** This use of a medication-maintenance model mimics the treatment situation and increases our ability to detect the effects of active medications, even those with slow onset of therapeutic effects. Laboratory research with human participants provides the necessary bridge from laboratory to clinic, and allows a relatively short, well controlled and safe alternative to the initial testing of a medication in an open label or even small controlled clinical trial. Combining the data from sensitive drug self-administration, drug discrimination and subjective effects measures will allow us to understand more fully the interaction between NMDA antagonism or GABAergic effects and cocaine's effects, and consequently to inform **cocaine** medication development endeavors. Such data will provide important information about the underlying neural mechanisms of single and repeated dose **cocaine** use in humans. The overall strength of this protocol lies in our utilization of a controlled laboratory setting to examine the interactive effects of an NMDA antagonist (dextromethorphan), a GABA transaminase inhibitor (vigabatrin), and a GABA analog which potentiates GABA (gabapentin), with **cocaine** use, **cocaine** "craving," and the subjective, physiological and discriminative stimulus effects of **cocaine.**

Website: http://crisp.cit.nih.gov/crisp/Crisp_Query.Generate_Screen

- **Project Title: NOVEL PHARMACOTHERAPIES FOR COCAINE DEPENDENCE**

Principal Investigator & Institution: Levin, Frances R.; Q. J. Kennedy Associate Professor of Cli; New York State Psychiatric Institute 1051 Riverside Dr New York, Ny 100321098

Timing: Fiscal Year 2002; Project Start 30-SEP-1999; Project End 31-AUG-2004

Summary: This MDRU proposal is aimed at 1) testing novel pharmacotherapies for **cocaine** dependence, and 2) developing a systematic approach to implementing clinical trials for such testing. A substantial among of evidence has been collected indicating that dopamine mediates the actions of **cocaine** that are assumed to be related to its abuse liability. To date, targeting the dopamine systems has not been clinically fruitful, probably because of the complexity of cocaine's actions. We hypothesized that agents that module the dopamine system, such as the excitatory and inhibitory amino acids, may be more likely to be successful therapeutic agents for **cocaine** dependence. Theoretically, either increasing the inhibitory influence of GABA or decreasing the excitatory influence of the glutamate system on cocaine-induced increases in dopamine should reduce the reinforcing effects of **cocaine.** Therefore, we will test a series of glutamatergic antagonists and GABAergic agonists. To perturb the glutamate system, we will use memantine, a non-competitive NMDA antagonist GV-196771A, a glycine site antagonist; acamprosate, a partial agonist at the polyamine site; ACEA-1021, a glycine site antagonist; and LY-293558, an AMPA antagonist. To perturb the glutamate system, we will use a memantine, a non-competitive NMDA antagonist; GV- 196771A, a glycine site antagonist; and LY-293558, an AMPA antagonist. To perturb the GABA system, we will use gabapentin, a GABA analog; baclofen, a GABAB agonist; and abecarnil, a GABAA partial agonist. We are proposing a hierarchical series of clinical trials, studying medications at "late Phase II" (Project 1), "early Phase II" (Project 2), and "late Phase I" levels (Project 3). Project 1 will tet memantine and gabapentin, in sequential double-blind placebo-controlled trials (N=40/arm), each lasting 2.5 years. Project 2 will test GV 196771A and baclofen against placebo in a 3-arm double-blind placebo-controlled trial (N=20/arm), followed by a similar trial of acamprosate, abecarnil and placebo. Each trial will last 2.5 years. Project 3 will test, in successive years, in placebo-controlled double blind laboratory trials (N=20/study), acamprosate, abecarnil, ACEA 1021, and LY 293558. Projects 1 and 2 will begin in year 1, Project 3 will begin in year 2. This MDRU will have the capability to move among three models and compare data across them: 1) a placebo-controlled design in a classic trial; 2) an innovative outpatient 3-arm placebo-controlled design; and 3) the human laboratory. The believe this to be a rational and cost effective approach to testing potentially useful medications.

Website: http://crisp.cit.nih.gov/crisp/Crisp_Query.Generate_Screen

- **Project Title: NOVEL TREATMENTS FOR COCAINE DEPENDENCE**

Principal Investigator & Institution: Weiss, Friedbert; Associate Member; Scripps Research Institute Tpc7 La Jolla, Ca 92037

Timing: Fiscal Year 2004; Project Start 15-AUG-1991; Project End 28-FEB-2009

Summary: (provided by applicant): This proposal seeks to continue studies conducted during previous funding periods that were concerned with the development of behavioral methods modeling long-lasting vulnerability to relapse in rats, and the application of these models for the testing of pharmacological agents that modify cocaine-seeking behavior. Susceptibility to relapse presents a great challenge for the treatment of **cocaine** addiction. Major factors implicated in the high rates of relapse associated with **cocaine** and other drug addictions include conditioned responses to drug-related environmental stimuli and subjective reactions to stress. A growing literature suggests that metabotropic glutamate receptors (mGluRs) play a prominent role in mediating neurobehavioral effects of **cocaine** and other drugs of abuse. Emerging evidence also implicates mGluRs in the regulation of anxiety and behavioral responses to stress. Based on these findings one may hypothesize that mGluR-mediated neural events play a role in conditioned drug-seeking responses elicited by drug-related environmental stimuli as well as in drug-seeking behavior induced by stress. The objective of this proposal is (1) to test this hypothesis by studying the effects of novel, selective mGluR ligands on drug-seeking and the resistance to extinction of this behavior in reinstatement models of relapse, and (2) to establish whether specific mGluR subtypes represent potential treatment targets for addictive behavior associated with the exposure to drug cues and stress. The research plan is to first systematically characterize the effect of ligands for Group I and II mGluRs on cocaine-seeking behavior induced by a drug-associated contextual stimulus or acute footshock stress, and to verify pharmacologically a role of specific mGluR subtypes in reductions of cocaine-seeking behavior. The characterization of the potential of mGluR ligands to block conditioned or stress-induced cocaine-seeking then will be extended to drug-seeking associated with other classes of drugs including heroin and nicotine. Finally, the potential of mGluR ligands to attenuate drug-seeking will be further qualified by establishing whether these agents preferentially modify behavior directed at obtaining drug reinforcers or exert general suppressant effects on motivated behavior, using stimuli conditioned to conventional reinforcers with high, but qualitatively divergent incentive value. These studies are expected to provide novel information on the role of specific mGluRs in the regulation of conditioned or stress-induced drug-seeking behavior as well as their role in incentive motivation, in general. This information will be directly relevant for the development of treatments targeting the mGluR system.

Website: http://crisp.cit.nih.gov/crisp/Crisp_Query.Generate_Screen

- **Project Title: PET IMAGING--COMORBID COCAINE DEPENDENCE AND DEPRESSION**

Principal Investigator & Institution: Rubin, Eric;; New York State Psychiatric Institute 1051 Riverside Dr New York, Ny 100321098

Timing: Fiscal Year 2002; Project Start 30-SEP-1998; Project End 31-AUG-2004

Summary: (Applicant's Abstract) Comorbidity of **cocaine** dependence and major depressive disorder (MDD) poses an important clinical challenge. The relatively high incidence of such comorbidity and a variety of previous investigations raise intriguing questions about neurobiological connections between these disorders. We will use positron emission tomography (PET) of human brain metabolism, before and after treatment of the comorbid disorders, as a window into such neurobiological relationships. Our team combines expertise in advanced functional brain imaging with experience in the diagnosis and treatment of comorbid MDD and **cocaine** dependence. Subjects for this study will be carefully screened volunteers in four samples: cocaine-dependent (CD) only, MDD alone, CD comorbid with MDD, and normal controls. Equal numbers of males and females will be recruited to assess gender differences. The MDD and CD+MDD groups will be treated for 12 weeks with venlafaxine, an antidepressant which our pilot data indicates is effective in the comorbid population. Specific hypotheses about the profile of cerebral metabolism in these groups will be examined as follows: 1) at baseline in all groups, 2) following treatment, when baseline and post-treatment scans will be compared to identify brain sites potentially involved in treatment effects, and 3) following treatment, when baseline scans for responders and non-responders in each treatment group will be correlated with treatment outcome to identify pre-treatment metabolic features which predict responsiveness. We will apply advanced quantitative procedures for examining global, regional, and "network" brain metabolism, and will correlate these measures with standardized measures of treatment success. This methodologic rigor will contribute to understanding the pathophysiology and treatment of patients with comorbid depression and **cocaine** dependence.

Website: http://crisp.cit.nih.gov/crisp/Crisp_Query.Generate_Screen

- **Project Title: PHARMACOTHERAPY FOR COCAINE DEPENDENCE**

Principal Investigator & Institution: Grabowski, John G.; Professor; Psychiatry and Behavioral Scis; University of Texas Hlth Sci Ctr Houston Box 20036 Houston, Tx 77225

Timing: Fiscal Year 2003; Project Start 01-MAY-2003; Project End 28-FEB-2006

Summary: (provided by applicant): **Cocaine** dependence has diverse adverse consequences and has proven difficult to treat. Behavioral interventions, including Community Reinforcement Model and Cognitive Behavior Therapy/Relapse Prevention have proven effective. Medications that might serve as effective adjuncts have been elusive. Recent primate self-administration data (Negus, 2002), several recent reports, and completion/analysis of a recent large clinical trial support further study of the agonist/ replacement approach. Still, target medications, dose, and duration must be further evaluated. This application proposes a large (140 S's, 35/group), long duration (6 month) rigorous blind randomized clinical trial. Sustained release d-amphetamine will be examined across dose range. of PBO, 45 mg, 60 mg, or 80 mg administered in identical capsules. Rigorous compliance measures using riboflavin, urine screens, and MEMS dispensing bottles will be applied. Consent will be followed by a 10 day period in which BZ positive urine screens must be provided and during which Intake and Evaluation will proceed. Medication run-up of 10 days will be followed by 20 weeks of stable medication. A dose reduction period and four weeks of behavior therapy alone will follow, Post treatment follow-up will be at 1 and 3 months. Intake evaluation will include standardized measures (.e.g. ASI, SCID, HAM A/D, Craving Questionnaire; HIV, EKG, TB, urine screens). There will be repeated weekly measures with thrice weekly urine screens. EKGs will be bi-weekly. Manual Driven Cognitive Behavior Therapy will be weekly. Blood samples will be obtained at regular intervals during run-up, maintenance, dose reduction and in the final three non-medication weeks. This design incorporates both major features and details in accord with NIDA's consensus review (January 2002) on optimal strategies for agonist evaluation.

Website: http://crisp.cit.nih.gov/crisp/Crisp_Query.Generate_Screen

- **Project Title: PIPERDYL ANALOGS AS COCAINE PHARMACOTHERAPY**

Principal Investigator & Institution: Harp, Jill; Assistant Professor; Winston-Salem State University 601 Martin Luther King Jr Dr Winston-Salem, Nc 27110

Timing: Fiscal Year 2002; Project Start 30-SEP-2002; Project End 29-SEP-2007

Summary: Cocaine abuse and dependence is a substantial public health threat in the United States and around the world. The widespread use of **cocaine** and other psychostimulants has stimulated extensive efforts to develop treatment programs for this type of addiction. One of the top priorities of the National Institute on Drug Abuse is to find a medication to reduce the effects of **cocaine** and to use this medication as one part of a comprehensive treatment program. The objective of this research proposal is to synthesize and test drugs that may aid in the fight against addiction to **cocaine,** amphetamines and other stimulants. **Cocaine** analogs, called tropanes, have been studied extensively. These drugs have high potency for blocking the dopamine transporter and last a long time, which is desirable for a therapeutic drug, but they are also self-administered by animals, and this ability to be reinforcing makes them less desirable. Removal of the two-carbon bridge of these tropanes gives rise to piperidines. Some piperidines have been shown to act as dopamine reuptake inhibitors without being reinforcing, or addictive. Thus, the central hypothesis of this proposal is that piperidine derivatives of **cocaine** analogs will be high potency inhibitors of the dopamine transporter (DAT) and the serotonin transporter. It is proposed that piperidine derivatives of tropanes reported to have high affinities for the dopamine transporter (DAT) and serotonin transporter (SERT or 5-HTT) will serve as excellent leads for medication development. The synthesis will be accomplished using established pathways and allows for easy entry and purification of all compounds. In vitro testing will include determination of IC50 and Ki values for all piperidines synthesized and their DAT/5-HT selectivity values. In addition, the ability of the new compounds to prevent induced monoamine release following methamphetamine application in vitro will be determined. Finally, in vivo behavioral place preference studies will be performed with the compounds to assess their reinforcing properties. The long-range goal of the project is to submit compounds that have appropriate profiles and lack abuse potential to the NIDA Division of Treatment Research and Development for further consideration as potential therapeutic agents for **cocaine** addiction.

Website: http://crisp.cit.nih.gov/crisp/Crisp_Query.Generate_Screen

- **Project Title: PREDICTORS: MEDICATION ADHERENCE IN HIV+ COCAINE ABUSERS**

Principal Investigator & Institution: Hinkin, Charles H.; Associate Professor; Psychiatry & Biobehav Sciences; University of California Los Angeles 10920 Wilshire Blvd., Suite 1200 Los Angeles, Ca 90024

Timing: Fiscal Year 2002; Project Start 05-JUL-2001; Project End 30-JUN-2005

Summary: Predictors of Medication Adherence and Antiretroviral Resistance Among HIV-Infected **Cocaine** Abusers Although Highly Active Antiretroviral Therapy (HAART) has been shown to dramatically reduce morbidity and mortality among HIV- infected individuals, without rigorous medication adherence viral replication will ensue and antiretroviral resistant HIV mutations will arise. Among HIV+ patients, there is growing evidence that those especially likely to demonstrate poor adherence are those who evidence significant neuropsychological impairment and those who are **cocaine** abusing/dependent. Using a structural equation modeling approach, the proposed study will investigate the impact of **cocaine** abuse, neurocognitive dysfunction, psychiatric disorder, psychosocial factors, demographic characteristics, and medication regimen complexity on medication adherence in a multiethnic sample of HIV+ **cocaine** abusing patients. Adherence will be objectively determined by use of computerized Medication Event Monitoring System (MEMS) caps, pill counts, adherence questionnaires, and self-report. Specific aims include: (1) how **cocaine** abuse/dependence affects medication adherence in HIV+ individuals, and how this interacts with time other variables of interest; (2) whether **cocaine** abuse and pattern of adherence failure are associated with the development of antiretroviral resistant HIV mutations, as indexed through genotypic resistance assays; (3) the predictive relationship between medication adherence and factors such as neurocognition, psychiatric status, risk taking, medical decision making and other critical psychosocial and sociocultural factors; and (4) the development of a taxonomy of risk factors and protective factors that will reliably identify subtypes of adherers/non-aderers. These questions will be investigated by our multidisciplinary team in a diverse sample of 300 HIV+ **cocaine** abusing/dependent adults. A comprehensive battery of psychosocial measures and neuropsychological tests will be administered at baseline and subjects adherence to their prescribed medical regimen will be monitored on a monthly basis for 6 months with the MEMS caps methodology. A blood sample will also be taken at baseline and at study completion, and assayed to determine whether antiretroviral resistant HIV mutations develop. It is expected that results from this study will help to identify those dually diagnosed HIV+ patients that are especially likely to be non- adherent and to inform targets for interventions that will enhance treatment adherence in this high risk population.

Website: http://crisp.cit.nih.gov/crisp/Crisp_Query.Generate_Screen

- **Project Title: PROCESS OF CHANGE IN DRUG ABUSE BY SCHIZOPHRENICS**

Principal Investigator & Institution: Bellack, Alan S.; Professor; Psychiatry; University of Maryland Balt Prof School Baltimore, Md 21201

Timing: Fiscal Year 2002; Project Start 20-APR-1999; Project End 31-MAR-2004

Summary: Substance abuse by individuals with schizophrenia has reached epidemic proportions, yet little is known about why they use substances or how they can be helped to decrease use. The most widely accepted conceptualization of their substance abuse treatment needs is adapted from Prochaska and DiClemente's Transtheoretical Model (TTM). This model has proven to be quite robust in explaining the process of change in a variety of less impaired substance abusing populations, and several instruments have proven to be reliable and valid for assessing central components of the model. However, the TTM assumes intentional behavior change and full participation in the process of change by the substance abuser. Schizophrenia is marked by a number of symptomatic, neurocognitive, and psychosocial characteristics that would make it difficult for many individuals to successfully perform these complex activities, thereby raising questions about the applicability of the model for this population. Notably, patients with schizophrenia have significant impairments in cognitive function, including attention, memory, and higher level "executive" abilities, that may limit their ability to analyze the pros and cons of substance use, retain a focus on goals for decreased use over time, and form realistic efficacy expectations based on past experience. The disorder also is frequently associated with avolition and anhedonia, which may interfere with the ability to sustain motivation to reduce use. The overall purpose of this project is to examine attitudes about substance use, motivation to reduce use, and the process of change among schizophrenia patients who meet DSM-IV criteria for current **Cocaine** Dependence or are in Early Remission. The specific focus is the validity of the TTM for this population, and the adequacy of the standard measures of stages and processes of change developed for less impaired groups. Four groups of subjects will be assessed at Baseline, 3-, 6-, 9-, and 12-months: 70 Schizophrenia patients with current **Cocaine** Dependence, 70 Schizophrenia patients who are in Early Remission from **Cocaine,** 70 patients with Major Depression and current **Cocaine** Dependence, and 70 patients with Major Depression who are in Early Remission from **Cocaine.**.

Website: http://crisp.cit.nih.gov/crisp/Crisp_Query.Generate_Screen

- **Project Title: PTSD AND DRUG DEPENDENCE: NEUROIMAGING OF REWARD CIRCUI***

Principal Investigator & Institution: Elman, Igor E.;; Mc Lean Hospital (Belmont, Ma) Belmont, Ma 02478

Timing: Fiscal Year 2004; Project Start 01-JUN-2004; Project End 31-MAY-2008

Summary: (provided by applicant): This proposal, entitled "PTSD and drug dependence: neuroimaging of reward circuitry" is a response to NIDA Request for R01 Applications (#DA-04-001; Stress and Drug Abuse: Epidemiology, Etiology, Prevention and Treatment). The primary goal of this proposal is to investigate brain reward function as a potential neuropathological basis for substance use disorders (SUDs) comorbidity in posttraumatic stress disorder (PTSD). Basic neuroscience and clinical findings suggest that brain reward circuitry is altered by chronic stress exposure in ways that may be important for facilitating SUDs. We hypothesize that: 1) functionally impaired brain reward mechanisms may comprise a neural substrate underlying core PTSD symptoms of reduced reactivity to natural rewarding stimuli or emotional numbing and that 2) this neural substrate is further altered by the presence of comorbid SUDs. The proposed project is designed to test these hypotheses integrating functional magnetic resonance imaging, psychopharmacology and cognitive psychology to empirically measure reward responses in PTSD, **cocaine** dependence, PTSD with comorbid **cocaine** dependence and in health. The proposed experiments have already been successfully performed in separate cohorts of healthy volunteers and piloted in PTSD subjects with and without **cocaine** dependence. The published data and preliminary results suggest unique patterns of hemodynamic responses in the nucleus accumbens (NAc) and related structures during reward processing along with PTSD-related abnormalities in performance on a behavioral probe of reward function. Three distinct experimental paradigms to be used in this project include a) low doses of an FDA-approved euphorigenic drug, morphine, which can be safely administered to drug-naive subjects, b) social reward in the form of visual processing of attractive faces and c) monetary incentive stimuli incorporated into a gambling task. We expect to find that in PTSD patients the magnitude of the NAc's activation in response to the three rewarding stimuli will be smaller relative to healthy controls, but larger than in individuals with comorbid PTSD and **cocaine** dependence. This research plan will provide important leads for understanding and preventing the development of SUDs in the context of chronic stress exposure or PTSD. Furthermore our project may offer insights on the pathogenesis of emotional numbing symptoms, which cause severe disability not only in PTSD patients, but also in those suffering from other neuropsychiatric conditions such as SUDs, schizophrenia and major depression.

Website: http://crisp.cit.nih.gov/crisp/Crisp_Query.Generate_Screen

- **Project Title: ROLE OF PROTEOGLYCANS IN COCAINE DEPENDENCE**

Principal Investigator & Institution: Sanna, Pietro P.; Associate Professor; Scripps Research Institute Tpc7 La Jolla, Ca 92037

Timing: Fiscal Year 2003; Project Start 15-AUG-2003; Project End 31-JUL-2005

Summary: (provided by applicant): In humans, chronic use of **cocaine** is often associated with a binge-like, uncontrollable pattern of use with overall tolerance and acute withdrawal. This **cocaine** withdrawal is characterized by severe depressive symptoms combined with irritability, anxiety, and anhedonia, lasting several hours to several days that may be one of the major motivating factors in the maintenance of the cocaine-dependence cycle. We have observed that the expression of Syndecan-3, a proteoglycan previously implicated in feeding behavior, is dramatically increased in the hypothalamus during withdrawal in animals self-administering **cocaine** and it was significantly higher in animals with an escalating pattern of **cocaine** self-administration. The present CEBRA proposal is aimed at investigating the role of hypothalamic Syndecan in **cocaine** intake. To this aim we propose to use adeno-associated (AAV) viral vectors expressing Syndecan -1, a peripheral form of Syndecan that is not cleaved by brain proteases and mimics the overexpression of Syndecan-3; constitutively shed Syndecan-1 ectodomain; or small interfering RNAs (siRNA) targeting Syndecan-3. The effect of hypothalamic injection of these constructs will be studied on **cocaine** self-administration in animals with an escalating pattern of **cocaine** self-administration in comparison to animals that self-administer consistent low levels of **cocaine.** The elucidation of the neurobiological bases for the transition from non-dependent drug use to addiction is of crucial importance for the development of novel and more effective therapeutic approaches.

Website: http://crisp.cit.nih.gov/crisp/Crisp_Query.Generate_Screen

- **Project Title: SCOR APPLICATION ON SEX, STRESS, AND COCAINE ADDICTION**

Principal Investigator & Institution: Sinha, Rajita; Associate Professor; Psychiatry; Yale University 47 College Street, Suite 203 New Haven, Ct 065208047

Timing: Fiscal Year 2002; Project Start 30-SEP-2002; Project End 31-AUG-2007

Summary: (provided by applicant): **Cocaine** addiction is a chronic relapsing disorder with devastating psychosocial, health and societal consequences. Emerging data clearly indicate the importance of studying sex-specific effects in **cocaine** dependence - a growing problem for women in this country. Stress has been identified as one of the key factors in increasing the vulnerability to develop **cocaine** dependence in women. Women also report stress and negative mood as playing a pivotal role in the continued drug use and relapse cycle. While there have been attempts to understand the mechanisms underlying the association between stress and **cocaine** addiction, systematic research on sex-specific factors that contribute to this association has been rare. The goal of this Center is to use interdisciplinary approaches of examination: (A) to assess the effects of early life stress, sex hormones and stress hormones on **cocaine** reinforcement and the risk of developing **cocaine** dependence; and (B) to understand the contribution of sex-based factors in the association between stress and **cocaine** relapse. These goals will be achieved using multidisciplinary laboratory and clinical research conducted in animals and in humans. A greater understanding of the interactions between sex, stress and **cocaine** dependence will be significant in the development of sex-specific prevention and treatment approaches that will specifically affect the health of women with **cocaine** dependence. The following specific aims will be achieved by the SCOR: (1) To establish a collaborative multidisciplinary research Center that will address the study of sex-specific factors in the relationship between stress and **cocaine** addiction. (2) To conduct a series of programmatic animal and human research studies aimed at understanding sex-specific factors in the relationship between stress and **cocaine** addiction. (3) To develop a collaborative research program that will utilize SCOR core resources to facilitate the investigation of sex-specific factors in ongoing independently-funded research at Yale relating to the etiology, neurobiology and treatment of **cocaine** addiction. (4) To assist a range of young investigators from different disciplines in conducting sex-specific research on stress and **cocaine** addiction through mentorship activities of Center staff.

Website: http://crisp.cit.nih.gov/crisp/Crisp_Query.Generate_Screen

- **Project Title: SEROTONIN AND COCAINE DEPENDENCE:TREATMENT IMPLICATIONS**

Principal Investigator & Institution: Patkar, Ashwin A.; Psychiatry and Human Behavior; Thomas Jefferson University Office of Research Administration Philadelphia, Pa 191075587

Timing: Fiscal Year 2003; Project Start 01-JUL-2003; Project End 31-MAR-2006

Summary: (provided by applicant): The proposal is being submitted for review under the R21 (exploratory grant) mechanism. Despite considerable efforts, medications with sound neurobiological rationale have not proven to be consistently effective in the treatment of **cocaine** dependence (CD). Based on findings from an ongoing study titled 'serotonergic function and treatment outcome in cocaine', the proposed research examines the hypothesis that there are inter-individual differences in neurobiological function, specifically serotonergic (5HT) function, among CD individuals, and that these differences influence the effectiveness of serotonergic pharmacotherapies. In a relatively novel pharmacological approach, the hypothesis will be examined in a 2 X 2 experimental design by randomly assigning 80 CD patients to 12 weeks of double-blind treatment with either paroxetine, a selective serotonergic reuptake inhibitor, or placebo. Subsequently these patients will be divided into lower 5HT and higher 5HT function groups based upon pre-treatment values of platelet tritiated paroxetine binding a measure of serotonin transporter sites and the during treatment and end-of-treatment outcome measures will be compared across the subject groups. The outcome measures will reflect abstinence from drugs and retention in treatment. Also, whether changes in paroxetine binding values during treatment are associated with reduced impulsivity and aggression and with outcome measures will be determined. The data analysis will examine the main effects of medication and 5HT function and then test the Treatment X 5HT interaction that is central to our main hypothesis. The rate of platelet 5HT uptake will also be examined as an additional index of the serotonin transporter. Relationships between this measure and outcome measures will be also explored. The findings may help to better understand the relationships between peripheral measures of 5HT function and clinical and outcome measures among **cocaine** patients. Moreover, the results may help to improve pharmacological strategies for the treatment of **cocaine** dependence.

Website: http://crisp.cit.nih.gov/crisp/Crisp_Query.Generate_Screen

- **Project Title: SEROTONIN TREATMENT OF COCAINE DEPENDENCE**

Principal Investigator & Institution: Strain, Eric C.; Professor; Psychiatry and Behavioral Scis; Johns Hopkins University 3400 N Charles St Baltimore, Md 21218

Timing: Fiscal Year 2002; Project Start 30-SEP-1996; Project End 31-MAR-2006

Summary: (Applicant's Abstract) This is a competitive renewal application to continue to study the efficacy of serotonergic medications in the outpatient treatment of **cocaine** dependence. The originally funded study examined tryptophan, the precursor of serotonin, in the treatment of **cocaine** abuse, and hence the grant was titled "Tryptophan and Behavior Therapy for **Cocaine** Abuse." Since this renewal shifts focus from tryptophan to another medication that alters serotonin functioning (fluoxetine), it has been re-titled "Serotonin Treatment of **Cocaine** Dependence." While several studies have reported on clinical experience in the use of fluoxetine for the treatment of **cocaine** use, most of these studies have methodological limitations (e.g., small sample sizes, heterogeneous study populations, failure to ensure compliance in taking medication, inadequate patient motivation). Importantly, there have now been several well conducted, controlled studies suggesting fluoxetine can be effective in the treatment of **cocaine** abuse - when medication compliance is assured, and when it is combined with incentives that provide motivation to stop using **cocaine.** Further, pilot subjects tested in our clinic with the currently proposed methods have shown positive responses. This proposal builds upon prior studies in its design and extends the methods used with our pilot subjects. It also continues the theme begun with the first study - that is, enhancing serotonergic functioning as a means of decreasing the reinforcing effects of **cocaine.** The current proposal again tests medication efficacy in the context of voucher incentives that provide motivation to stop **cocaine** use, but now has new design features in response to experience from the first clinical trial. Specifically, this proposal is to test fluoxetine in methadone maintained patients with concurrent **cocaine** dependence. There are several reasons for utilizing methadone maintained patients: compliance taking medication can be assured, retention rates are high, and concurrent **cocaine** dependence is common. The design is a 2 x 2, with patients randomly assigned to receive either double blind fluoxetine or placebo, and either voucher incentives or no voucher incentives. Voucher incentives can be effective in decreasing **cocaine** use, but studies have shown only about one-half of patients respond to this intervention. The main hypothesis to be tested in this study is that the combination of fluoxetine with vouchers will produce enhanced effects on decreasing **cocaine** use, compared to outcomes produced by the treatments alone. The principal logic underlying this study is that fluoxetine will weaken (but not necessarily eliminate) **cocaine** effects, and that this will translate into higher success rates under a behavior therapy that provides incentives for abstinence. These results will provide valuable new information about the ability of fluoxetine to enhance the effectiveness of an effective behavioral treatment intervention, and can lead to new and innovative treatment approaches for **cocaine** abusing patients.

Website: http://crisp.cit.nih.gov/crisp/Crisp_Query.Generate_Screen

- **Project Title: SEROTONIN, IMPULSIVITY AND COCAINE DEPENDENCE TREATMENT**

Principal Investigator & Institution: Moeller, Frederick G.; Associate Professor; Psychiatry and Behavioral Scis; University of Texas Hlth Sci Ctr Houston Box 20036 Houston, Tx 77225

Timing: Fiscal Year 2002; Project Start 20-SEP-1996; Project End 31-MAR-2005

Summary: This is a resubmission of a competing renewal of RO1 DA08425, Serotonin and Aggression in **Cocaine** Dependence. The title of renewal has been changed to reflect the newly defined emphasis on the impact of impulsivity on the treatment of **cocaine** dependence. **Cocaine** Dependence is associated with higher levels of impulsivity, both clinically and as measured by questionnaires and laboratory measures. We have found that impulsivity is associated with a poor outcome in the treatment of **cocaine** dependence. Further, there is evidence from our group and others that impulsivity is associated with decreased functioning of the neurotransmitter serotonin, and that serotonergic medication increases response to contingency management treatment for **cocaine** dependence. In light of the above data, we propose a treatment study to determine whether the serotonin reuptake inhibitor citalopram improves response to contingency management treatment of **cocaine** dependence. We also propose to measure serotonin and impulsivity to determine whether baseline serotonin function, and changes in impulsivity predict response to treatment. The Specific Aims of this proposal are: Aim 1. To determine whether chronic administration of the 5-HT re-uptake inhibitor citalopram improves response to contingency management treatment of **cocaine** dependence. Aim 2. To measure pretreatment Serotonin (5-HT) function using a citalopram neuroendocrine challenge and determine the relationship between 5-HT function and response to treatment in **cocaine** dependent subjects. Aim 3. To measure impulsivity in subjects undergoing treatment for **cocaine** dependence using laboratory tasks to determine if changes in impulsivity predict response to treatment for **cocaine** dependence.

Website: http://crisp.cit.nih.gov/crisp/Crisp_Query.Generate_Screen

- **Project Title: SUBSTANCE USE: FAMILY, FRIEND, AND COMMUNITY FACTORS**

Principal Investigator & Institution: Sterk, Claire E.; Professor and Chair; Behavioral Scis & Hlth Educ; Emory University 1784 North Decatur Road Atlanta, Ga 30322

Timing: Fiscal Year 2002; Project Start 01-JUN-2001; Project End 31-MAY-2006

Summary: (Applicant's Abstract) The specific aim of this application for a K02 award is to advance the applicant's quantitative skills, which in turn will allow her to build on the qualitative and quantitative skills she already has as well as on the largely qualitative contributions she has made to the substance abuse field. Much of her work in the substance abuse field has been qualitative in nature or been limited to less advanced quantitative approaches. Ultimately, the candidate anticipates that an extensive knowledge of advanced qualitative and quantitative skills will allow her to continue to make contributions to the field. In the research plan, the applicant proposes to build on her ongoing research on intergenerational substance abuse among mothers and daughters. Although research on familial, friend, and community factors on substance abuse exists, many questions remain regarding the complex relationship between risk and protective factors at all three of these levels. In the proposed research, the candidate aims: (1) to determine familial patterns of substance use, abuse and dependence among cocaine-dependent young adults (ages 18-25), their parents and their siblings. This includes the role of specific family members, familial aggregation, familial use patterns of specific drugs, and the development of familial substance use; (2) to explore the association between **cocaine** dependence and comorbid psychopathology, particularly depression, anxiety, antisocial personality disorder, and post-traumatic stress syndrome; (3) to examine the role of specific community factors in the development of substance use, abuse, and dependence. These factors involve local drug market forces, such as the availability, price and purity of **cocaine** and other drugs; community norms regarding substance use, and other relevant community characteristics; and (4) to investigate the dynamics of risk and protective factors at the individual, familial, and community levels. The development and training component of the application includes course work in advanced statistical techniques. This further training will allow the applicant to continue to build on her existing expertise and to continue to make contributions to the field by adding quantitative approaches to her largely qualitative work. The requested release time from teaching and administrative responsibilities will allow the candidate to enhance her research career.

Website: http://crisp.cit.nih.gov/crisp/Crisp_Query.Generate_Screen

- **Project Title: TREATING COCAINE ABUSE: A BEHAVIORAL APPROACH**

Principal Investigator & Institution: Higgins, Stephen T.; Professor; Psychiatry; University of Vermont & St Agric College 340 Waterman Building Burlington, Vt 05405

Timing: Fiscal Year 2002; Project Start 30-SEP-1994; Project End 31-AUG-2004

Summary: Cocaine dependence remains a major U.S. public health problem for which effective treatments are sorely needed. Towards that end, our group has been researching a multicomponent, outpatient treatment for **cocaine** dependence. The treatment integrates two key components: a voucher-based incentive program and Community Reinforcement Approach therapy. This treatment is one of the few reliably efficacious interventions for retaining cocaine-dependent adults in outpatient treatment and for engendering **cocaine** abstinence. The studies proposed in this competing continuation programmatically extend this treatment approach. Our current focus is on understanding how to increase post-treatment **cocaine** abstinence. Interestingly, evidence from us and others indicates that increasing during-treatment abstinence may be the most effective strategy for improving longer-term abstinence in cocaine-dependent outpatients. Experimental and correlational data from our clinic, for example, indicate that sustaining three or months of continuous **cocaine** abstinence during treatment increases greater than 3-fold the odds of **cocaine** abstinence at follow-up. Our prior trials also indicate clearly that the voucher-based incentive program is the most effective element in this multicomponent treatment for increasing during-treatment abstinence. Hence, the proposed studies will experimentally analyze how changes in the value of the voucher-based incentive program as well as length of treatment with it affects during-treatment and post-treatment **cocaine** abstinence. Additionally, while strong evidence exists supporting the efficacy of this voucher program, there is a striking dearth of information available on how alterations in its basic parameters affect outcome. Thus, the proposed trials also will provide practically important new parametric information on this intervention. We have proposed two trials. Trial 1 will use a randomized, parallel-groups design to examine the during- and post-treatment effects of this multicomponent treatment with the vouchers set at one-half, full, and twice their usual monetary value. Trial 2 will use the same design, but instead of manipulating the value of the vouchers, the length of time that patients receive them will be set at one-half, full, and twice the usual duration. Overall, these clinical trials will further understanding of cocaine-dependence treatment in at least two ways: First, they will rigorously evaluate the hypothesis that increasing during-treatment abstinence increases longer-term **cocaine** abstinence. If that hypothesis is supported, it will provide a concrete target for facilitating longer-term **cocaine** abstinence in future treatment efforts. Secondly, the trials will provide rigorous, experimental analyses of the relationships between the value of voucher-based incentives and length of treatment with them and treatment outcome. Such information is essential to a thorough evaluation of this emerging treatment technology.

Website: http://crisp.cit.nih.gov/crisp/Crisp_Query.Generate_Screen

- **Project Title: TREATMENT FOR BLACK PARENTING COCAINE DEPENDENT WOMEN**

Principal Investigator & Institution: Durant, Lauren E.; Psychiatry; Duke University Durham, Nc 27710

Timing: Fiscal Year 2003; Project Start 20-SEP-2003; Project End 30-JUN-2008

Summary: (provided by applicant): This Mentored Patient-Oriented Research Career Development Award (RCA--K23) application will support the career development of the candidate to become a clinical trials interventionist for substance abuse treatments with an emphasis on treatments appropriate for communities of color. Dr. Robert L. Hubbard of Duke University Medical Center and Duke Clinical Research Institute will be the primary mentor. The candidate will adapt the Community Reinforcement Approach (CRA), an efficacious treatment for **cocaine** dependence, for a difficult-to-treat group: Black parenting **cocaine** dependent women. In Study Phase I, Standard CRA will be modified based on recommendations from the available maternal treatment literature, interviews with clients and clinic staff and two small open pilot tests of Modified CRA. In Study Phase II, Modified CRA will be tested for feasibility and efficacy in a single blind, randomized clinical trial. Fifty participants will be randomized to Modified CRA or Treatment as Usual in an outpatient comprehensive Family Care Program. The primary endpoint will be retention--the proportion of participants retained for 12 weeks of treatment. The secondary endpoint will be abstinence--the proportion of urine samples negative for **cocaine** metabolite (benzoylecognine). This RCT will also (1) generate effect sizes for future effectiveness trials of Modified CRA for Black parenting **cocaine** dependent women and 2) result in supplemental appendices that detail translational and technology transfer issues in the implementation of Modified CRA in a woman-focused outpatient community treatment setting. The career training plan hinges on an advanced Masters Program in Clinical Trials at the Duke Clinical Research Institute and a set of coordinated mentorships in clinical trials, technology transfer, and culturally relevant treatment approaches for substance related disorders. Related career development activities will include leadership and participation in NIDA Clinical Trials Network protocols, publications of survey data assessing the needs of maternal populations, and participation in minority career development seminars at the Center for AIDS Prevention Research in San Francisco, and at Duke University Medical Center. The research and didactic elements of this K23 in hand, the applicant will emerge as an independent investigator capable of designing and implementing clinical interventions to improve substance abuse treatments not only for Black parenting women but for difficult-to-treat communities of color.

Website: http://crisp.cit.nih.gov/crisp/Crisp_Query.Generate_Screen

- **Project Title: TREATMENT OF COCAINE-INDUCED 5-HT DYSFUNCTION**

Principal Investigator & Institution: Van De Kar, Louis D.; Professor; Pharmacol & Exper Therapeutics; Loyola University Chicago Lewis Towers, 13Th Fl Chicago, Il 60611

Timing: Fiscal Year 2002; Project Start 01-FEB-2001; Project End 31-JAN-2006

Summary: The long term objective of this program is to find novel treatments for the mood disorders associated with **cocaine** withdrawal. A major problem with **cocaine** abuse is the return to **cocaine** use after a period of abstinence (relapse). contributing factor to **cocaine** relapse is withdrawal-induced anxiety and depression which stimulate re-administration as form of self-medication. Withdrawal from **cocaine** results in supersensitivity of serotonin-2A (5-HT2A) receptors. 5-HT2A receptor supersensitivity is associated with depression and anxiety. Therefore, treating 5-HT2A receptor supersensitivity may alleviate the anxiety and depression that contribute to **cocaine** relapse. However, to date, no studies have investigated the mechanisms responsible for cocaine-induced 5-HT2A receptor supersensitivity. The proposed studies will investigate the mechanisms through which withdrawal from **cocaine** induces supersensitivity of 5-HT2A receptor-mediated secretion of hormones. In addition, two potential therapeutic approaches will be tested to reverse the supersensitivity of post-synaptic 5-HT2A receptors during **cocaine** withdrawal. Our hypothesis is that the cocaine-induced changes in sensitivity of 5-HT2A receptors are due to changes in specific components of the intracellular signaling cascade. The proposed studies will investigate signaling mechanisms underlying the supersensitivity of 5-HT2A receptor systems in the hypothalamic paraventricular nucleus after withdrawal from **cocaine** and their response to treatment. Aim 1 will determine the minimum number of **cocaine** injection days that will produce supersensitivity of 5-HT2A receptor signaling. One of the characteristics of drug dependence is that a drug must be administered repeatedly before withdrawal effects appear. Aim 2 will determine the onset of supersensitivity of 5-HT2A receptors after exposure to **cocaine** and to determine whether these effects are irreversible. This study also will establish the treatment parameters to be used in aims 3-4. The **cocaine** withdrawal effect may be a compensatory supersensitivity of 5-HT2A receptors due to reduced 5-HT release. Thus, Aim 3 will determine how the **cocaine** withdrawal effects on 5-HT2A receptors can be reversed by increasing the levels of 5-HT in the synapse with selective monoamine oxidase-A (MAO-A) inhibitors. Aim 4 will determine how the **cocaine** withdrawal effects on 5-HT2A receptors can be reversed by 5-HT2A antagonists. Our results from these studies on the treatment with selective 5-HT2A antagonists and MAO-A inhibitors may lead to novel therapeutic approaches to reverse the supersensitivity of 5-HT2A receptors and hence treat mood disorders associated with **cocaine** withdrawal and relapse.

Website: http://crisp.cit.nih.gov/crisp/Crisp_Query.Generate_Screen

- **Project Title: TREATMENT OF DRUG DEPENDENCE AND PSYCHIATRIC ILLNESS**

Principal Investigator & Institution: Weiss, Roger D.; Professor of Psychiatry and Clinical Dir; Mc Lean Hospital (Belmont, Ma) Belmont, Ma 02478

Timing: Fiscal Year 2002; Project Start 20-JUL-2002; Project End 31-MAR-2007

Summary: (provided by the applicant) The primary aim of this K02 competing renewal application is to further the applicant?s scientific development in the area of treatment of drug dependent patients, particularly those who are "dually diagnosed" with drug abuse and coexisting psychiatric illness. Two major hypotheses guide the applicant?s current and planned research. The first is that since drug dependent and dually diagnosed patients are a heterogeneous group, identifying meaningful subgroups of patients and targeting specific therapies to these subgroups will improve treatment outcome. The second major hypothesis is that studying the integration of different treatment approaches (e.g., the combination of pharmacotherapy and psychotherapy) can lead to improved treatment for drug dependent patients. This application is designed to strengthen the applicant?s involvement in five funded projects as PI or Co-Investigator. The following funded projects are currently being pursued by the applicant: 1) a NIDA Behavioral Therapies Development Project to compare two different forms of group therapy for patients with bipolar disorder and substance dependence (DA09400, PI); 2) a multi-site randomized controlled trial evaluating combinations of pharmacotherapy and behavioral therapies in the treatment of alcohol dependence (AA11756, Site PI); 3) a multi-site study examining the genetics of **cocaine** dependence (DA12849, Site PI); 4) a NIDA-funded project examining the potential efficacy of CDP-choline in the treatment of **cocaine** dependence (DA11098, Co-Investigator); and 5) a multicenter NIMH-funded project to examine optimal treatments for individuals with bipolar disorder, for which the applicant will examine treatments for those patients with coexisting substance use disorder (MH80001, Substance Abuse Pathway Leader and Co-Investigator). The applicant proposes to expand his research capabilities by learning more about genetics and statistical methods through guided tutorials. Finally, the applicant will mentor younger investigators in their drug abuse research careers and serve the field in general through work as a reviewer on the NIDA Treatment Research IRG and participation in national organizations and editorial boards of addiction journals.

Website: http://crisp.cit.nih.gov/crisp/Crisp_Query.Generate_Screen

- **Project Title: VIRTUALITY REALITY CUE EXPOSURE FOR CRACK COCAINE**

Principal Investigator & Institution: Rothbaum, Barbara O.;; Virtually Better, Inc. 2450 Lawrenceville Hwy, Ste 101 Decatur, Ga 300333226

Timing: Fiscal Year 2003; Project Start 01-JUL-2003; Project End 30-JUN-2004

Summary: (provided by applicant): Virtual reality (VR) integrates real-time computer graphics and body tracking devices to immerse a participant in a computer-generated virtual environment. VR exposure therapy has been successful in the treatment of anxiety disorders. This Phase I STTR project applies VR to the treatment of substance use disorders (SUDs). The economic, social, physical, and psychological impact of SUDs is devastating. Treatments of most SUDs are promising, although the success rate with crack **cocaine** users is not encouraging. In the largest study of psychosocial treatments of **cocaine** dependence, 50 percent of participants were still using **cocaine** at the 6-month assessment. Drug craving is important in perpetuating drug dependence and is associated with relapse. Environmental cues previously associated with crack **cocaine** use have consistently induced craving in human laboratory research, often called cue reactivity studies. The ability of these environmental cues to precipitate craving and physiologic activity in drug dependent individuals is thought to be a result of classical conditioning in which drug related stimuli, through repeated pairing with drug use, acquire the ability to elicit specific drug related responses. It follows, then, that repeatedly presenting drug related environmental cues not followed by drug should lead to a reduction in the reactivity through the process of extinction. Although it is clear that craving is likely to be a classically conditioned phenomenon that is related to relapse, limitations of the cue reactivity laboratory procedures currently in use may restrict the therapeutic utility of these approaches. Therefore, we propose to develop a new medium for providing cue exposure treatment for crack **cocaine** dependence. We propose to construct a virtual crack house with four virtual environments (rooms) designed to elicit crack **cocaine** craving to be used in cue exposure procedures. The specific aims of the proposed project include: 1) The development of virtual environments to support cue exposure therapy for crack **cocaine** dependence; and 2) The preliminary testing of the **cocaine** virtual environments developed compared to neutral environments as to their ability to elicit craving in crack **cocaine** users in an open clinical design with 10 crack **cocaine** dependent participants. The long-term objectives to be achieved in Phase II include the development and testing of the treatment of crack **cocaine** dependence using VR cue exposure therapy in a controlled design.

Website: http://crisp.cit.nih.gov/crisp/Crisp_Query.Generate_Screen

E-Journals: PubMed Central[19]

PubMed Central (PMC) is a digital archive of life sciences journal literature developed and managed by the National Center for Biotechnology Information (NCBI) at the U.S. National Library of Medicine (NLM).[20] Access to this growing archive of e-journals is free and unrestricted.[21] To search, go to **http://www.pubmedcentral.nih.gov/index.html#search**, and type "cocaine dependence" (or synonyms) into the search box. This search gives you access to full-text articles. The following is a sample of items found for cocaine dependence in the PubMed Central database:

- **Acetylcholine enhancement in the nucleus accumbens prevents addictive behaviors of cocaine and morphine.** by Hikida T, Kitabatake Y, Pastan I, Nakanishi S.; 2003 May 13; http://www.pubmedcentral.gov/articlerender.fcgi?tool=pmcentrez&artid=156344

- **Heroin and cocaine co-use in a group of injection drug users in Montreal.** by Leri F, Stewart J, Tremblay A, Bruneau J.; 2004 Jan; http://www.pubmedcentral.gov/articlerender.fcgi?tool=pmcentrez&artid=305269

- **Molecular mechanisms of cocaine reward: Combined dopamine and serotonin transporter knockouts eliminate cocaine place preference.** by Sora I, Hall FS, Andrews AM, Itokawa M, Li XF, Wei HB, Wichems C, Lesch KP, Murphy DL, Uhl GR.; 2001 Apr 24; http://www.pubmedcentral.gov/articlerender.fcgi?tool=pmcentrez&artid=33204

The National Library of Medicine: PubMed

One of the quickest and most comprehensive ways to find academic studies in both English and other languages is to use PubMed, maintained by the National Library of Medicine. The advantage of PubMed over previously mentioned sources is that it covers a greater number of domestic and foreign

---

[19] Adapted from the National Library of Medicine: **http://www.pubmedcentral.nih.gov/about/intro.html**.

[20] With PubMed Central, NCBI is taking the lead in preservation and maintenance of open access to electronic literature, just as NLM has done for decades with printed biomedical literature. PubMed Central aims to become a world-class library of the digital age.

[21] The value of PubMed Central, in addition to its role as an archive, lies the availability of data from diverse sources stored in a common format in a single repository. Many journals already have online publishing operations, and there is a growing tendency to publish material online only, to the exclusion of print.

references. It is also free to the public.[22] If the publisher has a Web site that offers full text of its journals, PubMed will provide links to that site, as well as to sites offering other related data. User registration, a subscription fee, or some other type of fee may be required to access the full text of articles in some journals.

To generate your own bibliography of studies dealing with cocaine dependence, simply go to the PubMed Web site at **www.ncbi.nlm.nih.gov/pubmed**. Type "cocaine dependence" (or synonyms) into the search box, and click "Go." The following is the type of output you can expect from PubMed for "cocaine dependence" (hyperlinks lead to article summaries):

- **A comparison of contingency management and cognitive-behavioral approaches during methadone maintenance treatment for cocaine dependence.**
  Author(s): Rawson RA, Huber A, McCann M, Shoptaw S, Farabee D, Reiber C, Ling W.
  Source: Archives of General Psychiatry. 2002 September; 59(9): 817-24.
  http://www.ncbi.nlm.nih.gov/entrez/query.fcgi?cmd=Retrieve&db=pubmed&dopt=Abstract&list_uids=12215081

- **A controlled trial of fluoxetine in crack cocaine dependence.**
  Author(s): Batki SL, Washburn AM, Delucchi K, Jones RT.
  Source: Drug and Alcohol Dependence. 1996 June; 41(2): 137-42.
  http://www.ncbi.nlm.nih.gov/entrez/query.fcgi?cmd=Retrieve&db=pubmed&dopt=Abstract&list_uids=8809502

- **A double-blind, placebo-controlled outpatient trial of pergolide for cocaine dependence.**
  Author(s): Malcolm R, Kajdasz DK, Herron J, Anton RF, Brady KT.
  Source: Drug and Alcohol Dependence. 2000 August 1; 60(2): 161-8.
  http://www.ncbi.nlm.nih.gov/entrez/query.fcgi?cmd=Retrieve&db=pubmed&dopt=Abstract&list_uids=10940543

---

[22] PubMed was developed by the National Center for Biotechnology Information (NCBI) at the National Library of Medicine (NLM) at the National Institutes of Health (NIH). The PubMed database was developed in conjunction with publishers of biomedical literature as a search tool for accessing literature citations and linking to full-text journal articles at Web sites of participating publishers. Publishers that participate in PubMed supply NLM with their citations electronically prior to or at the time of publication.

- **A historically controlled trial of tyrosine for cocaine dependence.**
  Author(s): Galloway GP, Frederick SL, Thomas S, Hayner G, Staggers FE, Wiehl WO, Sajo E, Amodia D, Stewart P.
  Source: J Psychoactive Drugs. 1996 July-September; 28(3): 305-9.
  http://www.ncbi.nlm.nih.gov/entrez/query.fcgi?cmd=Retrieve&db=pubmed&dopt=Abstract&list_uids=8895116

- **A laboratory procedure for evaluation of pharmacotherapy for cocaine dependence.**
  Author(s): Kranzler H, Bauer L.
  Source: Nida Res Monogr. 1989; 95: 324-5. No Abstract Available.
  http://www.ncbi.nlm.nih.gov/entrez/query.fcgi?cmd=Retrieve&db=pubmed&dopt=Abstract&list_uids=2640979

- **A model for pharmacological research-treatment of cocaine dependence.**
  Author(s): Montoya ID, Hess JM, Preston KL, Gorelick DA.
  Source: Journal of Substance Abuse Treatment. 1995 November-December; 12(6): 415-21. Review.
  http://www.ncbi.nlm.nih.gov/entrez/query.fcgi?cmd=Retrieve&db=pubmed&dopt=Abstract&list_uids=8749725

- **A multicenter trial of bupropion for cocaine dependence in methadone-maintained patients.**
  Author(s): Margolin A, Kosten TR, Avants SK, Wilkins J, Ling W, Beckson M, Arndt IO, Cornish J, Ascher JA, Li SH, et al.
  Source: Drug and Alcohol Dependence. 1995 December; 40(2): 125-31.
  http://www.ncbi.nlm.nih.gov/entrez/query.fcgi?cmd=Retrieve&db=pubmed&dopt=Abstract&list_uids=8745134

- **A national 5-year follow-up of treatment outcomes for cocaine dependence.**
  Author(s): Simpson DD, Joe GW, Broome KM.
  Source: Archives of General Psychiatry. 2002 June; 59(6): 538-44.
  http://www.ncbi.nlm.nih.gov/entrez/query.fcgi?cmd=Retrieve&db=pubmed&dopt=Abstract&list_uids=12044196

- **A national evaluation of treatment outcomes for cocaine dependence.**
  Author(s): Simpson DD, Joe GW, Fletcher BW, Hubbard RL, Anglin MD.
  Source: Archives of General Psychiatry. 1999 June; 56(6): 507-14.
  http://www.ncbi.nlm.nih.gov/entrez/query.fcgi?cmd=Retrieve&db=pubmed&dopt=Abstract&list_uids=10359464

- **A pilot trial of amantadine for ambulatory withdrawal for cocaine dependence.**
  Author(s): Morgan C, Kosten T, Gawin F, Kleber H.
  Source: Nida Res Monogr. 1988; 81: 81-5. No Abstract Available.
  http://www.ncbi.nlm.nih.gov/entrez/query.fcgi?cmd=Retrieve&db=pu
  bmed&dopt=Abstract&list_uids=3136395

- **A pilot trial of olanzapine for the treatment of cocaine dependence.**
  Author(s): Kampman KM, Pettinati H, Lynch KG, Sparkman T, O'Brien CP.
  Source: Drug and Alcohol Dependence. 2003 June 5; 70(3): 265-73.
  http://www.ncbi.nlm.nih.gov/entrez/query.fcgi?cmd=Retrieve&db=pu
  bmed&dopt=Abstract&list_uids=12757964

- **A pilot trial of piracetam and ginkgo biloba for the treatment of cocaine dependence.**
  Author(s): Kampman K, Majewska MD, Tourian K, Dackis C, Cornish J, Poole S, O'Brien C.
  Source: Addictive Behaviors. 2003 April; 28(3): 437-48.
  http://www.ncbi.nlm.nih.gov/entrez/query.fcgi?cmd=Retrieve&db=pu
  bmed&dopt=Abstract&list_uids=12628617

- **A quasi-experimental comparison of the effectiveness of 6- versus 12-hour per week outpatient treatments for cocaine dependence.**
  Author(s): Alterman AI, Snider EC, Cacciola JS, May DJ, Parikh G, Maany I, Rosenbaum PR.
  Source: The Journal of Nervous and Mental Disease. 1996 January; 184(1): 54-6.
  http://www.ncbi.nlm.nih.gov/entrez/query.fcgi?cmd=Retrieve&db=pu
  bmed&dopt=Abstract&list_uids=8551291

- **A randomized controlled study of the effectiveness of intensive outpatient treatment for cocaine dependence.**
  Author(s): Gottheil E, Weinstein SP, Sterling RC, Lundy A, Serota RD.
  Source: Psychiatric Services (Washington, D.C.). 1998 June; 49(6): 782-7.
  http://www.ncbi.nlm.nih.gov/entrez/query.fcgi?cmd=Retrieve&db=pu
  bmed&dopt=Abstract&list_uids=9634157

- **A randomized controlled trial of auricular acupuncture for cocaine dependence.**
  Author(s): Avants SK, Margolin A, Holford TR, Kosten TR.
  Source: Archives of Internal Medicine. 2000 August 14-28; 160(15): 2305-12.
  http://www.ncbi.nlm.nih.gov/entrez/query.fcgi?cmd=Retrieve&db=pubmed&dopt=Abstract&list_uids=10927727

- **A randomized controlled trial of auricular acupuncture for cocaine dependence: treatments vs outcomes.**
  Author(s): Giglio JC.
  Source: Archives of Internal Medicine. 2001 March 26; 161(6): 894-5; Author Reply 895.
  http://www.ncbi.nlm.nih.gov/entrez/query.fcgi?cmd=Retrieve&db=pubmed&dopt=Abstract&list_uids=11268238

- **A randomized, double-blind, placebo-controlled study of ritanserin pharmacotherapy for cocaine dependence.**
  Author(s): Cornish JW, Maany I, Fudala PJ, Ehrman RN, Robbins SJ, O'Brien CP.
  Source: Drug and Alcohol Dependence. 2001 January 1; 61(2): 183-9.
  http://www.ncbi.nlm.nih.gov/entrez/query.fcgi?cmd=Retrieve&db=pubmed&dopt=Abstract&list_uids=11137283

- **A screening trial of amantadine as a medication for cocaine dependence.**
  Author(s): Shoptaw S, Kintaudi PC, Charuvastra C, Ling W.
  Source: Drug and Alcohol Dependence. 2002 May 1; 66(3): 217-24.
  http://www.ncbi.nlm.nih.gov/entrez/query.fcgi?cmd=Retrieve&db=pubmed&dopt=Abstract&list_uids=12062456

- **A two-rate hypothesis for patterns of retention in psychosocial treatments of cocaine dependence: findings from a study of African-American men and a review of the published data.**
  Author(s): Pena JM, Franklin RR, Rice JC, Foulks EF, Bland IJ, Shervington D, James A.
  Source: The American Journal on Addictions / American Academy of Psychiatrists in Alcoholism and Addictions. 1999 Fall; 8(4): 319-31. Review.
  http://www.ncbi.nlm.nih.gov/entrez/query.fcgi?cmd=Retrieve&db=pubmed&dopt=Abstract&list_uids=10598215

- **Acute dually diagnosed inpatients: the use of self-report symptom severity instruments in persons with depressive disorders and cocaine dependence.**
  Author(s): Kush FR, Sowers W.
  Source: Journal of Substance Abuse Treatment. 1997 January-February; 14(1): 61-6.
  http://www.ncbi.nlm.nih.gov/entrez/query.fcgi?cmd=Retrieve&db=pubmed&dopt=Abstract&list_uids=9218238

- **Adverse outcomes in a controlled trial of pergolide for cocaine dependence.**
  Author(s): Malcolm R, Herron J, Sutherland SE, Brady KT.
  Source: Journal of Addictive Diseases : the Official Journal of the Asam, American Society of Addiction Medicine. 2001; 20(1): 81-92.
  http://www.ncbi.nlm.nih.gov/entrez/query.fcgi?cmd=Retrieve&db=pubmed&dopt=Abstract&list_uids=11286433

- **Agonist-like or antagonist-like treatment for cocaine dependence with methadone for heroin dependence: two double-blind randomized clinical trials.**
  Author(s): Grabowski J, Rhoades H, Stotts A, Cowan K, Kopecky C, Dougherty A, Moeller FG, Hassan S, Schmitz J.
  Source: Neuropsychopharmacology : Official Publication of the American College of Neuropsychopharmacology. 2004 May; 29(5): 969-81.
  http://www.ncbi.nlm.nih.gov/entrez/query.fcgi?cmd=Retrieve&db=pubmed&dopt=Abstract&list_uids=15039761

- **Allelic association of the D2 dopamine receptor gene with cocaine dependence.**
  Author(s): Noble EP, Blum K, Khalsa ME, Ritchie T, Montgomery A, Wood RC, Fitch RJ, Ozkaragoz T, Sheridan PJ, Anglin MD, et al.
  Source: Drug and Alcohol Dependence. 1993 October; 33(3): 271-85. Erratum In: Drug Alcohol Depend 1993 December; 34(1): 83-4.
  http://www.ncbi.nlm.nih.gov/entrez/query.fcgi?cmd=Retrieve&db=pubmed&dopt=Abstract&list_uids=8261891

- **Amantadine for treatment of cocaine dependence in methadone-maintained patients.**
  Author(s): Handelsman L, Chordia PL, Escovar IL, Marion IJ, Lowinson JH.
  Source: The American Journal of Psychiatry. 1988 April; 145(4): 533.
  http://www.ncbi.nlm.nih.gov/entrez/query.fcgi?cmd=Retrieve&db=pubmed&dopt=Abstract&list_uids=3348463

- **Amantadine in the early treatment of cocaine dependence: a double-blind, placebo-controlled trial.**
  Author(s): Kampman K, Volpicelli JR, Alterman A, Cornish J, Weinrieb R, Epperson L, Sparkman T, O'Brien CP.
  Source: Drug and Alcohol Dependence. 1996 May; 41(1): 25-33.
  http://www.ncbi.nlm.nih.gov/entrez/query.fcgi?cmd=Retrieve&db=pubmed&dopt=Abstract&list_uids=8793307

- **Amlodipine treatment of cocaine dependence.**
  Author(s): Malcolm R, Brady KT, Moore J, Kajdasz D.
  Source: J Psychoactive Drugs. 1999 April-June; 31(2): 117-20.
  http://www.ncbi.nlm.nih.gov/entrez/query.fcgi?cmd=Retrieve&db=pubmed&dopt=Abstract&list_uids=10437993

- **An extreme case of cocaine dependence and marked improvement with methylphenidate treatment.**
  Author(s): Khantzian EJ.
  Source: The American Journal of Psychiatry. 1983 June; 140(6): 784-5.
  http://www.ncbi.nlm.nih.gov/entrez/query.fcgi?cmd=Retrieve&db=pubmed&dopt=Abstract&list_uids=6846640

- **Anger management group treatment for cocaine dependence: preliminary outcomes.**
  Author(s): Reilly PM, Shopshire MS.
  Source: The American Journal of Drug and Alcohol Abuse. 2000 May; 26(2): 161-77.
  http://www.ncbi.nlm.nih.gov/entrez/query.fcgi?cmd=Retrieve&db=pubmed&dopt=Abstract&list_uids=10852354

- **Antidepressants for cocaine dependence.**
  Author(s): Lima MS, Reisser AA, Soares BG, Farrell M.
  Source: Cochrane Database Syst Rev. 2003; (2): Cd002950. Review.
  http://www.ncbi.nlm.nih.gov/entrez/query.fcgi?cmd=Retrieve&db=pubmed&dopt=Abstract&list_uids=12804445

- **Antidepressants for cocaine dependence.**
  Author(s): Cochrane Database Syst Rev. 2003;(2):CD003352
  Source: Cochrane Database Syst Rev. 2001; (4): Cd002950. Review. Update In:
  http://www.ncbi.nlm.nih.gov/entrez/query.fcgi?cmd=Retrieve&db=pubmed&dopt=Abstract&list_uids=12804461

- **Antisocial personality disorder and cocaine dependence: their effects on behavioral and electroencephalographic measures of time estimation.**
  Author(s): Bauer LO.
  Source: Drug and Alcohol Dependence. 2001 June 1; 63(1): 87-95.
  http://www.ncbi.nlm.nih.gov/entrez/query.fcgi?cmd=Retrieve&db=pubmed&dopt=Abstract&list_uids=11297834

- **Antisocial personality disorder as a prognostic factor for pharmacotherapy of cocaine dependence.**
  Author(s): Leal J, Ziedonis D, Kosten T.
  Source: Drug and Alcohol Dependence. 1994 March; 35(1): 31-5.
  http://www.ncbi.nlm.nih.gov/entrez/query.fcgi?cmd=Retrieve&db=pubmed&dopt=Abstract&list_uids=8082553

- **Apathy syndrome in cocaine dependence.**
  Author(s): Kalechstein AD, Newton TF, Leavengood AH.
  Source: Psychiatry Research. 2002 January 31; 109(1): 97-100.
  http://www.ncbi.nlm.nih.gov/entrez/query.fcgi?cmd=Retrieve&db=pubmed&dopt=Abstract&list_uids=11850056

- **Applying behavioral concepts and principles to the treatment of cocaine dependence.**
  Author(s): Higgins ST, Budney AJ, Bickel WK.
  Source: Drug and Alcohol Dependence. 1994 January; 34(2): 87-97. Review.
  http://www.ncbi.nlm.nih.gov/entrez/query.fcgi?cmd=Retrieve&db=pubmed&dopt=Abstract&list_uids=8026305

- **Are neuroadaptations in D3 dopamine receptors linked to the development of cocaine dependence?**
  Author(s): Mash DC.
  Source: Molecular Psychiatry. 1997 January; 2(1): 7-8.
  http://www.ncbi.nlm.nih.gov/entrez/query.fcgi?cmd=Retrieve&db=pubmed&dopt=Abstract&list_uids=9154209

- **Aspirin or amiloride for cerebral perfusion defects in cocaine dependence.**
  Author(s): Kosten TR, Gottschalk PC, Tucker K, Rinder CS, Dey HM, Rinder HM.
  Source: Drug and Alcohol Dependence. 2003 August 20; 71(2): 187-94.
  http://www.ncbi.nlm.nih.gov/entrez/query.fcgi?cmd=Retrieve&db=pubmed&dopt=Abstract&list_uids=12927657

- **Baseline prediction of 7-month cocaine abstinence for cocaine dependence patients.**
  Author(s): Alterman AI, McKay JR, Mulvaney FD, Cnaan A, Cacciola JS, Tourian KA, Rutherford MJ, Merikle EP.
  Source: Drug and Alcohol Dependence. 2000 June 1; 59(3): 215-21.
  http://www.ncbi.nlm.nih.gov/entrez/query.fcgi?cmd=Retrieve&db=pubmed&dopt=Abstract&list_uids=10812282

- **Behavioral treatments of cocaine dependence.**
  Author(s): Grabowski J, Higgins ST, Kirby KC.
  Source: Nida Res Monogr. 1993; 135: 133-49. Review. No Abstract Available.
  http://www.ncbi.nlm.nih.gov/entrez/query.fcgi?cmd=Retrieve&db=pubmed&dopt=Abstract&list_uids=8289893

- **Bromocriptine for cocaine dependence. A controlled clinical trial.**
  Author(s): Handelsman L, Rosenblum A, Palij M, Magura S, Foote J, Lovejoy M, Stimmel B.
  Source: The American Journal on Addictions / American Academy of Psychiatrists in Alcoholism and Addictions. 1997 Winter; 6(1): 54-64.
  http://www.ncbi.nlm.nih.gov/entrez/query.fcgi?cmd=Retrieve&db=pubmed&dopt=Abstract&list_uids=9097872

- **Buprenorphine treatment for concurrent heroin and cocaine dependence: phase I study.**
  Author(s): Mendelson JH, Mello NK, Teoh SK, Kuehnle J, Sintavanarong P, Dooley-Coufos K.
  Source: Nida Res Monogr. 1991; 105: 196-202. No Abstract Available.
  http://www.ncbi.nlm.nih.gov/entrez/query.fcgi?cmd=Retrieve&db=pubmed&dopt=Abstract&list_uids=1875999

- **Cannabis diagnosis of patients receiving treatment for cocaine dependence.**
  Author(s): Miller NS, Klahr AL, Gold MS, Sweeney K, Cocores JA, Sweeney DR.
  Source: Journal of Substance Abuse. 1990; 2(1): 107-11.
  http://www.ncbi.nlm.nih.gov/entrez/query.fcgi?cmd=Retrieve&db=pubmed&dopt=Abstract&list_uids=2136098

- **Carbamazepine for cocaine dependence.**
  Author(s): Lima AR, Lima MS, Soares BG, Farrell M.
  Source: Cochrane Database Syst Rev. 2002; (2): Cd002023. Review.
  http://www.ncbi.nlm.nih.gov/entrez/query.fcgi?cmd=Retrieve&db=pubmed&dopt=Abstract&list_uids=12076433

- **Carbamazepine for cocaine dependence.**
  Author(s): Cochrane Database Syst Rev. 2003;(2):CD002950
  Source: Cochrane Database Syst Rev. 2001; (4): Cd002023. Review. Update In:
  http://www.ncbi.nlm.nih.gov/entrez/query.fcgi?cmd=Retrieve&db=pubmed&dopt=Abstract&list_uids=12804445

- **Carbamazepine for cocaine dependence.**
  Author(s): Lima AR, Lima MS, Soares BG, Churchill R, Farrell M.
  Source: Cochrane Database Syst Rev. 2000; (2): Cd002023. Review. Update In:
  http://www.ncbi.nlm.nih.gov/entrez/query.fcgi?cmd=Retrieve&db=pubmed&dopt=Abstract&list_uids=10796844

- **Carbamazepine in the treatment of cocaine dependence: subtyping by affective disorder.**
  Author(s): Brady KT, Sonne SC, Malcolm RJ, Randall CL, Dansky BS, Simpson K, Roberts JS, Brondino M.
  Source: Experimental and Clinical Psychopharmacology. 2002 August; 10(3): 276-85.
  http://www.ncbi.nlm.nih.gov/entrez/query.fcgi?cmd=Retrieve&db=pubmed&dopt=Abstract&list_uids=12233988

- **Carbamazepine treatment for cocaine dependence.**
  Author(s): Cornish JW, Maany I, Fudala PJ, Neal S, Poole SA, Volpicelli P, O'Brien CP.
  Source: Drug and Alcohol Dependence. 1995 June; 38(3): 221-7.
  http://www.ncbi.nlm.nih.gov/entrez/query.fcgi?cmd=Retrieve&db=pubmed&dopt=Abstract&list_uids=7555622

- **Carbamazepine treatment of cocaine dependence in methadone maintenance patients with dual opiate-cocaine addiction.**
  Author(s): Kuhn KL, Halikas JA, Kemp KD.
  Source: Nida Res Monogr. 1989; 95: 316-7.
  http://www.ncbi.nlm.nih.gov/entrez/query.fcgi?cmd=Retrieve&db=pubmed&dopt=Abstract&list_uids=2640978

- **Carbamazepine treatment of cocaine dependence: a placebo-controlled trial.**
  Author(s): Kranzler HR, Bauer LO, Hersh D, Klinghoffer V.
  Source: Drug and Alcohol Dependence. 1995 June; 38(3): 203-11.
  http://www.ncbi.nlm.nih.gov/entrez/query.fcgi?cmd=Retrieve&db=pubmed&dopt=Abstract&list_uids=7555620

- **Cautionary note on methylphenidate for cocaine dependence.**
  Author(s): Crowley TJ.
  Source: The American Journal of Psychiatry. 1984 February; 141(2): 327-8.
  http://www.ncbi.nlm.nih.gov/entrez/query.fcgi?cmd=Retrieve&db=pubmed&dopt=Abstract&list_uids=6691513

- **Changes in brain glucose metabolism in cocaine dependence and withdrawal.**
  Author(s): Volkow ND, Fowler JS, Wolf AP, Hitzemann R, Dewey S, Bendriem B, Alpert R, Hoff A.
  Source: The American Journal of Psychiatry. 1991 May; 148(5): 621-6.
  http://www.ncbi.nlm.nih.gov/entrez/query.fcgi?cmd=Retrieve&db=pubmed&dopt=Abstract&list_uids=2018164

- **Chemical aversion therapy in the treatment of cocaine dependence as part of a multimodal treatment program: treatment outcome.**
  Author(s): Frawley PJ, Smith JW.
  Source: Journal of Substance Abuse Treatment. 1990; 7(1): 21-9.
  http://www.ncbi.nlm.nih.gov/entrez/query.fcgi?cmd=Retrieve&db=pubmed&dopt=Abstract&list_uids=2313768

- **Choreoathetoid movements in cocaine dependence.**
  Author(s): Bartzokis G, Beckson M, Wirshing DA, Lu PH, Foster JA, Mintz J.
  Source: Biological Psychiatry. 1999 June 15; 45(12): 1630-5.
  http://www.ncbi.nlm.nih.gov/entrez/query.fcgi?cmd=Retrieve&db=pubmed&dopt=Abstract&list_uids=10376125

- **Classically conditioned responses in opioid and cocaine dependence: a role in relapse?**
  Author(s): Childress AR, McLellan AT, Ehrman R, O'Brien CP.
  Source: Nida Res Monogr. 1988; 84: 25-43.
  http://www.ncbi.nlm.nih.gov/entrez/query.fcgi?cmd=Retrieve&db=pubmed&dopt=Abstract&list_uids=3147384

- **Clinical outcomes following cocaine infusion in nontreatment-seeking individuals with cocaine dependence.**
  Author(s): Elman I, Krause S, Karlsgodt K, Schoenfeld DA, Gollub RL, Breiter HC, Gastfriend DR.
  Source: Biological Psychiatry. 2001 March 15; 49(6): 553-5.
  http://www.ncbi.nlm.nih.gov/entrez/query.fcgi?cmd=Retrieve&db=pubmed&dopt=Abstract&list_uids=11257241

- **Clinical trail of multiple treatment agents for cocaine dependence: a placebo-control; elimination study.**
  Author(s): Tennant F.
  Source: Nida Res Monogr. 1991; 105: 512-3. No Abstract Available.
  http://www.ncbi.nlm.nih.gov/entrez/query.fcgi?cmd=Retrieve&db=pubmed&dopt=Abstract&list_uids=1876104

- **Cocaine dependence treatment on an inpatient detoxification unit.**
  Author(s): Wallace BC.
  Source: Journal of Substance Abuse Treatment. 1987; 4(2): 85-92.
  http://www.ncbi.nlm.nih.gov/entrez/query.fcgi?cmd=Retrieve&db=pubmed&dopt=Abstract&list_uids=3041012

- **Cocaine dependence with and without comorbid depression: a comparison of patient characteristics.**
  Author(s): Schmitz JM, Stotts AL, Averill PM, Rothfleisch JM, Bailley SE, Sayre SL, Grabowski J.
  Source: Drug and Alcohol Dependence. 2000 August 1; 60(2): 189-98.
  http://www.ncbi.nlm.nih.gov/entrez/query.fcgi?cmd=Retrieve&db=pubmed&dopt=Abstract&list_uids=10940546

- **Cocaine dependence with and without post-traumatic stress disorder: a comparison of substance use, trauma history and psychiatric comorbidity.**
  Author(s): Back S, Dansky BS, Coffey SF, Saladin ME, Sonne S, Brady KT.
  Source: The American Journal on Addictions / American Academy of Psychiatrists in Alcoholism and Addictions. 2000 Winter; 9(1): 51-62.
  http://www.ncbi.nlm.nih.gov/entrez/query.fcgi?cmd=Retrieve&db=pubmed&dopt=Abstract&list_uids=10914293

- **Cocaine dependence with and without PTSD among subjects in the National Institute on Drug Abuse Collaborative Cocaine Treatment Study.**
  Author(s): Najavits LM, Gastfriend DR, Barber JP, Reif S, Muenz LR, Blaine J, Frank A, Crits-Christoph P, Thase M, Weiss RD.
  Source: The American Journal of Psychiatry. 1998 February; 155(2): 214-9.
  http://www.ncbi.nlm.nih.gov/entrez/query.fcgi?cmd=Retrieve&db=pubmed&dopt=Abstract&list_uids=9464200

- **Cocaine dependence.**
  Author(s): Gawin FH, Ellinwood EH Jr.
  Source: Annual Review of Medicine. 1989; 40: 149-61. Review.
  http://www.ncbi.nlm.nih.gov/entrez/query.fcgi?cmd=Retrieve&db=pubmed&dopt=Abstract&list_uids=2658744

- **Cocaine dependence. A clinical syndrome requiring neuroprotection.**
  Author(s): Herning RI, King DE, Better W, Cadet JL.
  Source: Annals of the New York Academy of Sciences. 1997 October 15; 825: 323-7.
  http://www.ncbi.nlm.nih.gov/entrez/query.fcgi?cmd=Retrieve&db=pubmed&dopt=Abstract&list_uids=9369997

- **Cocaine dependence: a disease of the brain's reward centers.**
  Author(s): Dackis CA, O'Brien CP.
  Source: Journal of Substance Abuse Treatment. 2001 October; 21(3): 111-7. Review.
  http://www.ncbi.nlm.nih.gov/entrez/query.fcgi?cmd=Retrieve&db=pubmed&dopt=Abstract&list_uids=11728784

- **Cocaine dependence: alcohol and other drug dependence and withdrawal characteristics.**
  Author(s): Miller NS, Summers GL, Gold MS.
  Source: Journal of Addictive Diseases : the Official Journal of the Asam, American Society of Addiction Medicine. 1993; 12(1): 25-35.
  http://www.ncbi.nlm.nih.gov/entrez/query.fcgi?cmd=Retrieve&db=pubmed&dopt=Abstract&list_uids=8381028

- **Cocaine withdrawal severity and urine toxicology results from treatment entry predict outcome in medication trials for cocaine dependence.**
  Author(s): Kampman KM, Volpicelli JR, Mulvaney F, Rukstalis M, Alterman AI, Pettinati H, Weinrieb RM, O'Brien CP.
  Source: Addictive Behaviors. 2002 March-April; 27(2): 251-60.
  http://www.ncbi.nlm.nih.gov/entrez/query.fcgi?cmd=Retrieve&db=pubmed&dopt=Abstract&list_uids=11817766

- **Cocaine withdrawal symptoms and initial urine toxicology results predict treatment attrition in outpatient cocaine dependence treatment.**
  Author(s): Kampman KM, Alterman AI, Volpicelli JR, Maany I, Muller ES, Luce DD, Mulholland EM, Jawad AF, Parikh GA, Mulvaney FD, Weinrieb RM, O'Brien CP.
  Source: Psychology of Addictive Behaviors : Journal of the Society of Psychologists in Addictive Behaviors. 2001 March; 15(1): 52-9.
  http://www.ncbi.nlm.nih.gov/entrez/query.fcgi?cmd=Retrieve&db=pubmed&dopt=Abstract&list_uids=11255939

- **Cocaine-primed craving and its relationship to depressive symptomatology in individuals with cocaine dependence.**
  Author(s): Elman I, Karlsgodt KH, Gastfriend DR, Chabris CF, Breiter HC.
  Source: Journal of Psychopharmacology (Oxford, England). 2002 June; 16(2): 163-7.
  http://www.ncbi.nlm.nih.gov/entrez/query.fcgi?cmd=Retrieve&db=pubmed&dopt=Abstract&list_uids=12095075

- **Combination of the dopaminergic agent, phentermine, and the serotonergic agent, fenfluramine, in the treatment of cocaine dependence.**
  Author(s): Kampman KM, Volpicelli J.
  Source: Journal of Substance Abuse Treatment. 1997 July-August; 14(4): 401-4.
  http://www.ncbi.nlm.nih.gov/entrez/query.fcgi?cmd=Retrieve&db=pubmed&dopt=Abstract&list_uids=9368218

- **Combinations of treatment modalities and therapeutic outcome for cocaine dependence.**
  Author(s): Khalsa ME, Paredes A, Anglin MD, Potepan P, Potter C.
  Source: Nida Res Monogr. 1993; 135: 237-59. No Abstract Available.
  http://www.ncbi.nlm.nih.gov/entrez/query.fcgi?cmd=Retrieve&db=pubmed&dopt=Abstract&list_uids=8289900

- **Community reinforcement approach for combined opioid and cocaine dependence. Patterns of engagement in alternate activities.**
  Author(s): Cochrane Database Syst Rev. 2001;(4):CD002023
  Source: Journal of Substance Abuse Treatment. 2000 April; 18(3): 255-61.
  http://www.ncbi.nlm.nih.gov/entrez/query.fcgi?cmd=Retrieve&db=pubmed&dopt=Abstract&list_uids=11687133

- **Community reinforcement approach for combined opioid and cocaine dependence. Patterns of engagement in alternate activities.**
  Author(s): Schottenfeld RS, Pantalon MV, Chawarski MC, Pakes J.
  Source: Journal of Substance Abuse Treatment. 2000 April; 18(3): 255-61.
  http://www.ncbi.nlm.nih.gov/entrez/query.fcgi?cmd=Retrieve&db=pubmed&dopt=Abstract&list_uids=10742639

- **Comparison of amantadine and desipramine combined with psychotherapy for treatment of cocaine dependence.**
  Author(s): Weddington WW Jr, Brown BS, Haertzen CA, Hess JM, Mahaffey JR, Kolar AF, Jaffe JH.
  Source: The American Journal of Drug and Alcohol Abuse. 1991 June; 17(2): 137-52.
  http://www.ncbi.nlm.nih.gov/entrez/query.fcgi?cmd=Retrieve&db=pubmed&dopt=Abstract&list_uids=1862788

- **Comparison of amantadine and desipramine combined with psychotherapy for treatment of cocaine dependence.**
  Author(s): Weddington WW, Brown BS, Haertzen CA, Hess JM, Kolar AF, Mahaffey JR.
  Source: Nida Res Monogr. 1989; 95: 483-4. No Abstract Available.
  http://www.ncbi.nlm.nih.gov/entrez/query.fcgi?cmd=Retrieve&db=pubmed&dopt=Abstract&list_uids=2701321

- **Congruence of the MCMI-II and MCMI-III in cocaine dependence.**
  Author(s): Marlowe DB, Festinger DS, Kirby KC, Rubenstein DF, Platt JJ.
  Source: Journal of Personality Assessment. 1998 August; 71(1): 15-28.
  http://www.ncbi.nlm.nih.gov/entrez/query.fcgi?cmd=Retrieve&db=pubmed&dopt=Abstract&list_uids=9807228

- **Continuing care for cocaine dependence: comprehensive 2-year outcomes.**
  Author(s): McKay JR, Alterman AI, Cacciola JS, O'Brien CP, Koppenhaver JM, Shepard DS.
  Source: Journal of Consulting and Clinical Psychology. 1999 June; 67(3): 420-7.
  http://www.ncbi.nlm.nih.gov/entrez/query.fcgi?cmd=Retrieve&db=pubmed&dopt=Abstract&list_uids=10369063

- **Coping and social skills training for alcohol and cocaine dependence.**
  Author(s): Monti PM, O'Leary TA.
  Source: The Psychiatric Clinics of North America. 1999 June; 22(2): 447-70, Xi. Review.
  http://www.ncbi.nlm.nih.gov/entrez/query.fcgi?cmd=Retrieve&db=pubmed&dopt=Abstract&list_uids=10385943

- **Counselor prompts to increase condom taking during treatment for cocaine dependence.**
  Author(s): Kirby KC, Marlowe DB, Carrigan DR, Platt JJ.
  Source: Behavior Modification. 1998 January; 22(1): 29-44.
  http://www.ncbi.nlm.nih.gov/entrez/query.fcgi?cmd=Retrieve&db=pubmed&dopt=Abstract&list_uids=9567735

- **Day hospital versus inpatient cocaine dependence rehabilitation: an interim report.**
  Author(s): Alterman AI.
  Source: Nida Res Monogr. 1991; 105: 363-4. No Abstract Available.
  http://www.ncbi.nlm.nih.gov/entrez/query.fcgi?cmd=Retrieve&db=pubmed&dopt=Abstract&list_uids=1876041

- **Day treatment for cocaine dependence: incremental utility over outpatient counseling and voucher incentives.**
  Author(s): Marlowe DB, Kirby KC, Festinger DS, Merikle EP, Tran GQ, Platt JJ.
  Source: Addictive Behaviors. 2003 March; 28(2): 387-98.
  http://www.ncbi.nlm.nih.gov/entrez/query.fcgi?cmd=Retrieve&db=pubmed&dopt=Abstract&list_uids=12573690

- **Day versus inpatient treatment for cocaine dependence: an experimental comparison.**
  Author(s): Schneider R, Mittelmeier C, Gadish D.
  Source: J Ment Health Adm. 1996 Spring; 23(2): 234-45.
  http://www.ncbi.nlm.nih.gov/entrez/query.fcgi?cmd=Retrieve&db=pubmed&dopt=Abstract&list_uids=10172622

- **Depression as a prognostic factor for pharmacological treatment of cocaine dependence.**
  Author(s): Ziedonis DM, Kosten TR.
  Source: Psychopharmacology Bulletin. 1991; 27(3): 337-43.
  http://www.ncbi.nlm.nih.gov/entrez/query.fcgi?cmd=Retrieve&db=pubmed&dopt=Abstract&list_uids=1775608

- **Depressive symptomatology and cocaine-induced pituitary-adrenal axis activation in individuals with cocaine dependence.**
  Author(s): Elman I, Breiter HC, Gollub RL, Krause S, Kantor HL, Baumgartner WA, Gastfriend DR, Rosen BR.
  Source: Drug and Alcohol Dependence. 1999 August 2; 56(1): 39-45.
  http://www.ncbi.nlm.nih.gov/entrez/query.fcgi?cmd=Retrieve&db=pubmed&dopt=Abstract&list_uids=10462091

- **Desipramine treatment for cocaine dependence. Role of antisocial personality disorder.**
  Author(s): Arndt IO, McLellan AT, Dorozynsky L, Woody GE, O'Brien CP.
  Source: The Journal of Nervous and Mental Disease. 1994 March; 182(3): 151-6.
  http://www.ncbi.nlm.nih.gov/entrez/query.fcgi?cmd=Retrieve&db=pubmed&dopt=Abstract&list_uids=8113775

- **Desipramine treatment for relapse prevention in cocaine dependence.**
  Author(s): McElroy SL, Weiss RD, Mendelson JH, Teoh SK, McAfee B, Mello NK.
  Source: Nida Res Monogr. 1989; 95: 57-63. No Abstract Available.
  http://www.ncbi.nlm.nih.gov/entrez/query.fcgi?cmd=Retrieve&db=pubmed&dopt=Abstract&list_uids=2701323

- **Desipramine treatment of cocaine dependence in methadone-maintained patients.**
  Author(s): Arndt IO, Dorozynsky L, Woody GE, McLellan AT, O'Brien CP.
  Source: Archives of General Psychiatry. 1992 November; 49(11): 888-93.
  http://www.ncbi.nlm.nih.gov/entrez/query.fcgi?cmd=Retrieve&db=pubmed&dopt=Abstract&list_uids=1444727

- **Determining a diagnostic cut-off on the Severity of Dependence Scale (SDS) for cocaine dependence.**
  Author(s): Kaye S, Darke S.
  Source: Addiction (Abingdon, England). 2002 June; 97(6): 727-31.
  http://www.ncbi.nlm.nih.gov/entrez/query.fcgi?cmd=Retrieve&db=pubmed&dopt=Abstract&list_uids=12084142

- **Developing and evaluating new treatments for alcoholism and cocaine dependence.**
  Author(s): O'Brien CP, Alterman A, Childress AR, McLellan AT.
  Source: Recent Dev Alcohol. 1992; 10: 303-25. Review.
  http://www.ncbi.nlm.nih.gov/entrez/query.fcgi?cmd=Retrieve&db=pubmed&dopt=Abstract&list_uids=1589603

- **Dextroamphetamine for cocaine-dependence treatment: a double-blind randomized clinical trial.**
  Author(s): Cochrane Database Syst Rev. 2002;(2):CD002023
  Source: Journal of Clinical Psychopharmacology. 2001 October; 21(5): 522-6.
  http://www.ncbi.nlm.nih.gov/entrez/query.fcgi?cmd=Retrieve&db=pubmed&dopt=Abstract&list_uids=12076433

- **Diethylpropion pharmacotherapeutic adjuvant therapy for inpatient treatment of cocaine dependence: a test of the cocaine-agonist hypothesis.**
  Author(s): Alim TN, Rosse RB, Vocci FJ Jr, Lindquist T, Deutsch SI.
  Source: Clinical Neuropharmacology. 1995 April; 18(2): 183-95.
  http://www.ncbi.nlm.nih.gov/entrez/query.fcgi?cmd=Retrieve&db=pubmed&dopt=Abstract&list_uids=8635177

- **Dissociation of "conscious desire" (craving) from and relapse in alcohol and cocaine dependence.**
  Author(s): Miller NS, Gold MS.
  Source: Annals of Clinical Psychiatry : Official Journal of the American Academy of Clinical Psychiatrists. 1994 June; 6(2): 99-106.
  http://www.ncbi.nlm.nih.gov/entrez/query.fcgi?cmd=Retrieve&db=pubmed&dopt=Abstract&list_uids=7804394

- **Disulfiram treatment for cocaine dependence in methadone-maintained opioid addicts.**
  Author(s): Petrakis IL, Carroll KM, Nich C, Gordon LT, McCance-Katz EF, Frankforter T, Rounsaville BJ.
  Source: Addiction (Abingdon, England). 2000 February; 95(2): 219-28.
  http://www.ncbi.nlm.nih.gov/entrez/query.fcgi?cmd=Retrieve&db=pubmed&dopt=Abstract&list_uids=10723850

- **Disulfiram versus placebo for cocaine dependence in buprenorphine-maintained subjects: a preliminary trial.**
  Author(s): George TP, Chawarski MC, Pakes J, Carroll KM, Kosten TR, Schottenfeld RS.
  Source: Biological Psychiatry. 2000 June 15; 47(12): 1080-6.
  http://www.ncbi.nlm.nih.gov/entrez/query.fcgi?cmd=Retrieve&db=pubmed&dopt=Abstract&list_uids=10862808

- **Divalproex loading in the treatment of cocaine dependence.**
  Author(s): Myrick H, Henderson S, Brady KT, Malcom R, Measom M.
  Source: J Psychoactive Drugs. 2001 July-September; 33(3): 283-7.
  http://www.ncbi.nlm.nih.gov/entrez/query.fcgi?cmd=Retrieve&db=pubmed&dopt=Abstract&list_uids=11718321

- **Dopamine agonists for cocaine dependence.**
  Author(s): Soares BG, Lima MS, Reisser AA, Farrell M.
  Source: Cochrane Database Syst Rev. 2003; (2): Cd003352. Review.
  http://www.ncbi.nlm.nih.gov/entrez/query.fcgi?cmd=Retrieve&db=pubmed&dopt=Abstract&list_uids=12804461

- **Dopamine agonists for cocaine dependence.**
  Author(s): Soares BG, Lima MS, Reisser AA, Farrell M.
  Source: Cochrane Database Syst Rev. 2001; (4): Cd003352. Review. Update In:
  http://www.ncbi.nlm.nih.gov/entrez/query.fcgi?cmd=Retrieve&db=pubmed&dopt=Abstract&list_uids=11687193

- **Double-blind comparison of amantadine and bromocriptine for ambulatory withdrawal from cocaine dependence.**
  Author(s): Tennant FS Jr, Sagherian AA.
  Source: Archives of Internal Medicine. 1987 January; 147(1): 109-12.
  http://www.ncbi.nlm.nih.gov/entrez/query.fcgi?cmd=Retrieve&db=pubmed&dopt=Abstract&list_uids=3541819

- **Double-blind comparison of carbamazepine and placebo for treatment of cocaine dependence.**
  Author(s): Montoya ID, Levin FR, Fudala PJ, Gorelick DA.
  Source: Drug and Alcohol Dependence. 1995 June; 38(3): 213-9.
  http://www.ncbi.nlm.nih.gov/entrez/query.fcgi?cmd=Retrieve&db=pubmed&dopt=Abstract&list_uids=7555621

- **Double-blind comparison of desipramine and placebo in withdrawal from cocaine dependence.**
  Author(s): Tennant FS Jr, Tarver AL.
  Source: Nida Res Monogr. 1984; 55: 159-63.
  http://www.ncbi.nlm.nih.gov/entrez/query.fcgi?cmd=Retrieve&db=pubmed&dopt=Abstract&list_uids=6443373

- **Double-blind placebo-controlled trial of methylphenidate in the treatment of adult ADHD patients with comorbid cocaine dependence.**
  Author(s): Schubiner H, Saules KK, Arfken CL, Johanson CE, Schuster CR, Lockhart N, Edwards A, Donlin J, Pihlgren E.
  Source: Experimental and Clinical Psychopharmacology. 2002 August; 10(3): 286-94.
  http://www.ncbi.nlm.nih.gov/entrez/query.fcgi?cmd=Retrieve&db=pubmed&dopt=Abstract&list_uids=12233989

- **Drug dreams in outpatients with bipolar disorder and cocaine dependence.**
  Author(s): Yee T, Perantie DC, Dhanani N, Brown ES.
  Source: The Journal of Nervous and Mental Disease. 2004 March; 192(3): 238-42.
  http://www.ncbi.nlm.nih.gov/entrez/query.fcgi?cmd=Retrieve&db=pubmed&dopt=Abstract&list_uids=15091306

- **Drugs for cocaine dependence: not easy.**
  Author(s): Hollister LE, Krajewski K, Rustin T, Gillespie H.
  Source: Archives of General Psychiatry. 1992 November; 49(11): 905-6.
  http://www.ncbi.nlm.nih.gov/entrez/query.fcgi?cmd=Retrieve&db=pubmed&dopt=Abstract&list_uids=1444730

- **Effect of cocaine dependence on plasma phenylalanine and tyrosine levels and on urinary MHPG excretion.**
  Author(s): Tennant FS Jr.
  Source: The American Journal of Psychiatry. 1985 October; 142(10): 1200-1.
  http://www.ncbi.nlm.nih.gov/entrez/query.fcgi?cmd=Retrieve&db=pubmed&dopt=Abstract&list_uids=4037134

- **Effectiveness of propranolol for cocaine dependence treatment may depend on cocaine withdrawal symptom severity.**
  Author(s): Kampman KM, Volpicelli JR, Mulvaney F, Alterman AI, Cornish J, Gariti P, Cnaan A, Poole S, Muller E, Acosta T, Luce D, O'Brien C.
  Source: Drug and Alcohol Dependence. 2001 June 1; 63(1): 69-78.
  http://www.ncbi.nlm.nih.gov/entrez/query.fcgi?cmd=Retrieve&db=pubmed&dopt=Abstract&list_uids=11297832

- **Evaluation of treatment for cocaine dependence.**
  Author(s): O'Brien CP, Alterman A, Walter D, Childress AR, McLellan AT.
  Source: Nida Res Monogr. 1989; 95: 78-84.
  http://www.ncbi.nlm.nih.gov/entrez/query.fcgi?cmd=Retrieve&db=pubmed&dopt=Abstract&list_uids=2701324

- **Event-related potential evidence for frontal cortex effects of chronic cocaine dependence.**
  Author(s): Biggins CA, MacKay S, Clark W, Fein G.
  Source: Biological Psychiatry. 1997 September 15; 42(6): 472-85.
  http://www.ncbi.nlm.nih.gov/entrez/query.fcgi?cmd=Retrieve&db=pubmed&dopt=Abstract&list_uids=9285083

- **Evolving conceptualizations of cocaine dependence.**
  Author(s): Gawin FH, Kleber HD.
  Source: Yale J Biol Med. 1988 March-April; 61(2): 123-36. Review.
  http://www.ncbi.nlm.nih.gov/entrez/query.fcgi?cmd=Retrieve&db=pubmed&dopt=Abstract&list_uids=3043925

- **Family history and diagnosis of alcohol dependence in cocaine dependence.**
  Author(s): Miller NS, Gold MS, Belkin BM, Klahr AL.
  Source: Psychiatry Research. 1989 August; 29(2): 113-21.
  http://www.ncbi.nlm.nih.gov/entrez/query.fcgi?cmd=Retrieve&db=pubmed&dopt=Abstract&list_uids=2798591

- **Features of cocaine dependence with concurrent alcohol abuse.**
  Author(s): Brady KT, Sonne S, Randall CL, Adinoff B, Malcolm R.
  Source: Drug and Alcohol Dependence. 1995 July; 39(1): 69-71.
  http://www.ncbi.nlm.nih.gov/entrez/query.fcgi?cmd=Retrieve&db=pubmed&dopt=Abstract&list_uids=7587977

- **Fifty-five years of cocaine dependence.**
  Author(s): Brown R, Middlefell R.
  Source: British Journal of Addiction. 1989 August; 84(8): 946.
  http://www.ncbi.nlm.nih.gov/entrez/query.fcgi?cmd=Retrieve&db=pu
  bmed&dopt=Abstract&list_uids=2775916

- **Fluoxetine for cocaine dependence in methadone maintenance.**
  Author(s): Balon R.
  Source: Journal of Clinical Psychopharmacology. 1994 October; 14(5): 360-
  1.
  http://www.ncbi.nlm.nih.gov/entrez/query.fcgi?cmd=Retrieve&db=pu
  bmed&dopt=Abstract&list_uids=7806696

- **Fluoxetine for cocaine dependence in methadone maintenance: quantitative plasma and urine cocaine/benzoylecgonine concentrations.**
  Author(s): Batki SL, Manfredi LB, Jacob P 3rd, Jones RT.
  Source: Journal of Clinical Psychopharmacology. 1993 August; 13(4): 243-
  50.
  http://www.ncbi.nlm.nih.gov/entrez/query.fcgi?cmd=Retrieve&db=pu
  bmed&dopt=Abstract&list_uids=8376611

- **Fluoxetine is ineffective for treatment of cocaine dependence or concurrent opiate and cocaine dependence: two placebo-controlled double-blind trials.**
  Author(s): Grabowski J, Rhoades H, Elk R, Schmitz J, Davis C, Creson D, Kirby K.
  Source: Journal of Clinical Psychopharmacology. 1995 June; 15(3): 163-74.
  http://www.ncbi.nlm.nih.gov/entrez/query.fcgi?cmd=Retrieve&db=pu
  bmed&dopt=Abstract&list_uids=7635993

- **Gabapentin in the treatment of cocaine dependence: a case series.**
  Author(s): Myrick H, Henderson S, Brady KT, Malcolm R.
  Source: The Journal of Clinical Psychiatry. 2001 January; 62(1): 19-23.
  http://www.ncbi.nlm.nih.gov/entrez/query.fcgi?cmd=Retrieve&db=pu
  bmed&dopt=Abstract&list_uids=11235923

- **Gender differences in cocaine craving among non-treatment-seeking individuals with cocaine dependence.**
  Author(s): Elman I, Karlsgodt KH, Gastfriend DR.
  Source: The American Journal of Drug and Alcohol Abuse. 2001 May; 27(2): 193-202.
  http://www.ncbi.nlm.nih.gov/entrez/query.fcgi?cmd=Retrieve&db=pubmed&dopt=Abstract&list_uids=11417935

- **Glutamatergic agents for cocaine dependence.**
  Author(s): Dackis C, O'Brien C.
  Source: Annals of the New York Academy of Sciences. 2003 November; 1003: 328-45. Review.
  http://www.ncbi.nlm.nih.gov/entrez/query.fcgi?cmd=Retrieve&db=pubmed&dopt=Abstract&list_uids=14684456

- **Goals and rationale for pharmacotherapeutic approach in treating cocaine dependence: insights from basic and clinical research.**
  Author(s): Kreek MJ.
  Source: Nida Res Monogr. 1997; 175: 5-35. Review. No Abstract Available.
  http://www.ncbi.nlm.nih.gov/entrez/query.fcgi?cmd=Retrieve&db=pubmed&dopt=Abstract&list_uids=9467791

- **Group counseling versus individualized relapse prevention aftercare following intensive outpatient treatment for cocaine dependence: initial results.**
  Author(s): McKay JR, Alterman AI, Cacciola JS, Rutherford MJ, O'Brien CP, Koppenhaver J.
  Source: Journal of Consulting and Clinical Psychology. 1997 October; 65(5): 778-88.
  http://www.ncbi.nlm.nih.gov/entrez/query.fcgi?cmd=Retrieve&db=pubmed&dopt=Abstract&list_uids=9337497

- **Homozygosity at the dopamine DRD3 receptor gene in cocaine dependence.**
  Author(s): Comings DE, Gonzalez N, Wu S, Saucier G, Johnson P, Verde R, MacMurray JP.
  Source: Molecular Psychiatry. 1999 September; 4(5): 484-7.
  http://www.ncbi.nlm.nih.gov/entrez/query.fcgi?cmd=Retrieve&db=pubmed&dopt=Abstract&list_uids=10523822

- **Impact of comorbid personality disorders and personality disorder symptoms on outcomes of behavioral treatment for cocaine dependence.**
  Author(s): Marlowe DB, Kirby KC, Festinger DS, Husband SD, Platt JJ.
  Source: The Journal of Nervous and Mental Disease. 1997 August; 185(8): 483-90.
  http://www.ncbi.nlm.nih.gov/entrez/query.fcgi?cmd=Retrieve&db=pubmed&dopt=Abstract&list_uids=9284861

- **Implications of recent research for program quality in cocaine dependence treatment.**
  Author(s): Carroll KM.
  Source: Substance Use & Misuse. 2000 October-December; 35(12-14): 2011-30. Review.
  http://www.ncbi.nlm.nih.gov/entrez/query.fcgi?cmd=Retrieve&db=pubmed&dopt=Abstract&list_uids=11138715

- **Incentives improve outcome in outpatient behavioral treatment of cocaine dependence.**
  Author(s): Higgins ST, Budney AJ, Bickel WK, Foerg FE, Donham R, Badger GJ.
  Source: Archives of General Psychiatry. 1994 July; 51(7): 568-76.
  http://www.ncbi.nlm.nih.gov/entrez/query.fcgi?cmd=Retrieve&db=pubmed&dopt=Abstract&list_uids=8031230

- **Increasing treatment adherence among outpatients with depression and cocaine dependence: results of a pilot study.**
  Author(s): Daley DC, Salloum IM, Zuckoff A, Kirisci L, Thase ME.
  Source: The American Journal of Psychiatry. 1998 November; 155(11): 1611-3.
  http://www.ncbi.nlm.nih.gov/entrez/query.fcgi?cmd=Retrieve&db=pubmed&dopt=Abstract&list_uids=9812129

- **Integrating psychotherapy and pharmacotherapy for cocaine dependence: results from a randomized clinical trial.**
  Author(s): Carroll KM, Rounsaville BJ, Nich C, Gordon L, Gawin F.
  Source: Nida Res Monogr. 1995; 150: 19-35. No Abstract Available.
  http://www.ncbi.nlm.nih.gov/entrez/query.fcgi?cmd=Retrieve&db=pubmed&dopt=Abstract&list_uids=8742770

- **Intimate violence and post-traumatic stress disorder among individuals with cocaine dependence.**
  Author(s): Dansky BS, Byrne CA, Brady KT.
  Source: The American Journal of Drug and Alcohol Abuse. 1999 May; 25(2): 257-68.
  http://www.ncbi.nlm.nih.gov/entrez/query.fcgi?cmd=Retrieve&db=pubmed&dopt=Abstract&list_uids=10395159

- **Lamotrigine in patients with bipolar disorder and cocaine dependence.**
  Author(s): Brown ES, Nejtek VA, Perantie DC, Orsulak PJ, Bobadilla L.
  Source: The Journal of Clinical Psychiatry. 2003 February; 64(2): 197-201.
  http://www.ncbi.nlm.nih.gov/entrez/query.fcgi?cmd=Retrieve&db=pubmed&dopt=Abstract&list_uids=12633129

- **Learned helplessness and cocaine dependence: an investigation.**
  Author(s): Sterling RC, Gottheil E, Weinstein SP, Lundy A, Serota RD.
  Source: Journal of Addictive Diseases : the Official Journal of the Asam, American Society of Addiction Medicine. 1996; 15(2): 13-24.
  http://www.ncbi.nlm.nih.gov/entrez/query.fcgi?cmd=Retrieve&db=pubmed&dopt=Abstract&list_uids=8703998

- **Looking back on cocaine dependence: reasons for recovery.**
  Author(s): Flynn PM, Joe GW, Broome KM, Simpson DD, Brown BS.
  Source: The American Journal on Addictions / American Academy of Psychiatrists in Alcoholism and Addictions. 2003 October-December; 12(5): 398-411.
  http://www.ncbi.nlm.nih.gov/entrez/query.fcgi?cmd=Retrieve&db=pubmed&dopt=Abstract&list_uids=14660154

- **Magnetic resonance imaging evidence of "silent" cerebrovascular toxicity in cocaine dependence.**
  Author(s): Bartzokis G, Beckson M, Hance DB, Lu PH, Foster JA, Mintz J, Ling W, Bridge P.
  Source: Biological Psychiatry. 1999 May 1; 45(9): 1203-11.
  http://www.ncbi.nlm.nih.gov/entrez/query.fcgi?cmd=Retrieve&db=pubmed&dopt=Abstract&list_uids=10331113

- **Management of clinical trials with new medications for cocaine dependence and abuse.**
  Author(s): Kiev A.
  Source: Nida Res Monogr. 1997; 175: 96-117. Review.
  http://www.ncbi.nlm.nih.gov/entrez/query.fcgi?cmd=Retrieve&db=pubmed&dopt=Abstract&list_uids=9467794

- **Mazindol treatment for cocaine dependence.**
  Author(s): Stine SM, Krystal JH, Kosten TR, Charney DS.
  Source: Drug and Alcohol Dependence. 1995 October; 39(3): 245-52.
  http://www.ncbi.nlm.nih.gov/entrez/query.fcgi?cmd=Retrieve&db=pubmed&dopt=Abstract&list_uids=8556974

- **Measuring adherence and competence of dynamic therapists in the treatment of cocaine dependence.**
  Author(s): Barber JP, Krakauer I, Calvo N, Badgio PC, Faude J.
  Source: The Journal of Psychotherapy Practice and Research. 1997 Winter; 6(1): 12-24.
  http://www.ncbi.nlm.nih.gov/entrez/query.fcgi?cmd=Retrieve&db=pubmed&dopt=Abstract&list_uids=9058557

- **Mediators of outcome of psychosocial treatments for cocaine dependence.**
  Author(s): Crits-Christoph P, Gibbons MB, Barber JP, Gallop R, Beck AT, Mercer D, Tu X, Thase ME, Weiss RD, Frank A.
  Source: Journal of Consulting and Clinical Psychology. 2003 October; 71(5): 918-25.
  http://www.ncbi.nlm.nih.gov/entrez/query.fcgi?cmd=Retrieve&db=pubmed&dopt=Abstract&list_uids=14516240

- **Methylphenidate (Ritalin) treatment of cocaine dependence--a preliminary report.**
  Author(s): Khantzian EJ, Gawin F, Kleber HD, Riordan CE.
  Source: Journal of Substance Abuse Treatment. 1984; 1(2): 107-12.
  http://www.ncbi.nlm.nih.gov/entrez/query.fcgi?cmd=Retrieve&db=pubmed&dopt=Abstract&list_uids=6536756

- **Monetary reinforcement of abstinence from cocaine among mentally ill patients with cocaine dependence.**
  Author(s): Shaner A, Roberts LJ, Eckman TA, Tucker DE, Tsuang JW, Wilkins JN, Mintz J.
  Source: Psychiatric Services (Washington, D.C.). 1997 June; 48(6): 807-10.
  http://www.ncbi.nlm.nih.gov/entrez/query.fcgi?cmd=Retrieve&db=pubmed&dopt=Abstract&list_uids=9175190

- **Neurometric QEEG studies of crack cocaine dependence and treatment outcome.**
  Author(s): Prichep LS, Alper K, Kowalik SC, Rosenthal M.
  Source: Journal of Addictive Diseases : the Official Journal of the Asam, American Society of Addiction Medicine. 1996; 15(4): 39-53.
  http://www.ncbi.nlm.nih.gov/entrez/query.fcgi?cmd=Retrieve&db=pubmed&dopt=Abstract&list_uids=8943581

- **Neurophysiological signs of cocaine dependence: increased electroencephalogram beta during withdrawal.**
  Author(s): Herning RI, Guo X, Better WE, Weinhold LL, Lange WR, Cadet JL, Gorelick DA.
  Source: Biological Psychiatry. 1997 June 1; 41(11): 1087-94.
  http://www.ncbi.nlm.nih.gov/entrez/query.fcgi?cmd=Retrieve&db=pubmed&dopt=Abstract&list_uids=9146819

- **New pharmacotherapies for cocaine dependence.. revisited.**
  Author(s): Meyer RE.
  Source: Archives of General Psychiatry. 1992 November; 49(11): 900-4. Review. Erratum In: Arch Gen Psychiatry 1993 January; 50(1): 16.
  http://www.ncbi.nlm.nih.gov/entrez/query.fcgi?cmd=Retrieve&db=pubmed&dopt=Abstract&list_uids=1444729

- **Nimodipine pharmacotherapeutic adjuvant therapy for inpatient treatment of cocaine dependence.**
  Author(s): Rosse RB, Alim TN, Fay-McCarthy M, Collins JP Jr, Vocci FJ Jr, Lindquist T, Jentgen C, Hess AL, Deutsch SI.
  Source: Clinical Neuropharmacology. 1994 August; 17(4): 348-58.
  http://www.ncbi.nlm.nih.gov/entrez/query.fcgi?cmd=Retrieve&db=pubmed&dopt=Abstract&list_uids=9316683

- **No association between D2 dopamine receptor (DRD2) alleles or haplotypes and cocaine dependence or severity of cocaine dependence in European- and African-Americans.**
  Author(s): Gelernter J, Kranzler H, Satel SL.
  Source: Biological Psychiatry. 1999 February 1; 45(3): 340-5.
  http://www.ncbi.nlm.nih.gov/entrez/query.fcgi?cmd=Retrieve&db=pubmed&dopt=Abstract&list_uids=10023512

- **No association between polymorphisms in the serotonin transporter gene and susceptibility to cocaine dependence among African-American individuals.**
  Author(s): Patkar AA, Berrettini WH, Hoehe M, Hill KP, Gottheil E, Thornton CC, Weinstein SP.
  Source: Psychiatric Genetics. 2002 September; 12(3): 161-4.
  http://www.ncbi.nlm.nih.gov/entrez/query.fcgi?cmd=Retrieve&db=pubmed&dopt=Abstract&list_uids=12218660

- **Old psychotherapies for cocaine dependence revisited.**
  Author(s): Carroll KM.
  Source: Archives of General Psychiatry. 1999 June; 56(6): 505-6.
  http://www.ncbi.nlm.nih.gov/entrez/query.fcgi?cmd=Retrieve&db=pubmed&dopt=Abstract&list_uids=10359463

- **One-year follow-up of psychotherapy and pharmacotherapy for cocaine dependence. Delayed emergence of psychotherapy effects.**
  Author(s): Carroll KM, Rounsaville BJ, Nich C, Gordon LT, Wirtz PW, Gawin F.
  Source: Archives of General Psychiatry. 1994 December; 51(12): 989-97.
  http://www.ncbi.nlm.nih.gov/entrez/query.fcgi?cmd=Retrieve&db=pubmed&dopt=Abstract&list_uids=7979888

- **Open trials as a method of prioritizing medications for inclusion in controlled trials for cocaine dependence.**
  Author(s): Kampman KM, Rukstalis M, Ehrman R, McGinnis DE, Gariti P, Volpicelli JR, Pettinati H, O'Brien CP.
  Source: Addictive Behaviors. 1999 March-April; 24(2): 287-91.
  http://www.ncbi.nlm.nih.gov/entrez/query.fcgi?cmd=Retrieve&db=pubmed&dopt=Abstract&list_uids=10336110

- **Open-label pilot study of bupropion plus bromocriptine for treatment of cocaine dependence.**
  Author(s): Montoya ID, Preston KL, Rothman R, Gorelick DA.
  Source: The American Journal of Drug and Alcohol Abuse. 2002; 28(1): 189-96.
  http://www.ncbi.nlm.nih.gov/entrez/query.fcgi?cmd=Retrieve&db=pubmed&dopt=Abstract&list_uids=11853133

- **Outcome related electrophysiological subtypes of cocaine dependence.**
  Author(s): Prichep LS, Alper KR, Sverdlov L, Kowalik SC, John ER, Merkin H, Tom ML, Howard B, Rosenthal MS.
  Source: Clin Electroencephalogr. 2002 January; 33(1): 8-20.
  http://www.ncbi.nlm.nih.gov/entrez/query.fcgi?cmd=Retrieve&db=pubmed&dopt=Abstract&list_uids=11795212

- **Overview of potential treatment medications for cocaine dependence.**
  Author(s): McCance EF.
  Source: Nida Res Monogr. 1997; 175: 36-72. Review. No Abstract Available.
  http://www.ncbi.nlm.nih.gov/entrez/query.fcgi?cmd=Retrieve&db=pubmed&dopt=Abstract&list_uids=9467792

- **Pemoline for the treatment of cocaine dependence in methadone-maintained patients.**
  Author(s): Margolin A, Avants SK, Kosten TR.
  Source: J Psychoactive Drugs. 1996 July-September; 28(3): 301-4.
  http://www.ncbi.nlm.nih.gov/entrez/query.fcgi?cmd=Retrieve&db=pubmed&dopt=Abstract&list_uids=8895115

- **Pergolide mesylate. Adverse events occurring in the treatment of cocaine dependence.**
  Author(s): Malcolm R, Moore JW, Kajdasz DK, Cochrane CE.
  Source: The American Journal on Addictions / American Academy of Psychiatrists in Alcoholism and Addictions. 1997 Spring; 6(2): 117-23.
  http://www.ncbi.nlm.nih.gov/entrez/query.fcgi?cmd=Retrieve&db=pubmed&dopt=Abstract&list_uids=9134073

- **Peripheral cocaine-blocking agents: new medications for cocaine dependence. An introduction to immunological and enzymatic approaches to treating cocaine dependence reported by Fox, Gorelick and Cohen in the immediately succeeding articles (see pages 153-174).**
  Author(s): Sparenborg S, Vocci F, Zukin S.
  Source: Drug and Alcohol Dependence. 1997 December 15; 48(3): 149-51.
  http://www.ncbi.nlm.nih.gov/entrez/query.fcgi?cmd=Retrieve&db=pubmed&dopt=Abstract&list_uids=9449012

- **Personality disorders in cocaine dependence.**
  Author(s): Weiss RD, Mirin SM, Griffin ML, Gunderson JG, Hufford C.
  Source: Comprehensive Psychiatry. 1993 May-June; 34(3): 145-9.
  http://www.ncbi.nlm.nih.gov/entrez/query.fcgi?cmd=Retrieve&db=pubmed&dopt=Abstract&list_uids=8339531

- **Pharmacologic approaches to the treatment of cocaine dependence.**
  Author(s): Taylor WA, Gold MS.
  Source: The Western Journal of Medicine. 1990 May; 152(5): 573-7. Review.
  http://www.ncbi.nlm.nih.gov/entrez/query.fcgi?cmd=Retrieve&db=pubmed&dopt=Abstract&list_uids=1971975

- **Pharmacologic treatments for heroin and cocaine dependence.**
  Author(s): Kleber HD.
  Source: The American Journal on Addictions / American Academy of Psychiatrists in Alcoholism and Addictions. 2003; 12 Suppl 2: S5-S18. Review.
  http://www.ncbi.nlm.nih.gov/entrez/query.fcgi?cmd=Retrieve&db=pubmed&dopt=Abstract&list_uids=12857659

- **Pharmacological and behavioral treatments of cocaine dependence: controlled studies.**
  Author(s): O'Brien CP, Childress AR, Arndt IO, McLellan AT, Woody GE, Maany I.
  Source: The Journal of Clinical Psychiatry. 1988 February; 49 Suppl: 17-22. Review.
  http://www.ncbi.nlm.nih.gov/entrez/query.fcgi?cmd=Retrieve&db=pubmed&dopt=Abstract&list_uids=3276670

- **Pharmacological approaches to cocaine dependence.**
  Author(s): Kosten TR.
  Source: Clinical Neuropharmacology. 1992; 15 Suppl 1 Pt A: 70A-71A.
  http://www.ncbi.nlm.nih.gov/entrez/query.fcgi?cmd=Retrieve&db=pubmed&dopt=Abstract&list_uids=1498999

- **Pharmacological treatment of cocaine dependence: a systematic review.**
  Author(s): de Lima MS, de Oliveira Soares BG, Reisser AA, Farrell M.
  Source: Addiction (Abingdon, England). 2002 August; 97(8): 931-49. Review.
  http://www.ncbi.nlm.nih.gov/entrez/query.fcgi?cmd=Retrieve&db=pubmed&dopt=Abstract&list_uids=12144591

- **Pharmacotherapies for cocaine dependence.**
  Author(s): O'Leary G, Weiss RD.
  Source: Current Psychiatry Reports. 2000 December; 2(6): 508-13. Review.
  http://www.ncbi.nlm.nih.gov/entrez/query.fcgi?cmd=Retrieve&db=pubmed&dopt=Abstract&list_uids=11123003

- **Pharmacotherapy of cerebral ischemia in cocaine dependence.**
  Author(s): Kosten TR.
  Source: Drug and Alcohol Dependence. 1998 January 1; 49(2): 133-44. Review.
  http://www.ncbi.nlm.nih.gov/entrez/query.fcgi?cmd=Retrieve&db=pubmed&dopt=Abstract&list_uids=9543650

- **Pilot randomized double blind placebo-controlled study of dexamphetamine for cocaine dependence.**
  Author(s): Shearer J, Wodak A, van Beek I, Mattick RP, Lewis J.
  Source: Addiction (Abingdon, England). 2003 August; 98(8): 1137-41.
  http://www.ncbi.nlm.nih.gov/entrez/query.fcgi?cmd=Retrieve&db=pubmed&dopt=Abstract&list_uids=12873248

- **Pituitary volume in men with concurrent heroin and cocaine dependence.**
  Author(s): Teoh SK, Mendelson JH, Woods BT, Mello NK, Hallgring E, Anfinsen P, Douglas A, Mercer G.
  Source: The Journal of Clinical Endocrinology and Metabolism. 1993 June; 76(6): 1529-32.
  http://www.ncbi.nlm.nih.gov/entrez/query.fcgi?cmd=Retrieve&db=pubmed&dopt=Abstract&list_uids=8501161

- **Platelet abnormalities associated with cerebral perfusion defects in cocaine dependence.**
  Author(s): Kosten TR, Tucker K, Gottschalk PC, Rinder CS, Rinder HM.
  Source: Biological Psychiatry. 2004 January 1; 55(1): 91-7.
  http://www.ncbi.nlm.nih.gov/entrez/query.fcgi?cmd=Retrieve&db=pubmed&dopt=Abstract&list_uids=14706430

- **Posttraumatic stress disorder and cocaine dependence. Order of onset.**
  Author(s): Brady KT, Dansky BS, Sonne SC, Saladin ME.
  Source: The American Journal on Addictions / American Academy of Psychiatrists in Alcoholism and Addictions. 1998 Spring; 7(2): 128-35.
  http://www.ncbi.nlm.nih.gov/entrez/query.fcgi?cmd=Retrieve&db=pubmed&dopt=Abstract&list_uids=9598216

- **Potentially functional polymorphism in the promoter region of prodynorphin gene may be associated with protection against cocaine dependence or abuse.**
  Author(s): Chen AC, LaForge KS, Ho A, McHugh PF, Kellogg S, Bell K, Schluger RP, Leal SM, Kreek MJ.
  Source: American Journal of Medical Genetics. 2002 May 8; 114(4): 429-35.
  http://www.ncbi.nlm.nih.gov/entrez/query.fcgi?cmd=Retrieve&db=pubmed&dopt=Abstract&list_uids=11992566

- **Predicting treatment-outcome in cocaine dependence from admission urine drug screen and peripheral serotonergic measures.**
  Author(s): Patkar AA, Thornton CC, Berrettini WH, Gottheil E, Weinstein SP, Hill KP.
  Source: Journal of Substance Abuse Treatment. 2002 July; 23(1): 33-40.
  http://www.ncbi.nlm.nih.gov/entrez/query.fcgi?cmd=Retrieve&db=pubmed&dopt=Abstract&list_uids=12127466

- **Predictors of dropout from psychosocial treatment of cocaine dependence.**
  Author(s): Siqueland L, Crits-Christoph P, Frank A, Daley D, Weiss R, Chittams J, Blaine J, Luborsky L.
  Source: Drug and Alcohol Dependence. 1998 September 1; 52(1): 1-13.
  http://www.ncbi.nlm.nih.gov/entrez/query.fcgi?cmd=Retrieve&db=pubmed&dopt=Abstract&list_uids=9788001

- **Prevalence of hyperthyroidism in veterans hospitalized for severe cocaine dependence.**
  Author(s): Burke WM, Dhopesh VP.
  Source: The American Journal of Medicine. 1993 July; 95(1): 113-4.
  http://www.ncbi.nlm.nih.gov/entrez/query.fcgi?cmd=Retrieve&db=pubmed&dopt=Abstract&list_uids=8328487

- **Psychological approaches for the treatment of cocaine dependence--a neurobehavioral approach.**
  Author(s): Rawson RA, Obert JL, McCann MJ, Ling W.
  Source: Journal of Addictive Diseases : the Official Journal of the Asam, American Society of Addiction Medicine. 1991; 11(2): 97-119.
  http://www.ncbi.nlm.nih.gov/entrez/query.fcgi?cmd=Retrieve&db=pubmed&dopt=Abstract&list_uids=1811763

- **Psychomotor and electroencephalographic sequelae of cocaine dependence.**
  Author(s): Bauer LO.
  Source: Nida Res Monogr. 1996; 163: 66-93. Review.
  http://www.ncbi.nlm.nih.gov/entrez/query.fcgi?cmd=Retrieve&db=pubmed&dopt=Abstract&list_uids=8809854

- **Psychopharmacologic treatment of cocaine dependence.**
  Author(s): Blaine JD, Ling W.
  Source: Psychopharmacology Bulletin. 1992; 28(1): 11-4.
  http://www.ncbi.nlm.nih.gov/entrez/query.fcgi?cmd=Retrieve&db=pubmed&dopt=Abstract&list_uids=1609036

- **Psychosocial stress and the duration of cocaine use in non-treatment seeking individuals with cocaine dependence.**
  Author(s): Karlsgodt KH, Lukas SE, Elman I.
  Source: The American Journal of Drug and Alcohol Abuse. 2003 August; 29(3): 539-51.
  http://www.ncbi.nlm.nih.gov/entrez/query.fcgi?cmd=Retrieve&db=pubmed&dopt=Abstract&list_uids=14510039

- **Psychosocial treatments for cocaine dependence.**
  Author(s): Hennessy GO, De Menil V, Weiss RD.
  Source: Current Psychiatry Reports. 2003 October; 5(5): 362-4. Review.
  http://www.ncbi.nlm.nih.gov/entrez/query.fcgi?cmd=Retrieve&db=pubmed&dopt=Abstract&list_uids=13678556

- **Psychosocial treatments for cocaine dependence: National Institute on Drug Abuse Collaborative Cocaine Treatment Study.**
  Author(s): Crits-Christoph P, Siqueland L, Blaine J, Frank A, Luborsky L, Onken LS, Muenz LR, Thase ME, Weiss RD, Gastfriend DR, Woody GE, Barber JP, Butler SF, Daley D, Salloum I, Bishop S, Najavits LM, Lis J, Mercer D, Griffin ML, Moras K, Beck AT.
  Source: Archives of General Psychiatry. 1999 June; 56(6): 493-502.
  http://www.ncbi.nlm.nih.gov/entrez/query.fcgi?cmd=Retrieve&db=pubmed&dopt=Abstract&list_uids=10359461

- **Psychosocial treatments for cocaine dependence: rethinking lessons learned.**
  Author(s): Strain EC.
  Source: Archives of General Psychiatry. 1999 June; 56(6): 503-4.
  http://www.ncbi.nlm.nih.gov/entrez/query.fcgi?cmd=Retrieve&db=pubmed&dopt=Abstract&list_uids=10359462

- **Psychotherapy for cocaine dependence.**
  Author(s): O'Brien CP, McLellan AT, Alterman A, Childress AR.
  Source: Ciba Found Symp. 1992; 166: 207-16; Discussion 216-23.
  http://www.ncbi.nlm.nih.gov/entrez/query.fcgi?cmd=Retrieve&db=pubmed&dopt=Abstract&list_uids=1638915

- **Quantitative EEG correlates of crack cocaine dependence.**
  Author(s): Alper KR, Chabot RJ, Kim AH, Prichep LS, John ER.
  Source: Psychiatry Research. 1990 December; 35(2): 95-105.
  http://www.ncbi.nlm.nih.gov/entrez/query.fcgi?cmd=Retrieve&db=pubmed&dopt=Abstract&list_uids=2100807

- **Quantitative electroencephalographic characteristics of crack cocaine dependence.**
  Author(s): Prichep LS, Alper KR, Kowalik S, Merkin H, Tom M, John ER, Rosenthal MS.
  Source: Biological Psychiatry. 1996 November 15; 40(10): 986-93.
  http://www.ncbi.nlm.nih.gov/entrez/query.fcgi?cmd=Retrieve&db=pubmed&dopt=Abstract&list_uids=8915557

- **Quantitative medial temporal lobe brain morphology and hypothalamic-pituitary-adrenal axis function in cocaine dependence: a preliminary report.**
  Author(s): Jacobsen LK, Giedd JN, Kreek MJ, Gottschalk C, Kosten TR.
  Source: Drug and Alcohol Dependence. 2001 March 1; 62(1): 49-56.
  http://www.ncbi.nlm.nih.gov/entrez/query.fcgi?cmd=Retrieve&db=pubmed&dopt=Abstract&list_uids=11173167

- **Quantitative morphology of the caudate and putamen in patients with cocaine dependence.**
  Author(s): Jacobsen LK, Giedd JN, Gottschalk C, Kosten TR, Krystal JH.
  Source: The American Journal of Psychiatry. 2001 March; 158(3): 486-9.
  http://www.ncbi.nlm.nih.gov/entrez/query.fcgi?cmd=Retrieve&db=pubmed&dopt=Abstract&list_uids=11229995

- **Quetiapine in bipolar disorder and cocaine dependence.**
  Author(s): Brown ES, Nejtek VA, Perantie DC, Bobadilla L.
  Source: Bipolar Disorders. 2002 December; 4(6): 406-11.
  http://www.ncbi.nlm.nih.gov/entrez/query.fcgi?cmd=Retrieve&db=pubmed&dopt=Abstract&list_uids=12519101

- **Racial identity and its assessment in a sample of African-American men in treatment for cocaine dependence.**
  Author(s): Pena JM, Bland IJ, Shervington D, Rice JC, Foulks EF.
  Source: The American Journal of Drug and Alcohol Abuse. 2000 February; 26(1): 97-112.
  http://www.ncbi.nlm.nih.gov/entrez/query.fcgi?cmd=Retrieve&db=pubmed&dopt=Abstract&list_uids=10718166

- **Randomized placebo-controlled trial of baclofen for cocaine dependence: preliminary effects for individuals with chronic patterns of cocaine use.**
  Author(s): Shoptaw S, Yang X, Rotheram-Fuller EJ, Hsieh YC, Kintaudi PC, Charuvastra VC, Ling W.
  Source: The Journal of Clinical Psychiatry. 2003 December; 64(12): 1440-8.
  http://www.ncbi.nlm.nih.gov/entrez/query.fcgi?cmd=Retrieve&db=pubmed&dopt=Abstract&list_uids=14728105

- **Randomized trial of buprenorphine for treatment of concurrent opiate and cocaine dependence.**
  Author(s): Montoya ID, Gorelick DA, Preston KL, Schroeder JR, Umbricht A, Cheskin LJ, Lange WR, Contoreggi C, Johnson RE, Fudala PJ.
  Source: Clinical Pharmacology and Therapeutics. 2004 January; 75(1): 34-48.
  http://www.ncbi.nlm.nih.gov/entrez/query.fcgi?cmd=Retrieve&db=pubmed&dopt=Abstract&list_uids=14749690

- **Reduced frontal white matter integrity in cocaine dependence: a controlled diffusion tensor imaging study.**
  Author(s): Lim KO, Choi SJ, Pomara N, Wolkin A, Rotrosen JP.
  Source: Biological Psychiatry. 2002 June 1; 51(11): 890-5.
  http://www.ncbi.nlm.nih.gov/entrez/query.fcgi?cmd=Retrieve&db=pubmed&dopt=Abstract&list_uids=12022962

- **Relapse prevention treatment for cocaine dependence: group vs. individual format.**
  Author(s): Schmitz JM, Oswald LM, Jacks SD, Rustin T, Rhoades HM, Grabowski J.
  Source: Addictive Behaviors. 1997 May-June; 22(3): 405-18.
  http://www.ncbi.nlm.nih.gov/entrez/query.fcgi?cmd=Retrieve&db=pubmed&dopt=Abstract&list_uids=9183510

- **Replacement medication for cocaine dependence: methylphenidate.**
  Author(s): Grabowski J, Roache JD, Schmitz JM, Rhoades H, Creson D, Korszun A.
  Source: Journal of Clinical Psychopharmacology. 1997 December; 17(6): 485-8.
  http://www.ncbi.nlm.nih.gov/entrez/query.fcgi?cmd=Retrieve&db=pubmed&dopt=Abstract&list_uids=9408812

- **'Research' versus 'real-world' patients: representativeness of participants in clinical trials of treatments for cocaine dependence.**
  Author(s): Carroll KM, Nich C, McLellan AT, McKay JR, Rounsaville BJ.
  Source: Drug and Alcohol Dependence. 1999 April 1; 54(2): 171-7.
  http://www.ncbi.nlm.nih.gov/entrez/query.fcgi?cmd=Retrieve&db=pubmed&dopt=Abstract&list_uids=10217557

- **Retention in psychosocial treatment of cocaine dependence: predictors and impact on outcome.**
  Author(s): Siqueland L, Crits-Christoph P, Gallop R, Barber JP, Griffin ML, Thase ME, Daley D, Frank A, Gastfriend DR, Blaine J, Connolly MB, Gladis M.
  Source: The American Journal on Addictions / American Academy of Psychiatrists in Alcoholism and Addictions. 2002 Winter; 11(1): 24-40.
  http://www.ncbi.nlm.nih.gov/entrez/query.fcgi?cmd=Retrieve&db=pubmed&dopt=Abstract&list_uids=11876581

- **Risperidone decreases craving and relapses in individuals with schizophrenia and cocaine dependence.**
  Author(s): Smelson DA, Losonczy MF, Davis CW, Kaune M, Williams J, Ziedonis D.
  Source: Canadian Journal of Psychiatry. Revue Canadienne De Psychiatrie. 2002 September; 47(7): 671-5.
  http://www.ncbi.nlm.nih.gov/entrez/query.fcgi?cmd=Retrieve&db=pubmed&dopt=Abstract&list_uids=12355680

- **Risperidone for the treatment of cocaine dependence: randomized, double-blind trial.**
  Author(s): Grabowski J, Rhoades H, Silverman P, Schmitz JM, Stotts A, Creson D, Bailey R.
  Source: Journal of Clinical Psychopharmacology. 2000 June; 20(3): 305-10.
  http://www.ncbi.nlm.nih.gov/entrez/query.fcgi?cmd=Retrieve&db=pubmed&dopt=Abstract&list_uids=10831016

- **Ritanserin in the treatment of cocaine dependence.**
  Author(s): Johnson BA, Chen YR, Swann AC, Schmitz J, Lesser J, Ruiz P, Johnson P, Clyde C.
  Source: Biological Psychiatry. 1997 November 15; 42(10): 932-40.
  http://www.ncbi.nlm.nih.gov/entrez/query.fcgi?cmd=Retrieve&db=pubmed&dopt=Abstract&list_uids=9359980

- **Secular trends in New York City hospital discharge diagnoses of congenital syphilis and cocaine dependence, 1982-88.**
  Author(s): Webber MP, Hauser WA.
  Source: Public Health Reports (Washington, D.C. : 1974). 1993 May-June; 108(3): 279-84.
  http://www.ncbi.nlm.nih.gov/entrez/query.fcgi?cmd=Retrieve&db=pubmed&dopt=Abstract&list_uids=8497564

- **Self-regulation factors in cocaine dependence--a clinical perspective.**
  Author(s): Khantzian EJ.
  Source: Nida Res Monogr. 1991; 110: 211-26. No Abstract Available.
  http://www.ncbi.nlm.nih.gov/entrez/query.fcgi?cmd=Retrieve&db=pu
  bmed&dopt=Abstract&list_uids=1944499

- **Serum prolactin levels and treatment outcome in cocaine dependence.**
  Author(s): Weiss RD, Hufford C, Mendelson JH.
  Source: Biological Psychiatry. 1994 April 15; 35(8): 573-4.
  http://www.ncbi.nlm.nih.gov/entrez/query.fcgi?cmd=Retrieve&db=pu
  bmed&dopt=Abstract&list_uids=8038302

- **Severity of cocaine dependence as a predictor of relapse to cocaine use.**
  Author(s): Weiss RD, Griffin ML, Hufford C.
  Source: The American Journal of Psychiatry. 1992 November; 149(11):
  1595-6.
  http://www.ncbi.nlm.nih.gov/entrez/query.fcgi?cmd=Retrieve&db=pu
  bmed&dopt=Abstract&list_uids=1415833

- **Social network therapy for cocaine dependence.**
  Author(s): Galanter M.
  Source: Adv Alcohol Subst Abuse. 1986 Winter; 6(2): 159-75.
  http://www.ncbi.nlm.nih.gov/entrez/query.fcgi?cmd=Retrieve&db=pu
  bmed&dopt=Abstract&list_uids=3604789

- **Structured interview versus self-report test vantages for the assessment
  of personality pathology in cocaine dependence.**
  Author(s): Marlowe DB, Husband SD, Bonieskie LM, Kirby KC, Platt JJ.
  Source: Journal of Personality Disorders. 1997 Summer; 11(2): 177-90.
  http://www.ncbi.nlm.nih.gov/entrez/query.fcgi?cmd=Retrieve&db=pu
  bmed&dopt=Abstract&list_uids=9203112

- **Subclinical neurological and neurovascular deficits in cocaine
  dependence. Gender and psychosocial considerations.**
  Author(s): King DE, Herning RI, Cadet JL.
  Source: Annals of the New York Academy of Sciences. 1997 October 15;
  825: 328-31.
  http://www.ncbi.nlm.nih.gov/entrez/query.fcgi?cmd=Retrieve&db=pu
  bmed&dopt=Abstract&list_uids=9369998

- **Subject-collateral reports of drinking in inpatient alcoholics with comorbid cocaine dependence.**
  Author(s): Stasiewicz PR, Stalker RG.
  Source: The American Journal of Drug and Alcohol Abuse. 1999 May; 25(2): 319-29.
  http://www.ncbi.nlm.nih.gov/entrez/query.fcgi?cmd=Retrieve&db=pubmed&dopt=Abstract&list_uids=10395163

- **Temporal progression of cocaine dependence symptoms in the US National Comorbidity Survey.**
  Author(s): Shaffer HJ, Eber GB.
  Source: Addiction (Abingdon, England). 2002 May; 97(5): 543-54.
  http://www.ncbi.nlm.nih.gov/entrez/query.fcgi?cmd=Retrieve&db=pubmed&dopt=Abstract&list_uids=12033655

- **The Addiction Severity Index in clinical efficacy trials of medications for cocaine dependence.**
  Author(s): Cacciola JS, Alterman AI, O'Brien CP, McLellan AT.
  Source: Nida Res Monogr. 1997; 175: 182-91. Review.
  http://www.ncbi.nlm.nih.gov/entrez/query.fcgi?cmd=Retrieve&db=pubmed&dopt=Abstract&list_uids=9467798

- **The cocaine epidemic: treatment options for cocaine dependence.**
  Author(s): Chychula NM, Okore C.
  Source: The Nurse Practitioner. 1990 August; 15(8): 33-40. Review.
  http://www.ncbi.nlm.nih.gov/entrez/query.fcgi?cmd=Retrieve&db=pubmed&dopt=Abstract&list_uids=2204847

- **The diagnosis of alcohol and cannabis dependence (addiction) in cocaine dependence (addiction).**
  Author(s): Miller NS, Gold MS, Klahr AL.
  Source: Int J Addict. 1990 July; 25(7): 735-44.
  http://www.ncbi.nlm.nih.gov/entrez/query.fcgi?cmd=Retrieve&db=pubmed&dopt=Abstract&list_uids=2272719

- **The diagnosis of alcohol and cannabis dependence in cocaine dependence.**
  Author(s): Miller NS, Gold MS, Belkin BM.
  Source: Adv Alcohol Subst Abuse. 1990; 8(3-4): 33-42.
  http://www.ncbi.nlm.nih.gov/entrez/query.fcgi?cmd=Retrieve&db=pubmed&dopt=Abstract&list_uids=2343796

- **The effectiveness of two intensities of psychosocial treatment for cocaine dependence.**
  Author(s): Coviello DM, Alterman AI, Rutherford MJ, Cacciola JS, McKay JR, Zanis DA.
  Source: Drug and Alcohol Dependence. 2001 January 1; 61(2): 145-54.
  http://www.ncbi.nlm.nih.gov/entrez/query.fcgi?cmd=Retrieve&db=pubmed&dopt=Abstract&list_uids=11137279

- **The prevalence of marijuana (cannabis) use and dependence in cocaine dependence.**
  Author(s): Miller NS, Klahr AL, Gold MS, Sweeney K, Cocores JA.
  Source: N Y State J Med. 1990 October; 90(10): 491-2.
  http://www.ncbi.nlm.nih.gov/entrez/query.fcgi?cmd=Retrieve&db=pubmed&dopt=Abstract&list_uids=2234615

- **The role of alcohol in cocaine dependence.**
  Author(s): Khalsa H, Paredes A, Anglin MD.
  Source: Recent Dev Alcohol. 1992; 10: 7-35.
  http://www.ncbi.nlm.nih.gov/entrez/query.fcgi?cmd=Retrieve&db=pubmed&dopt=Abstract&list_uids=1317049

- **The role of multifamily therapy in promoting retention in treatment of alcohol and cocaine dependence.**
  Author(s): Conner KR, Shea RR, McDermott MP, Grolling R, Tocco RV, Baciewicz G.
  Source: The American Journal on Addictions / American Academy of Psychiatrists in Alcoholism and Addictions. 1998 Winter; 7(1): 61-73.
  http://www.ncbi.nlm.nih.gov/entrez/query.fcgi?cmd=Retrieve&db=pubmed&dopt=Abstract&list_uids=9522008

- **The role of therapist characteristics in training effects in cognitive, supportive-expressive, and drug counseling therapies for cocaine dependence.**
  Author(s): Siqueland L, Crits-Christoph P, Barber JP, Butler SF, Thase M, Najavits L, Onken LS.
  Source: The Journal of Psychotherapy Practice and Research. 2000 Summer; 9(3): 123-30.
  http://www.ncbi.nlm.nih.gov/entrez/query.fcgi?cmd=Retrieve&db=pubmed&dopt=Abstract&list_uids=10896736

- **The self-medication hypothesis of addictive disorders: focus on heroin and cocaine dependence.**
  Author(s): Khantzian EJ.
  Source: The American Journal of Psychiatry. 1985 November; 142(11): 1259-64. Review.
  http://www.ncbi.nlm.nih.gov/entrez/query.fcgi?cmd=Retrieve&db=pubmed&dopt=Abstract&list_uids=3904487

- **The significance of a coexisting opioid use disorder in cocaine dependence: an empirical study.**
  Author(s): Weiss RD, Martinez-Raga J, Hufford C.
  Source: The American Journal of Drug and Alcohol Abuse. 1996 May; 22(2): 173-84.
  http://www.ncbi.nlm.nih.gov/entrez/query.fcgi?cmd=Retrieve&db=pubmed&dopt=Abstract&list_uids=8727053

- **The validity of self-reported drug use in non-treatment seeking individuals with cocaine dependence: correlation with biochemical assays.**
  Author(s): Elman I, Krause S, Breiter HC, Gollub RL, Heintges J, Baumgartner WA, Rosen BR, Gastfriend DR.
  Source: The American Journal on Addictions / American Academy of Psychiatrists in Alcoholism and Addictions. 2000 Summer; 9(3): 216-21.
  http://www.ncbi.nlm.nih.gov/entrez/query.fcgi?cmd=Retrieve&db=pubmed&dopt=Abstract&list_uids=11000917

- **Training in cognitive, supportive-expressive, and drug counseling therapies for cocaine dependence.**
  Author(s): Crits-Christoph P, Siqueland L, Chittams J, Barber JP, Beck AT, Frank A, Liese B, Luborsky L, Mark D, Mercer D, Onken LS, Najavits LM, Thase ME, Woody G.
  Source: Journal of Consulting and Clinical Psychology. 1998 June; 66(3): 484-92.
  http://www.ncbi.nlm.nih.gov/entrez/query.fcgi?cmd=Retrieve&db=pubmed&dopt=Abstract&list_uids=9642886

- **Treating cocaine dependence: new challenges for the therapeutic community.**
  Author(s): Zweben JE.
  Source: J Psychoactive Drugs. 1986 July-September; 18(3): 239-45.
  http://www.ncbi.nlm.nih.gov/entrez/query.fcgi?cmd=Retrieve&db=pubmed&dopt=Abstract&list_uids=3772649

- **Treating crack cocaine dependence: the critical role of relapse prevention.**
  Author(s): Wallace BC.
  Source: J Psychoactive Drugs. 1992 April-June; 24(2): 213-22. Review.
  http://www.ncbi.nlm.nih.gov/entrez/query.fcgi?cmd=Retrieve&db=pubmed&dopt=Abstract&list_uids=1507002

- **Treating crack cocaine dependence: the critical role of relapse prevention.**
  Author(s): Wallace BC.
  Source: J Psychoactive Drugs. 1990 April-June; 22(2): 149-58. Review.
  http://www.ncbi.nlm.nih.gov/entrez/query.fcgi?cmd=Retrieve&db=pubmed&dopt=Abstract&list_uids=2197391

- **Treatment of cocaine dependence in methadone maintenance clients: a pilot study comparing the efficacy of desipramine and amantadine.**
  Author(s): Kolar AF, Brown BS, Weddington WW, Haertzen CC, Michaelson BS, Jaffe JH.
  Source: Int J Addict. 1992; 27(7): 849-68.
  http://www.ncbi.nlm.nih.gov/entrez/query.fcgi?cmd=Retrieve&db=pubmed&dopt=Abstract&list_uids=1319961

- **Treatment of cocaine dependence through the principles of behavior analysis and behavioral pharmacology.**
  Author(s): Higgins ST, Budney AJ.
  Source: Nida Res Monogr. 1993; 137: 97-121. Review. No Abstract Available.
  http://www.ncbi.nlm.nih.gov/entrez/query.fcgi?cmd=Retrieve&db=pubmed&dopt=Abstract&list_uids=8289930

- **Treatment of heroin and cocaine dependence in general practice.**
  Author(s): Hewetson J.
  Source: Nurs Times. 1967 April 21; 63(16): 516-8. No Abstract Available.
  http://www.ncbi.nlm.nih.gov/entrez/query.fcgi?cmd=Retrieve&db=pubmed&dopt=Abstract&list_uids=6021960

- **Urine testing during treatment of cocaine dependence.**
  Author(s): Burke WM, Ravi NV, Dhopesh V, Vandegrift B, Maany I, McLellan AT.
  Source: Nida Res Monogr. 1989; 95: 320-1. No Abstract Available.
  http://www.ncbi.nlm.nih.gov/entrez/query.fcgi?cmd=Retrieve&db=pubmed&dopt=Abstract&list_uids=2701299

- **Use of a cue exposure paradigm for the evaluation of a potential pharmacotherapeutic agents for cocaine dependence.**
  Author(s): Kranzler HR, Bauer LO.
  Source: Addictive Behaviors. 1993 November-December; 18(6): 599-60.
  http://www.ncbi.nlm.nih.gov/entrez/query.fcgi?cmd=Retrieve&db=pubmed&dopt=Abstract&list_uids=8178699

- **Use of cocaine-discrimination techniques for preclinical evaluation of candidate therapeutics for cocaine dependence.**
  Author(s): Spealman RD.
  Source: Nida Res Monogr. 1992; 119: 175-9. Review. No Abstract Available.
  http://www.ncbi.nlm.nih.gov/entrez/query.fcgi?cmd=Retrieve&db=pubmed&dopt=Abstract&list_uids=1435975

- **Using cue reactivity to evaluate medications for treatment of cocaine dependence: a critical review.**
  Author(s): Modesto-Lowe V, Kranzler HR.
  Source: Addiction (Abingdon, England). 1999 November; 94(11): 1639-51. Review.
  http://www.ncbi.nlm.nih.gov/entrez/query.fcgi?cmd=Retrieve&db=pubmed&dopt=Abstract&list_uids=10892004

- **Validation of the criteria for DSM diagnosis of cocaine abuse and cocaine dependence.**
  Author(s): Friedman AS, Cacciola J.
  Source: The American Journal of Drug and Alcohol Abuse. 1998 February; 24(1): 169-77.
  http://www.ncbi.nlm.nih.gov/entrez/query.fcgi?cmd=Retrieve&db=pubmed&dopt=Abstract&list_uids=9513636

- **Why publish three negative articles on carbamazepine as a medication for the treatment of cocaine dependence?**
  Author(s): Johanson CE.
  Source: Drug and Alcohol Dependence. 1995 June; 38(3): 201-2.
  http://www.ncbi.nlm.nih.gov/entrez/query.fcgi?cmd=Retrieve&db=pubmed&dopt=Abstract&list_uids=7555619

Vocabulary Builder

The following vocabulary builder provides definitions of words used in this chapter that have not been defined in previous chapters:

Adjustment: The dynamic process wherein the thoughts, feelings, behavior, and biophysiological mechanisms of the individual continually change to adjust to the environment. [NIH]

Antagonism: Interference with, or inhibition of, the growth of a living organism by another living organism, due either to creation of unfavorable conditions (e. g. exhaustion of food supplies) or to production of a specific antibiotic substance (e. g. penicillin). [NIH]

Applicability: A list of the commodities to which the candidate method can be applied as presented or with minor modifications. [NIH]

Aspartate: A synthetic amino acid. [NIH]

Attenuated: Strain with weakened or reduced virulence. [NIH]

Attenuation: Reduction of transmitted sound energy or its electrical equivalent. [NIH]

Audiologist: Study of hearing including treatment of persons with hearing defects. [NIH]

Blot: To transfer DNA, RNA, or proteins to an immobilizing matrix such as nitrocellulose. [NIH]

Catecholamine: A group of chemical substances manufactured by the adrenal medulla and secreted during physiological stress. [NIH]

Compulsion: In psychology, an irresistible urge, sometimes amounting to obsession to perform a particular act which usually is carried out against the performer's will or better judgment. [NIH]

Cortisol: A steroid hormone secreted by the adrenal cortex as part of the body's response to stress. [NIH]

Cytokine: Small but highly potent protein that modulates the activity of many cell types, including T and B cells. [NIH]

Deletion: A genetic rearrangement through loss of segments of DNA (chromosomes), bringing sequences, which are normally separated, into close proximity. [NIH]

Discrimination: The act of qualitative and/or quantitative differentiation between two or more stimuli. [NIH]

Dysphoric: A feeling of unpleasantness and discomfort. [NIH]

EEG: A graphic recording of the changes in electrical potential associated with the activity of the cerebral cortex made with the electroencephalogram. [NIH]

Electrode: Component of the pacing system which is at the distal end of the lead. It is the interface with living cardiac tissue across which the stimulus is transmitted. [NIH]

Enzymatic: Phase where enzyme cuts the precursor protein. [NIH]

Epitope: A molecule or portion of a molecule capable of binding to the combining site of an antibody. For every given antigenic determinant, the body can construct a variety of antibody-combining sites, some of which fit almost perfectly, and others which barely fit. [NIH]

Estrogen: One of the two female sex hormones. [NIH]

Excitatory: When cortical neurons are excited, their output increases and each new input they receive while they are still excited raises their output markedly. [NIH]

Genetics: The biological science that deals with the phenomena and mechanisms of heredity. [NIH]

Heterogeneity: The property of one or more samples or populations which implies that they are not identical in respect of some or all of their parameters, e. g. heterogeneity of variance. [NIH]

Hybridoma: A hybrid cell resulting from the fusion of a specific antibody-producing spleen cell with a myeloma cell. [NIH]

Infections: The illnesses caused by an organism that usually does not cause disease in a person with a normal immune system. [NIH]

Initiation: Mutation induced by a chemical reactive substance causing cell changes; being a step in a carcinogenic process. [NIH]

Insight: The capacity to understand one's own motives, to be aware of one's own psychodynamics, to appreciate the meaning of symbolic behavior. [NIH]

Ligands: A RNA simulation method developed by the MIT. [NIH]

Linkage: The tendency of two or more genes in the same chromosome to remain together from one generation to the next more frequently than expected according to the law of independent assortment. [NIH]

Medial: Lying near the midsaggital plane of the body; opposed to lateral.

[NIH]

Mesolimbic: Inner brain region governing emotion and drives. [NIH]

Metabotropic: A glutamate receptor which triggers an increase in production of 2 intracellular messengers: diacylglycerol and inositol 1, 4, 5-triphosphate. [NIH]

Modeling: A treatment procedure whereby the therapist presents the target behavior which the learner is to imitate and make part of his repertoire. [NIH]

Modification: A change in an organism, or in a process in an organism, that is acquired from its own activity or environment. [NIH]

Morphological: Relating to the configuration or the structure of live organs. [NIH]

MRNA: The RNA molecule that conveys from the DNA the information that is to be translated into the structure of a particular polypeptide molecule. [NIH]

Myopia: Astigmatism in which one principal meridian is myopic and the other enmetropic, or in which both meridians are myopic. [NIH]

Nuclei: A body of specialized protoplasm found in nearly all cells and containing the chromosomes. [NIH]

Pharmacodynamic: Is concerned with the response of living tissues to chemical stimuli, that is, the action of drugs on the living organism in the absence of disease. [NIH]

Pharmacokinetic: The mathematical analysis of the time courses of absorption, distribution, and elimination of drugs. [NIH]

Phenotypes: An organism as observed, i. e. as judged by its visually perceptible characters resulting from the interaction of its genotype with the environment. [NIH]

Physiology: The science that deals with the life processes and functions of organismus, their cells, tissues, and organs. [NIH]

Plasticity: In an individual or a population, the capacity for adaptation: a) through gene changes (genetic plasticity) or b) through internal physiological modifications in response to changes of environment (physiological plasticity). [NIH]

Polymerase: An enzyme which catalyses the synthesis of DNA using a single DNA strand as a template. The polymerase copies the template in the 5'-3'direction provided that sufficient quantities of free nucleotides, dATP and dTTP are present. [NIH]

Polymorphism: The occurrence together of two or more distinct forms in the same population. [NIH]

Postsynaptic: Nerve potential generated by an inhibitory hyperpolarizing stimulation. [NIH]

Potentiate: A degree of synergism which causes the exposure of the organism to a harmful substance to worsen a disease already contracted. [NIH]

Probe: An instrument used in exploring cavities, or in the detection and dilatation of strictures, or in demonstrating the potency of channels; an elongated instrument for exploring or sounding body cavities. [NIH]

Prodrug: A substance that gives rise to a pharmacologically active metabolite, although not itself active (i. e. an inactive precursor). [NIH]

Promoter: A chemical substance that increases the activity of a carcinogenic process. [NIH]

Protease: Any enzyme that catalyzes hydrolysis of a protein. [NIH]

Protocol: The detailed plan for a clinical trial that states the trial's rationale, purpose, drug or vaccine dosages, length of study, routes of administration, who may participate, and other aspects of trial design. [NIH]

Psychoactive: Those drugs which alter sensation, mood, consciousness or other psychological or behavioral functions. [NIH]

Reticular: Coarse-fibered, netlike dermis layer. [NIH]

Ritalin: Drug used to treat hyperactive children. [NIH]

Sayre: A metal splint used to immobilize the hip in hip joint disease. [NIH]

Schizophrenia: A mental disorder characterized by a special type of disintegration of the personality. [NIH]

Septal: An abscess occurring at the root of the tooth on the proximal surface. [NIH]

Sequencer: Device that reads off the order of nucleotides in a cloned gene. [NIH]

Sequencing: The determination of the order of nucleotides in a DNA or RNA chain. [NIH]

Specificity: Degree of selectivity shown by an antibody with respect to the number and types of antigens with which the antibody combines, as well as with respect to the rates and the extents of these reactions. [NIH]

Stimulus: That which can elicit or evoke action (response) in a muscle, nerve, gland or other excitable issue, or cause an augmenting action upon any function or metabolic process. [NIH]

Striatum: A higher brain's domain thus called because of its stripes. [NIH]

Suppression: A conscious exclusion of disapproved desire contrary with repression, in which the process of exclusion is not conscious. [NIH]

Temporal: One of the two irregular bones forming part of the lateral surfaces and base of the skull, and containing the organs of hearing. [NIH]

Therapeutics: The branch of medicine which is concerned with the treatment of diseases, palliative or curative. [NIH]

Threshold: For a specified sensory modality (e. g. light, sound, vibration), the lowest level (absolute threshold) or smallest difference (difference threshold, difference limen) or intensity of the stimulus discernible in prescribed conditions of stimulation. [NIH]

Transcriptase: An enzyme which catalyses the synthesis of a complementary mRNA molecule from a DNA template in the presence of a mixture of the four ribonucleotides (ATP, UTP, GTP and CTP). [NIH]

Translation: The process whereby the genetic information present in the linear sequence of ribonucleotides in mRNA is converted into a corresponding sequence of amino acids in a protein. It occurs on the ribosome and is unidirectional. [NIH]

Translational: The cleavage of signal sequence that directs the passage of the protein through a cell or organelle membrane. [NIH]

Vector: Plasmid or other self-replicating DNA molecule that transfers DNA between cells in nature or in recombinant DNA technology. [NIH]

Vitro: Descriptive of an event or enzyme reaction under experimental investigation occurring outside a living organism. Parts of an organism or microorganism are used together with artificial substrates and/or conditions. [NIH]

Vivo: Outside of or removed from the body of a living organism. [NIH]

Chapter 4. Patents on Cocaine Dependence

Overview

You can learn about innovations relating to cocaine dependence by reading recent patents and patent applications. Patents can be physical innovations (e.g. chemicals, pharmaceuticals, medical equipment) or processes (e.g. treatments or diagnostic procedures). The United States Patent and Trademark Office defines a patent as a grant of a property right to the inventor, issued by the Patent and Trademark Office.[23] Patents, therefore, are intellectual property. For the United States, the term of a new patent is 20 years from the date when the patent application was filed. If the inventor wishes to receive economic benefits, it is likely that the invention will become commercially available to patients with cocaine dependence within 20 years of the initial filing. It is important to understand, therefore, that an inventor's patent does not indicate that a product or service is or will be commercially available to patients with cocaine dependence. The patent implies only that the inventor has "the right to exclude others from making, using, offering for sale, or selling" the invention in the United States. While this relates to U.S. patents, similar rules govern foreign patents.

In this chapter, we show you how to locate information on patents and their inventors. If you find a patent that is particularly interesting to you, contact the inventor or the assignee for further information.

---

[23]Adapted from The U. S. Patent and Trademark Office:
http://www.uspto.gov/web/offices/pac/doc/general/whatis.htm.

Patent Applications on Cocaine Dependence

As of December 2000, U.S. patent applications are open to public viewing.[24] Applications are patent requests which have yet to be granted (the process to achieve a patent can take several years). The following patent applications have been filed since December 2000 relating to cocaine dependence:

- **Anti-cocaine catalytic antibody**

  Inventor(s): Landry, Donald W.; (New York, NY)

  Correspondence: John P. White; Cooper & Dunham LLP; 1185 Avenue of the Americas; New York; NY; 10036; US

  Patent Application Number: 20030077793

  Date filed: August 28, 2001

  Abstract: Disclosed are catalytic antibodies and polypeptides capable of degrading **cocaine.** Said catalytic antibodies and polypeptides are characterized by the amino acid sequence of their complementary determining regions and framework regions. The present invention also discloses a pharmaceutical composition and a method for decreasing the concentration and a method for decreasing the concentration of **cocaine** of a subject. Finally, the invention discloses pharmaceutical compositions and methods for treating **cocaine** overdose and addiction in subjects.

  Excerpt(s): Throughout this application, various publications are referenced by author and date. Full citations for these publications may be found listed alphabetically at the end of the specification immediately preceding Sequence Listing and the claims. The disclosures of these publications in their entireties are hereby incorporated by reference into this application in order to more fully describe the state of the art as known to those skilled therein as of the date of the invention described and claimed herein.... Catalytic antibodies have unique potential for the treatment of **cocaine** addiction and overdose. **Cocaine** reinforces self-administration by inhibiting a dopamine re-uptake transporter (1) in the mesolimbocortical "reward pathway". No antagonist to **cocaine** is known (2), perhaps reflecting the difficulties inherent in blocking a blocker. As an alternative to receptor-based therapeutics, a circulating agent could interrupt the delivery of **cocaine** to its binding site in the brain (3). An agent such as an antibody that merely bound the drug could be depleted stoichiometrically by complex formation but an enzyme that bound drug, transformed it and released product would be available for additional binding. Catalytic antibodies, a novel class of artificial enzyme, are

---

[24] This has been a common practice outside the United States prior to December 2000.

inducible for a wide array of reactions and their substrate specificity is programmable to small molecules such as **cocaine** (4).... It has previously described (9) the first catalytic antibodies to degrade **cocaine**, Mab 3B9 and Mab 6A12. The antibodies were elicited by an immunogenic conjugate (TSA 1) of a phosphonate monoester transition-state analog (Scheme 1). The rate acceleration of these first artificial **cocaine** esterases (10.sup.2-10.sup.3) corresponded in magnitude to their relative stabilization of the ground-state to the transition-state (.about.K.sub.m/K.sub.1). Catalytic antibodies with more potent catalytic mechanisms and with higher turnover rates are possible and, it has been estimated, necessary for clinical applications. Increased activity can be pursued either through repeated hybridoma generation or through mutagenesis of catalytic antibodies in hand. However, sequencing of the variable domains of Mab's 3B9 and 6A12 revealed 93% homology at the complementarity determining regions (see below). Such a lack of diversity has been noted previously for catalytic antibodies (10) and limits the opportunities for improving activity since a particular class of homologous catalytic antibodies may fail to optimize to the desired activity. A potential solution to this problem, that would not compromise the core structure of the analog, would be to vary the surfaces of the analog rendered inaccessible by attachment to carrier protein and thereby present distinct epitopes for immunorecognition. The syntheses of three analogs of **cocaine** hydrolysis with identical phosphonate replacements but differing constructions for the immunoconjugates is now reported. The kinetics and the structural diversity of the catalytic antibodies elicited by these analogs has been characterized. The preferred catalytic antibodies for mutagenesis studies have been identified.

Web site: http://appft1.uspto.gov/netahtml/PTO/search-bool.html

- **Cocaine receptor binding ligands**

Inventor(s): Abraham, Philip; (Cary, NC), Boja, John W.; (Baltimore, MD), Carroll, Frank I.; (Durham, NC), Kuhar, Michael J.; (Baltimore, MD), Lewin, Anita H.; (Chapel Hill, NC)

Correspondence: OBLON, SPIVAK, MCCLELLAND, MAIER & NEUSTADT, P.C.; 1940 DUKE STREET; ALEXANDRIA; VA; 22314; US

Patent Application Number: 20030203934

Date filed: October 25, 2002

Abstract: A class of binding ligands for **cocaine** receptors and other receptors in the brain. Specifically, a novel family of compounds shows high binding specificity and activity, and, in a radiolabeled form, can be used to bind to these receptors, for biochemical assays and imaging techniques. Such imaging is useful for determining effective doses of new drug candidates in human populations. In addition, the high specificity, slow onset and long duration of the action of these compounds at the receptors makes them particularly well suited for therapeutic uses, for example as substitute medication for psychostimulant abuse. Some of these compounds may be useful in treating Parkinson's Disease or depression, by virtue of their inhibitory properties at monoamine transporters.

Excerpt(s): This application is a continuation-in-part application of U.S. patent application Ser. No. 08/506,541, filed Jul. 24, 1995, which is a continuation-in-part of (1) U.S. patent application Ser. No. 07/972,472, filed Mar. 23, 1993, which issued May 9, 1995 as U.S. Pat. No. 5,413,779; (2) U.S. patent application Ser. No. 08/164,576, filed Dec. 10, 1993, which is in turn a continuation-in-part of U.S. patent application Ser. No. 07/792,648, filed Nov. 15, 1991, now U.S. Pat. No. 5,380,848, which is in turn a continuation-in-part of U.S. patent application Ser. No. 07/564,755, filed Aug. 9, 1990, now U.S. Pat. No. 5,128,118 and U.S. PCT Application PCT/US91/05553, filed Aug. 9, 1991, filed in the U.S. PCT Receiving Office and designating the United States; and (3) U.S. patent application Ser. No. 08/436,970, filed May 8, 1995, all of which are incorporated herein by reference in their entirety.... This invention is directed to a class of binding ligands for **cocaine** receptors and other receptors in the brain. Specifically, a novel family of compounds shows high binding specificity and activity, and, in a radiolabeled form, can be used to bind to these receptors, for biochemical assays and imaging techniques. Such imaging is useful for determining effective doses of new drug candidates in human populations. In addition, the high specificity, slow onset and long duration of the action of these compounds at the receptors makes them particularly well suited for therapeutic uses, for example as substitute medication for psychostimulant abuse. Some of these compounds may be useful in treating Parkinson's Disease or depression, by virtue of their inhibitory properties at monoamine transporters.... Sites of specific interest included **cocaine** receptors associated with dopamine (DA) transporter sites.

Web site: http://appft1.uspto.gov/netahtml/PTO/search-bool.html

- **Sigma receptor antagonists having anti-cocaine properties and uses thereof**

Inventor(s): Matsumoto, Rae R.; (Edmond, OK)

Correspondence: DUNLAP, CODDING & ROGERS P.C.; PO BOX 16370; OKLAHOMA CITY; OK; 73114; US

Patent Application Number: 20030171347

Date filed: June 21, 2002

Abstract: The present invention relates to novel sigma receptor antagonist compounds that have anti-cocaine properties. These sigma receptor antagonists are useful in the treatment of **cocaine** overdose and addiction as well as movement disorders. The sigma receptor antagonists of the present invention may also be used in the treatment of neurological, psychiatric, gastrointestinal, cardiovascular, endocrine and immune system disorders as well as for imaging procedures. The present invention also relates to novel pharmaceutical compounds incorporating sigma receptor antagonists which can be used to treat overdose and addiction resulting from the use of **cocaine** and/or other drugs of abuse.

Excerpt(s): Cocaine has been reported to be the third most commonly abused drug, after alcohol and marijuana. It is further responsible for more serious intoxications and deaths than any other illicit compound. Currently, no effective treatments exist for **cocaine** overdose and addiction. **Cocaine** interacts with sigma receptors and this interaction provides the target for pharmacological intervention. Drugs that interfere with cocaine's access to sigma receptors mitigate the actions of **cocaine.** The sigma receptor compounds disclosed and claimed herein have anti-cocaine action: they prevent the behavioral toxic and psychomotor stimulant effects of **cocaine....** Cocaine abuse and dependence have risen to epidemic proportions in recent years, and it remains a major public health problem. **Cocaine** has been reported to be the third most commonly abused drug, after alcohol and marijuana. In addition, **cocaine** overdose is responsible for more serious intoxications and deaths than any other illicit drug. Despite tremendous efforts in recent years to identify new treatment strategies to break the addictive process, existing treatments for **cocaine** addiction are very limited and there are no pharmacotherapies to address the problem of toxicity. In spite of the war on drugs, the prevalence of **cocaine** use remains high in the U.S. and as a consequence, there is an urgent need to develop effective pharmacotherapies to aid in breaking the cycle of abuse.

Web site: http://appft1.uspto.gov/netahtml/PTO/search-bool.html

Keeping Current

In order to stay informed about patents and patent applications dealing with cocaine dependence, you can access the U.S. Patent Office archive via the Internet at the following Web address: **http://www.uspto.gov/patft/index.html**. You will see two broad options: (1) Issued Patent, and (2) Published Applications. To see a list of issued patents, perform the following steps: Under "Issued Patents," click "Quick Search." Then, type "cocaine dependence" (or synonyms) into the "Term 1" box. After clicking on the search button, scroll down to see the various patents which have been granted to date on cocaine dependence.

You can also use this procedure to view pending patent applications concerning cocaine dependence. Simply go back to the following Web address: **http://www.uspto.gov/patft/index.html**. Select "Quick Search" under "Published Applications." Then proceed with the steps listed above.

CHAPTER 5. BOOKS ON COCAINE DEPENDENCE

Overview

This chapter provides bibliographic book references relating to cocaine dependence. You have many options to locate books on cocaine dependence. The simplest method is to go to your local bookseller and inquire about titles that they have in stock or can special order for you. Some patients, however, feel uncomfortable approaching their local booksellers and prefer online sources (e.g. **www.amazon.com** and **www.bn.com**). In addition to online booksellers, excellent sources for book titles on cocaine dependence include the Combined Health Information Database and the National Library of Medicine. Once you have found a title that interests you, visit your local public or medical library to see if it is available for loan.

Book Summaries: Federal Agencies

The Combined Health Information Database collects various book abstracts from a variety of healthcare institutions and federal agencies. To access these summaries, go directly to the following hyperlink: **http://chid.nih.gov/detail/detail.html**. You will need to use the "Detailed Search" option. To find book summaries, use the drop boxes at the bottom of the search page where "You may refine your search by." Select the dates and language you prefer. For the format option, select "Monograph/Book." Now type "cocaine dependence" (or synonyms) into the "For these words:" box. You will only receive results on books. You should check back periodically with this database which is updated every 3 months. The following is a typical result when searching for books on cocaine dependence:

- **Behavioral Treatments for Drug Abuse and Dependence**

  Contact: National Clearinghouse for Alcohol and Drug Information, Substance Abuse and Mental Health Service Administration, PO Box 2345, Rockville, MD, 20852-2345, (301) 468-2600, http://www.health.org. US Government Printing Office, PO Box 371954, Pittsburgh, PA, 15250-7954, (202) 512-1800, http://www.access.gpo.gov.

  Summary: This monograph reviews technical papers on the application of behavior treatment; methadone treatment; behavioral interventions; cure reactivity; **cocaine dependence**; cognitive therapy; harm reduction; multisystemic treatment of serious juvenile offenders; dialectical behavior therapy; substance abuse research; and clinical trials.

Book Summaries: Online Booksellers

Commercial Internet-based booksellers, such as Amazon.com and Barnes & Noble.com, offer summaries which have been supplied by each title's publisher. Some summaries also include customer reviews. Your local bookseller may have access to in-house and commercial databases that index all published books (e.g. Books in Print®). The following have been recently listed with online booksellers as relating to cocaine dependence (sorted alphabetically by title; follow the hyperlink to view more details at Amazon.com):

- **A millionaire's cocaine encounter** by William C. Smatt; ISBN: 0962649104;
  http://www.amazon.com/exec/obidos/ASIN/0962649104/icongroupinterna

- **A System Description of the Cocaine Trade MR-236** by Bonnie Dombey-Moore, et al; ISBN: 0833014803;
  http://www.amazon.com/exec/obidos/ASIN/0833014803/icongroupinterna

- **A Very Greedy Drug: Cocaine in Context** by Jason Ditton, et al; ISBN: 3718659034;
  http://www.amazon.com/exec/obidos/ASIN/3718659034/icongroupinterna

- **Acute Cocaine Intoxication: Current Methods of Treatment (Nida Research Monograph; 123)** by Heinz Sorer (Editor), National Institute on Drug Abuse; ISBN: 0160416701;
  http://www.amazon.com/exec/obidos/ASIN/0160416701/icongroupinterna

- **Addictions: Gambling, Smoking, Cocaine Use, and Others** by Margaret Oldroyd, Hyde; ISBN: 0070316457; http://www.amazon.com/exec/obidos/ASIN/0070316457/icongroupin terna

- **Adverse Health Consequences of Cocaine Abuse**; ISBN: 9241561076; http://www.amazon.com/exec/obidos/ASIN/9241561076/icongroupin terna

- **Allegations of a CIA connection to crack cocaine epidemic : hearings before the Select Committee on Intelligence of the United States Senate, One Hundred Fourth Congress, second session... Wednesday, October 23, 1996; Tuesday, November 26, 1996 (SuDoc Y 4.IN 8/19:S.HRG.104-865)**; ISBN: 0160551307; http://www.amazon.com/exec/obidos/ASIN/0160551307/icongroupin terna

- **Allegations of a CIA Connection to Crack Cocaine Epidemic: Hearings Before the Select Committee on Intelligence of the United States Senate One Hundred Fourth Congress Second Session on Allegations of a CIA co** by Arlen Spector (Editor); ISBN: 0788180460; http://www.amazon.com/exec/obidos/ASIN/0788180460/icongroupin terna

- **An Individual Drug Counseling Approach to Treat Cocaine Addition: The Collaborative Cocaine Treatment Study Model** by Delinda E. Mercer; ISBN: 016050144X; http://www.amazon.com/exec/obidos/ASIN/016050144X/icongroupin terna

- **An Industrial Geography of Cocaine (Latin American Studies: Social Sciences and Law)** by Christian M. Allen; ISBN: 0415949408; http://www.amazon.com/exec/obidos/ASIN/0415949408/icongroupin terna

- **Analytical Toxicology of Cocaine (62 Selected Articles Published in the Journal of Analytical Toxicology 1988-1994)** by Joseph R. Monforte (Editor); ISBN: 091247419X; http://www.amazon.com/exec/obidos/ASIN/091247419X/icongroupin terna

- **Annual report on cocaine use among arrestees (SuDoc J 28.15/2-5:)** by U.S. Dept of Justice; ISBN: B00011030K; http://www.amazon.com/exec/obidos/ASIN/B00011030K/icongroupi nterna

- **Assessment of Two Cost-Effectiveness Studies on Cocaine Control Policy (Compass Series)** by Charles F. Manski (Editor), et al; ISBN:

0309064775;
http://www.amazon.com/exec/obidos/ASIN/0309064775/icongroupin
terna

- **Billy Franklin's Tough Enough: The Cocaine Investigation of United States Senator Chuck Robb** by Billy Franklin, Judi Tull (Contributor); ISBN: 1878901192;
http://www.amazon.com/exec/obidos/ASIN/1878901192/icongroupin
terna

- **Biological Basis of Cocaine Addiction (Annals of the New York Academy of Sciences, Vol 937)** by Vanya Quinones-Jenab (Editor), Vanya Quiinones-Jenab; ISBN: 1573313025;
http://www.amazon.com/exec/obidos/ASIN/1573313025/icongroupin
terna

- **Black-tar heroin, meth, and cocaine continue to flood the United States from Mexico : hearing before the Subcommittee on Criminal Justice, Drug Policy, and Human Resources of the Committee on Government Reform, House of Representatives, One Hundred Sixth Congress, second session, June 30, 2000 (SuDoc Y 4.G 74/7:B 56)**; ISBN: 0160658128;
http://www.amazon.com/exec/obidos/ASIN/0160658128/icongroupin
terna

- **C.I.A. Cocaine in America?: A Veteran of the C.I.A. Drug War Tells All** by Kenneth C. Bucchi; ISBN: 1561713228;
http://www.amazon.com/exec/obidos/ASIN/1561713228/icongroupin
terna

- **Clean Start: An Outpatient Program for Initiating Cocaine Recovery** by William E. McAuliffe, Jeffrey Albert; ISBN: 0898621909;
http://www.amazon.com/exec/obidos/ASIN/0898621909/icongroupin
terna

- **Clinician's Guide to Cocaine Addiction: Theory, Research, and Treatment** by Thomas R. Kosten (Editor), Herbert D. Kleber (Editor); ISBN: 0898621925;
http://www.amazon.com/exec/obidos/ASIN/0898621925/icongroupin
terna

- **Coca and Cocaine Effects on People and Policy in Latin America**; ISBN: 0939521245;
http://www.amazon.com/exec/obidos/ASIN/0939521245/icongroupin
terna

- **Coca, Cocaine and the War on Drugs** by Catholic Institute for International Rel; ISBN: 1852871113;

http://www.amazon.com/exec/obidos/ASIN/1852871113/icongroupin
terna

- **Cocaine Solutions: Help for Cocaine Abusers and Their Families** by Jennifer Rice-Licare, Katharine Delaney-McLoughlin; ISBN: 0918393825;
http://www.amazon.com/exec/obidos/ASIN/0918393825/icongroupin
terna

- **Cocaine True, Cocaine Blue** by Eugene Richards (Photographer), et al; ISBN: 0893815438;
http://www.amazon.com/exec/obidos/ASIN/0893815438/icongroupin
terna

- **Commonly Abused Drugs : Marijuana, Cocaine & Crack (Family Forum Library)** by Alan Gadol (Author); ISBN: 1566880211;
http://www.amazon.com/exec/obidos/ASIN/1566880211/icongroupin
terna

- **Consumer Reference Book and Index About Cocaine and Its Dangerous Influences** by John C. Bartone, Jone C. Bartone; ISBN: 0788302817;
http://www.amazon.com/exec/obidos/ASIN/0788302817/icongroupin
terna

- **Crack & Cocaine (Junior Drug Awareness)** by Linda N. Bayer, Steven L. Jaffe; ISBN: 0791051773;
http://www.amazon.com/exec/obidos/ASIN/0791051773/icongroupin
terna

- **Crack & Cocaine Epidemic (Facts on)** by Clint Twist; ISBN: 0749600497;
http://www.amazon.com/exec/obidos/ASIN/0749600497/icongroupin
terna

- **Crack and Cocaine (Issues Series)** by David Browne; ISBN: 0531170470;
http://www.amazon.com/exec/obidos/ASIN/0531170470/icongroupin
terna

- **Crack and cocaine use in England and Wales**; ISBN: 0862527872;
http://www.amazon.com/exec/obidos/ASIN/0862527872/icongroupin
terna

- **Crack, Powder Cocaine & Heroin: Drug Purchase & Use Patterns in Six U. S. Cities** by K. Jack Riley; ISBN: 0788176277;
http://www.amazon.com/exec/obidos/ASIN/0788176277/icongroupin
terna

- **Crack: Cocaine Squared** by Christina Dye; ISBN: 0892302143;
http://www.amazon.com/exec/obidos/ASIN/0892302143/icongroupin
terna

- **Crack: Treating Cocaine Addiction** by George Medzerian; ISBN: 0830636226;
  http://www.amazon.com/exec/obidos/ASIN/0830636226/icongroupin terna

- **Crack: What You Should Know About the Cocaine Epidemic (Perigee)** by Calvin Chatlos, Lawrence D. Chilnick; ISBN: 0399513485;
  http://www.amazon.com/exec/obidos/ASIN/0399513485/icongroupin terna

- **Danger: Cocaine (The Drug Awareness Library)** by Ruth Chier; ISBN: 0823923371;
  http://www.amazon.com/exec/obidos/ASIN/0823923371/icongroupin terna

- **Dealer: A Soccer Star's Deliverance from the Cocaine Underworld** by Jon Kregel; ISBN: 082543033X;
  http://www.amazon.com/exec/obidos/ASIN/082543033X/icongroupin terna

- **Dealer: Portrait of a Cocaine Merchant.** by Richard. Woodley; ISBN: 0030865840;
  http://www.amazon.com/exec/obidos/ASIN/0030865840/icongroupin terna

- **Death Beat: A Colombian Journalist's Life Inside the Cocaine Wars** by Maria Jimena Duzan, et al; ISBN: 0060170573;
  http://www.amazon.com/exec/obidos/ASIN/0060170573/icongroupin terna

- **Development of Medications for the Treatment of Opiate and Cocaine Addictions: Issues for the Government and Private Sector** by Carolyn E. Fulco, et al; ISBN: 0309052440;
  http://www.amazon.com/exec/obidos/ASIN/0309052440/icongroupin terna

- **Dropback: A Story of the Intrigue and Villainy behind the Cocaine Trade** by Piet Van Alder; ISBN: 0964325675;
  http://www.amazon.com/exec/obidos/ASIN/0964325675/icongroupin terna

- **Drug Abuse: The Crack Cocaine Epidemic: Health Consequences and Treatment**; ISBN: 1568068018;
  http://www.amazon.com/exec/obidos/ASIN/1568068018/icongroupin terna

- **Drug control impact of DOD's detection and monitoring on cocaine flow : report to congressional requesters (SuDoc GA 1.13:NSIAD-91-297)** by U.S. General Accounting Office; ISBN: B00010COLW;

http://www.amazon.com/exec/obidos/ASIN/B00010COLW/icongrou
pinterna

- **Drugs and crack in Illinois : hearing before the Subcommittee on the Constitution of the Committee on the Judiciary, United States Senate, One Hundred First Congress, second session, on the growing problem of crack cocaine in the Chicago, IL, area (SuDoc Y 4.J 89/2:S.hrg.101-1279)**; ISBN: B0001072VO;
http://www.amazon.com/exec/obidos/ASIN/B0001072VO/icongroupi
nterna

- **Drugs and Money: Laundering Latin America's Cocaine Dollars** by Robert E. Grosse (Author); ISBN: 0275970426;
http://www.amazon.com/exec/obidos/ASIN/0275970426/icongroupin
terna

- **Estimation of cocaine availability, 1996-1999 (SuDoc PREX 26.2:C 64)** by U.S. Postal Service; ISBN: B000114W3Y;
http://www.amazon.com/exec/obidos/ASIN/B000114W3Y/icongroup
interna

- **Evaluation of analytical methodologies for non-intrusive drug testing : supercritical fluid extraction of cocaine from hair (SuDoc J 28.15/2:601-98)** by Janet F. Morrison; ISBN: B00010ZKW2;
http://www.amazon.com/exec/obidos/ASIN/B00010ZKW2/icongroup
interna

- **Facts on the Crack and Cocaine Epidemic (Facts on Series)** by Clint Twist; ISBN: 0531108228;
http://www.amazon.com/exec/obidos/ASIN/0531108228/icongroupin
terna

- **Federal Cocaine Sentencing Policy: Hearing Before the Subcommittee on Crime and Drugs of the Committee on the Judiciary, United States Senate, One Hun** by United States; ISBN: 016070166X;
http://www.amazon.com/exec/obidos/ASIN/016070166X/icongroupin
terna

- **Focus on Cocaine and Crack: A Drug-Alert Book (Drug Alert Series)** by Jeffrey Shulman, et al; ISBN: 0941477983;
http://www.amazon.com/exec/obidos/ASIN/0941477983/icongroupin
terna

- **Freud's Cocaine Papers** by Art O'Donoghue, Art Odonoghue; ISBN: 1879816105;
http://www.amazon.com/exec/obidos/ASIN/1879816105/icongroupin
terna

- **Gettin' Tall: Cocaine Use Within a Subculture of Canadian Professional Musicians: An Ethnographic Inquiry** by O'Bireck, Gary M. O'Bireck; ISBN: 1551300281;
  http://www.amazon.com/exec/obidos/ASIN/1551300281/icongroupin terna

- **Goodbye to the White Lady: Cocaine Addiction & Recovery: A Case of Hesitation, Heartache, and Renewal** by Cardwell C. Nuckols; ISBN: 0830633855;
  http://www.amazon.com/exec/obidos/ASIN/0830633855/icongroupin terna

- **Grandmothers As Caregivers: Raising the Children of the Crack Cocaine Epidemic (Family Caregiver Applications Series, Vol 2)** by Meredith Minkler, Kathleen M. Roe; ISBN: 0803948476;
  http://www.amazon.com/exec/obidos/ASIN/0803948476/icongroupin terna

- **Hearing on crack cocaine Tuesday, November 9, 1993, Thurgood Marshall Federal Judiciary Building, room C-415, One Columbia [i.e. Columbus] Circle, N.E., Washington, D.C (SuDoc Y 3.SE 5:14-993/11/9)**; ISBN: B00010L3RI;
  http://www.amazon.com/exec/obidos/ASIN/B00010L3RI/icongroupi nterna

- **Inside the Cocaine Cartel: The Riveting Eyewitness Account of Life Inside the Colombian Cartel** by Richard Smitten (Contributor), et al; ISBN: 156171254X;
  http://www.amazon.com/exec/obidos/ASIN/156171254X/icongroupin terna

- **Learn About Cocaine & Crack (#1345B)**; ISBN: 0894862081;
  http://www.amazon.com/exec/obidos/ASIN/0894862081/icongroupin terna

- **Life in the Fast Lane: Information About Amphetamines, Cocaine and 'crack'** by Charles Rutter; ISBN: 0946507112;
  http://www.amazon.com/exec/obidos/ASIN/0946507112/icongroupin terna

- **Lines Across Europe: Nature and Extent of Cocaine Use in Barcelona, Rotterdam and Turin** by B. Bieleman, et al; ISBN: 902651347X;
  http://www.amazon.com/exec/obidos/ASIN/902651347X/icongroupin terna

- **Maier's Cocaine Addiction/Der Kokainismus** by Oriana J. Kalant (Editor); ISBN: 0888681607;

http://www.amazon.com/exec/obidos/ASIN/0888681607/icongroupin
terna

- **Man Who Made It Snow: Inside the Cocaine Carte**; ISBN: 1561718890;
  http://www.amazon.com/exec/obidos/ASIN/1561718890/icongroupin
  terna

- **Medication development for the treatment of cocaine dependence :
  issues in clinical efficacy trials (SuDoc HE 20.3965:175)** by U.S. Dept of
  Health and Human Services; ISBN: B00010UUKY;
  http://www.amazon.com/exec/obidos/ASIN/B00010UUKY/icongroup
  interna

- **My Name Is Cocaine and Other Poems** by Lasan S. Darboe; ISBN:
  0754113264;
  http://www.amazon.com/exec/obidos/ASIN/0754113264/icongroupin
  terna

- **Need to Know: Cocaine (Need to Know)** by Rob Alcraft; ISBN:
  0431097755;
  http://www.amazon.com/exec/obidos/ASIN/0431097755/icongroupin
  terna

- **Need to Know: Pack A of 4: Heroin / Cocaine / LSD / Amphetamines
  (Need to Know)** by Rob Alcraft; ISBN: 0431097887;
  http://www.amazon.com/exec/obidos/ASIN/0431097887/icongroupin
  terna

- **Neurobiological models for evaluating mechanisms underlying cocaine
  addiction (SuDoc HE 20.3965:145)** by U.S. Dept of Health and Human
  Services; ISBN: B00010LVWA;
  http://www.amazon.com/exec/obidos/ASIN/B00010LVWA/icongrou
  pinterna

- **Neurotoxicity and neuropathology associated with cocaine abuse
  (SuDoc HE 20.3965:163)** by U.S. Dept of Health and Human Services;
  ISBN: B00010R3ZE;
  http://www.amazon.com/exec/obidos/ASIN/B00010R3ZE/icongroupi
  nterna

- **One Step over the Line: A No Nonsense Guide to Recognizing and
  Treating Cocaine Dependency** by Joanne Baum; ISBN: 0062500457;
  http://www.amazon.com/exec/obidos/ASIN/0062500457/icongroupin
  terna

- **Overview, report of investigation concerning allegations of connections
  between CIA and the Contras in cocaine trafficking to the United States
  (SuDoc PREX 3.2:2001042000)** by U.S. Postal Service; ISBN: B000112XB2;

http://www.amazon.com/exec/obidos/ASIN/B000112XB2/icongroupi
nterna

- **Prenatal Cocaine Exposure** by Richard J. Konkol (Editor), George D. Olsen (Editor); ISBN: 0849394651;
  http://www.amazon.com/exec/obidos/ASIN/0849394651/icongroupin
  terna

- **Prenatal Cocaine Exposure: Scientific Considerations and Policy Implications** by Suzanne L. Wenzel; ISBN: 0833030019;
  http://www.amazon.com/exec/obidos/ASIN/0833030019/icongroupin
  terna

- **Prenatal Cocaine Exposure: The South Looks for Answers (Sacus Special Report, 1991)** by Elizabeth F. Shores, Elizabeth Morsund (Illustrator); ISBN: 0942388038;
  http://www.amazon.com/exec/obidos/ASIN/0942388038/icongroupin
  terna

- **Prenatal Exposure to Drugs/Alcohol: Characteristics and Educational Implications of Fetal Alcohol Syndrome and Cocaine - Polydrug Effects** by Jeanette M. Soby; ISBN: 0398064369;
  http://www.amazon.com/exec/obidos/ASIN/0398064369/icongroupin
  terna

- **Price and purity of cocaine : the relationship to emergency room visits and death, and to drug use among arrestees (SuDoc PREX 1.2:C 64)** by U.S. Postal Service; ISBN: B00010CMM8;
  http://www.amazon.com/exec/obidos/ASIN/B00010CMM8/icongrou
  pinterna

- **Psychological Effects of Cocaine and Crack Addiction** by Ann Holmes, et al; ISBN: 0791048985;
  http://www.amazon.com/exec/obidos/ASIN/0791048985/icongroupin
  terna

- **Psychotherapy of Cocaine Addiction: Entering the Interpersonal World of the Cocaine Addict (Library of Substance Abuse and Addiction Treatment)** by Jeffrey, Ph.D. Faude, David, Ph.D. Mark; ISBN: 0765700727;
  http://www.amazon.com/exec/obidos/ASIN/0765700727/icongroupin
  terna

- **Recent Developments in Alcoholism: Alcohol and Cocaine Similarities and Differences: Clinical Pathology, Psychosocial Factors and Treatment, Pharmac** by Marc Galanter (Editor); ISBN: 0306441454;
  http://www.amazon.com/exec/obidos/ASIN/0306441454/icongroupin
  terna

- **Red Cocaine : The Drugging of America** by Joseph D. Douglass; ISBN: 096266460X;
  http://www.amazon.com/exec/obidos/ASIN/096266460X/icongroupin terna

- **Report of investigation : allegations of connections between CIA and the Contras in cocaine trafficking to the United States (SuDoc PREX 3.2:C 76/V.1-)** by U.S. Postal Service; ISBN: B00010Y36Q;
  http://www.amazon.com/exec/obidos/ASIN/B00010Y36Q/icongroupi nterna

- **Report on the Central Intelligence Agency's alleged involvement in crack cocaine trafficking in the Los Angeles area (SuDoc Y 4.IN 8/18:IN 8/10)**; ISBN: 0160604265;
  http://www.amazon.com/exec/obidos/ASIN/0160604265/icongroupin terna

- **Report to the Congress cocaine and federal sentencing policy (SuDoc Y 3.SE 5:2/2002017000)**; ISBN: B000116OVW;
  http://www.amazon.com/exec/obidos/ASIN/B000116OVW/icongrou pinterna

- **Response to the National Research Council's Assessment of Rand's Controlling Cocaine Study** by Jonathan P. Caulkins, et al; ISBN: 0833029118;
  http://www.amazon.com/exec/obidos/ASIN/0833029118/icongroupin terna

- **Restricted activity days and other problems associated with use of marijuana or cocaine among persons 18-44 years of age, United States, 1991 (SuDoc HE 20.6209/3:246)** by U.S. Dept of Health and Human Services; ISBN: B00010IY5C;
  http://www.amazon.com/exec/obidos/ASIN/B00010IY5C/icongroupi nterna

- **Scotland Yards Cocaine C** by Andrew Jennings (Author); ISBN: 0099879905;
  http://www.amazon.com/exec/obidos/ASIN/0099879905/icongroupin terna

- **Scotland Yard's Cocaine Connection** by Andrew Jennings, et al; ISBN: 022402521X;
  http://www.amazon.com/exec/obidos/ASIN/022402521X/icongroupin terna

- **Snow Job?: The War Against International Cocaine Trafficking** by Kevin Jack Riley; ISBN: 1560002425;

http://www.amazon.com/exec/obidos/ASIN/1560002425/icongroupin
terna

- **Snowfields: The War on Cocaine in the Andes** by Clare Hargreaves;
ISBN: 0841913285;
http://www.amazon.com/exec/obidos/ASIN/0841913285/icongroupin
terna

- **Soldier D: SAS - the Columbian Cocaine War** by David Monnery; ISBN:
189812504X;
http://www.amazon.com/exec/obidos/ASIN/189812504X/icongroupin
terna

- **Stopping the flood of cocaine with Operation Snowcap : is it working? :
thirteenth report (SuDoc Y 1.1/8:101-673)** by U.S. Congressional Budget
Office; ISBN: B000103NNA;
http://www.amazon.com/exec/obidos/ASIN/B000103NNA/icongroup
interna

- **Study mission to London World Ministerial Cocaine Conference,
Greece, and Morocco (April 5 to 17, 1990) : report of the Select
Committee on Narcotics Abuse and Control, One Hundred First
Congress, second session (SuDoc Y 4.N 16:101-2-8)**; ISBN: B000104IQG;
http://www.amazon.com/exec/obidos/ASIN/B000104IQG/icongroupi
nterna

- **Subcutaneously, my dear Watson : Sherlock Holmes and the cocaine
habit** by Jack Tracy, Jim Berkey; ISBN: 091873603X;
http://www.amazon.com/exec/obidos/ASIN/091873603X/icongroupin
terna

- **Subcutaneously, My Dear Watson: Sherlock Holmes and the Cocaine
Habit (91P)** by Jack Tracey; ISBN: 0918736021;
http://www.amazon.com/exec/obidos/ASIN/0918736021/icongroupin
terna

- **Tales of Cocaine Alley** by G. E. Martin; ISBN: 1414036345;
http://www.amazon.com/exec/obidos/ASIN/1414036345/icongroupin
terna

- **The 2002 Official Patient's Sourcebook on Cocaine Dependence: A
Revised and Updated Directory for the Internet Age** by Icon Health
Publications; ISBN: 0597832358;
http://www.amazon.com/exec/obidos/ASIN/0597832358/icongroupin
terna

- **The Addictive Behavorial Personalities and Crack Cocaine Addiction
Cycle: An Analysis of Being "Out of Control"** by Moses Calhoun; ISBN:
0805934189;

http://www.amazon.com/exec/obidos/ASIN/0805934189/icongroupin
terna

- **The All American Cocaine Story** by David Britt; ISBN: 0896380734;
http://www.amazon.com/exec/obidos/ASIN/0896380734/icongroupin
terna

- **The Biological Basis of Cocaine Addiction (Annals of the New York Academy of Sciences, V. 937)** by Vanya Quinones-Jenab (Editor), Vanya Quiinones-Jenab; ISBN: 1573313033;
http://www.amazon.com/exec/obidos/ASIN/1573313033/icongroupin
terna

- **The CIA-contra-crack cocaine controversy a review of the Justice Department's investigations and prosecutions (SuDoc J 1.2:99006533)** by U.S. Dept of Justice; ISBN: B00010Y8CU;
http://www.amazon.com/exec/obidos/ASIN/B00010Y8CU/icongroupi
nterna

- **The Cocaine Connection** by R. L. Brent (Author); ISBN: 0441113001;
http://www.amazon.com/exec/obidos/ASIN/0441113001/icongroupin
terna

- **The Cocaine Crisis** by David Allen (Editor); ISBN: 0306424827;
http://www.amazon.com/exec/obidos/ASIN/0306424827/icongroupin
terna

- **The Cocaine Eaters** by Brian Moser, Donald Tayler; ISBN: 9997555643;
http://www.amazon.com/exec/obidos/ASIN/9997555643/icongroupin
terna

- **The Cocaine Epidemic/633** by Michael H. Irwin; ISBN: 0882910183;
http://www.amazon.com/exec/obidos/ASIN/0882910183/icongroupin
terna

- **The cocaine pusher** by Chuma G. Ezenyirioha; ISBN: 9782582271;
http://www.amazon.com/exec/obidos/ASIN/9782582271/icongroupin
terna

- **The Cocaine Trilogy: Beam Me Up, Scotty / Stone Cowboy / Snowblind** by Michael Guinzburg, et al; ISBN: 0862419778;
http://www.amazon.com/exec/obidos/ASIN/0862419778/icongroupin
terna

- **The Cocaine War: Drugs, Politics, and the Environment** by Belen Boville Luca De Tena, et al; ISBN: 0875862934;
http://www.amazon.com/exec/obidos/ASIN/0875862934/icongroupin
terna

- **The Cocaine Whores** by Erich, V Von Neff, et al; ISBN: 1893084035; http://www.amazon.com/exec/obidos/ASIN/1893084035/icongroupin terna

- **The Emergence of Crack Cocaine Abuse** by Edith Fairman Cooper, Edith Fairman Copper; ISBN: 1590335120; http://www.amazon.com/exec/obidos/ASIN/1590335120/icongroupin terna

- **The Epidemiology of Cocaine Use and Abuse (Adm)** by Susan Schober (Editor), et al; ISBN: 016035854X; http://www.amazon.com/exec/obidos/ASIN/016035854X/icongroupin terna

- **The Last Run: The Dramatic True Story of an American Woman's Escape from a Colombian Cocaine Family** by Kay Wolff, Sybil Taylor; ISBN: 0425133567; http://www.amazon.com/exec/obidos/ASIN/0425133567/icongroupin terna

- **The Neurobiology of Cocaine Addiction: From Bench to Bedside (Journal of Addictive Diseases)** by Herman Joseph (Editor), et al; ISBN: 0789000318; http://www.amazon.com/exec/obidos/ASIN/0789000318/icongroupin terna

- **The Rise and Fall of a Violent Crime Wave: Crack Cocaine and the Social Construction of a Crime Problem** by Henry H. Brownstein; ISBN: 091157736X; http://www.amazon.com/exec/obidos/ASIN/091157736X/icongroupin terna

- **The South American cocaine trade an "industry" in transition (SuDoc J 24.2:97002519)** by U.S. Dept of Justice; ISBN: B00010SCZ4; http://www.amazon.com/exec/obidos/ASIN/B00010SCZ4/icongroupi nterna

- **The Steel Drug: Cocaine and Crack in Perspective** by Patricia G. Erickson, et al; ISBN: 0029096456; http://www.amazon.com/exec/obidos/ASIN/0029096456/icongroupin terna

- **The Steel Drug: Cocaine in Perspective** by Patricia G. Erickson; ISBN: 0669145726; http://www.amazon.com/exec/obidos/ASIN/0669145726/icongroupin terna

- **The Taming of Cocaine: Cocaine Use in European and American Cities (Criminological Studies)** by Tom Decorte; ISBN: 9054872845;

http://www.amazon.com/exec/obidos/ASIN/9054872845/icongroupin terna

- **The U.S. Sentencing Commission and cocaine sentencing policy : hearing before the Committee on the Judiciary, United States Senate, One Hundred Fourth Congress, first session... August 10, 1995 (SuDoc Y 4.J 89/2:S.HRG.104-154)**; ISBN: 0160476569; http://www.amazon.com/exec/obidos/ASIN/0160476569/icongroupin terna

- **Tips for teens : about crack and cocaine (SuDoc HE 20.402:T 49/COCAINE)** by U.S. Dept of Health and Human Services; ISBN: B00010S2XG; http://www.amazon.com/exec/obidos/ASIN/B00010S2XG/icongroupi nterna

- **Trafficking Cocaine - Colombian Drug Entrepreneurs in the Netherlands (STUDIES OF ORGANIZED CRIME Volume 1)** by Damian Zaitch; ISBN: 9041118845; http://www.amazon.com/exec/obidos/ASIN/9041118845/icongroupin terna

- **Trafficking: The Boom and Bust of the Air America Cocaine Ring** by Berkeley Rice; ISBN: 0684190249; http://www.amazon.com/exec/obidos/ASIN/0684190249/icongroupin terna

- **Treating Cocaine Dependency (#1464A)** by David Smith, Donald Wesson; ISBN: 0894862790; http://www.amazon.com/exec/obidos/ASIN/0894862790/icongroupin terna

- **Treatment of Cocaine Abuse : An Annotated Bibliography** by John J. Miletich (Author); ISBN: 0313278393; http://www.amazon.com/exec/obidos/ASIN/0313278393/icongroupin terna

- **Treatment of hardcore cocaine users (SuDoc GA 1.13:HEHS-95-179 R)** by U.S. General Accounting Office; ISBN: B00010TPMS; http://www.amazon.com/exec/obidos/ASIN/B00010TPMS/icongroup interna

- **Trends in demographic characteristics and patterns of drug use of clients admitted to drug abuse treatment programs for cocaine abuse in selected states cocaine client admissions, 1979-1984 (SuDoc HE 20.8202:C 64/3)** by U.S. Dept of Health and Human Services; ISBN: B00010BYB8;

http://www.amazon.com/exec/obidos/ASIN/B00010BYB8/icongroupi
nterna

- **Upon this "rock" cocaine Satan builds his church** by Cynthia A. Jackson;
  ISBN: 0963956302;
  http://www.amazon.com/exec/obidos/ASIN/0963956302/icongroupin
  terna

- **WASHTON: COCAINE - A CLINICIAN'S HANDBOOK (NOT
  HANDLED BY NY): A Clinician's Handbook** by A.M. Washton (Editor),
  M.S. Gold (Editor); ISBN: 0471916668;
  http://www.amazon.com/exec/obidos/ASIN/0471916668/icongroupin
  terna

Chapters on Cocaine Dependence

Frequently, cocaine dependence will be discussed within a book, perhaps
within a specific chapter. In order to find chapters that are specifically
dealing with cocaine dependence, an excellent source of abstracts is the
Combined Health Information Database. You will need to limit your search
to book chapters and cocaine dependence using the "Detailed Search"
option. Go directly to the following hyperlink:
http://chid.nih.gov/detail/detail.html. To find book chapters, use the drop
boxes at the bottom of the search page where "You may refine your search
by." Select the dates and language you prefer, and the format option "Book
Chapter." By making these selections and typing in "cocaine dependence"
(or synonyms) into the "For these words:" box, you will only receive results
on chapters in books.

General Home References

In addition to references for cocaine dependence, you may want a general
home medical guide that spans all aspects of home healthcare. The following
list is a recent sample of such guides (sorted alphabetically by title;
hyperlinks provide rankings, information, and reviews at Amazon.com):

- **Drugs (Health Issues)** by Sarah Lennard-Brown; Library Binding - 64
  pages (March 2002), Raintree/Steck Vaughn; ISBN: 0739847732;
  **http://www.amazon.com/exec/obidos/ASIN/0739847732/icongroupinter
  na**

- **The Encyclopedia of Drugs and Alcohol (Reference)** by Greg Roza;
  School & Library Binding - 199 pages (September 2001); Franklin Watts,

Incorporated; ISBN: 0531118991;
http://www.amazon.com/exec/obidos/ASIN/0531118991/icongroupinterna

Vocabulary Builder

The following vocabulary builder provides definitions of words used in this chapter that have not been defined in previous chapters:

Subculture: A culture derived from another culture or the aseptic division and transfer of a culture or a portion of that culture (inoculum) to fresh nutrient medium. [NIH]

CHAPTER 6. PERIODICALS AND NEWS ON COCAINE DEPENDENCE

Overview

Keeping up on the news relating to cocaine dependence can be challenging. Subscribing to targeted periodicals can be an effective way to stay abreast of recent developments on cocaine dependence. Periodicals include newsletters, magazines, and academic journals.

In this chapter, we suggest a number of news sources and present various periodicals that cover cocaine dependence beyond and including those which are published by patient associations mentioned earlier. We will first focus on news services, and then on periodicals. News services, press releases, and newsletters generally use more accessible language, so if you do chose to subscribe to one of the more technical periodicals, make sure that it uses language you can easily follow.

News Services and Press Releases

Well before articles show up in newsletters or the popular press, they may appear in the form of a press release or a public relations announcement. One of the simplest ways of tracking press releases on cocaine dependence is to search the news wires. News wires are used by professional journalists, and have existed since the invention of the telegraph. Today, there are several major "wires" that are used by companies, universities, and other organizations to announce new medical breakthroughs. In the following sample of sources, we will briefly describe how to access each service. These services only post recent news intended for public viewing.

PR Newswire

Perhaps the broadest of the wires is PR Newswire Association, Inc. To access this archive, simply go to **http://www.prnewswire.com**. Below the search box, select the option "The last 30 days." In the search box, type "cocaine dependence" or synonyms. The search results are shown by order of relevance. When reading these press releases, do not forget that the sponsor of the release may be a company or organization that is trying to sell a particular product or therapy. Their views, therefore, may be biased. The following is typical of press releases that can be found on PR Newswire:

- **Malden Detective and Three Others Charged with Participating in Cocaine Conspiracy, Reports U.S. Attorney**

  Summary: BOSTON, May 21 /PRNewswire/ -- A Detective with the Malden Police Department and three other men were arrested late yesterday on a federal Complaint charging them with conspiring to possess cocaine with intent to distribute.

  United States Attorney Michael J. Sullivan and Mark R. Trouville, Special Agent in Charge of the U.S. Drug Enforcement Administration in New England, announced that DAVID JORDAN, age 43, of 123 Spring Street in Stoneham, Massachusetts, JON MINOTTI, age 37, of 3 O'Grady Circle in Stoneham, Massachusetts, ANTHONY BUCCI, age 41, of 6 Maple Road in North Reading, Massachusetts, and FRANCIS MUOLO, age 39, of 11 Marble Street in Stoneham, Massachusetts, were each charged in a criminal Complaint with conspiracy to possess over 500 grams of cocaine with intent to distribute.

  An affidavit filed in support of the Complaint alleges that on December 24, 2003, MINOTTI, BUCCI, MUOLO, and JORDAN conspired to steal three kilograms of cocaine from a scheduled drug deal. It is alleged that MINOTTI made arrangements for a supplier to bring three kilograms of cocaine to a meeting at the Malden Medical Center parking lot where BUCCI was to purchase the cocaine. It is alleged that shortly after the supplier arrived with the cocaine, JORDAN, a Detective with the Malden Police Department, arrived on the scene, blocking the supplier's vehicle with his own. It is alleged that JORDAN identified himself as a police officer and that MINOTTI fled into nearby woods with the three kilograms of cocaine. It is alleged that JORDAN then allowed the supplier and BUCCI to leave the scene. It is alleged that, as had been previously arranged, MUOLO, who had been waiting in his car on the other side of the nearby woods, picked up MINOTTI after he had run through the woods with the cocaine.

According to the Complaint affidavit, at the time, DEA agents were involved in a drug investigation and had a wiretap on the drug supplier's telephone. As part of the separate investigation, the DEA agents were surveilling the supplier and observed the incident. Shortly after, the DEA began an investigation of JORDAN and his associates. The Complaint also alleges that after JORDAN became aware that law enforcement agents were investigating the drug supplier from whom the cocaine had been stolen, JORDAN spoke with DEA agents on several occasions attempting to find out the status of the investigation. It is also alleged that JORDAN made false statements to law enforcement about his involvement in the events that transpired in the Malden Medical Center parking lot on December 24, 2003.

The defendants are expected to have initial appearances at 2:00 pm this afternoon before U.S. Magistrate Judge Joyce London Alexander. If convicted, each defendant faces a mandatory minimum of 5 years' imprisonment and a maximum of 40 years' imprisonment, to be followed by 4 years of supervised release, and a $2 million fine.

The investigation is continuing.

The case was investigated by the U.S. Drug Enforcement Administration; and the Massachusetts State Police (including the Middlesex County District Attorney's Narcotics Unit), with the assistance of the U.S. Marshals Service; the Bureau of Alcohol, Tobacco, Firearms, and Explosives; and the Stoneham, Everett, and Malden Police Departments. It is being prosecuted by Assistant U.S. Attorney John J. Farley in Sullivan's Public Corruption and Special Prosecutions Unit.

Reuters Health

The Reuters' Medical News and Health eLine databases can be very useful in exploring news archives relating to cocaine dependence. While some of the listed articles are free to view, others can be purchased for a nominal fee. To access this archive, go to **http://www.reutershealth.com/en/index.html** and search by "cocaine dependence" (or synonyms). The following was recently listed in this archive for cocaine dependence:

- **Abuse drug and behavior therapy curb cocaine use**
  Source: Reuters Health eLine
  Date: March 01, 2004

- **Acupuncture ineffective as stand-alone treatment of cocaine dependence**
  Source: Reuters Industry Breifing
  Date: January 02, 2002

- **Mechanism of cocaine 'high' pinpointed in mice**
  Source: Reuters Health eLine
  Date: April 26, 2001

- **Longer treatment helps severe cocaine addiction**
  Source: Reuters Health eLine
  Date: June 15, 1999

- **Mu Opioid Receptor Upregulation Linked To Cocaine Craving**
  Source: Reuters Medical News
  Date: October 31, 1996

The NIH

Within MEDLINEplus, the NIH has made an agreement with the New York Times Syndicate, the AP News Service, and Reuters to deliver news that can be browsed by the public. Search news releases at **http://www.nlm.nih.gov/medlineplus/alphanews_a.html**. MEDLINEplus allows you to browse across an alphabetical index. Or you can search by date at **http://www.nlm.nih.gov/medlineplus/newsbydate.html**. Often, news items are indexed by MEDLINEplus within their search engine.

Business Wire

Business Wire is similar to PR Newswire. To access this archive, simply go to **http://www.businesswire.com**. You can scan the news by industry category or company name.

Market Wire

Market Wire is more focused on technology than the other wires. To browse the latest press releases by topic, such as alternative medicine, biotechnology, fitness, healthcare, legal, nutrition, and pharmaceuticals, log on to Market Wire's Medical/Health channel at the following hyperlink **http://www.marketwire.com/mw/release_index?channel=MedicalHealth**. Market Wire's home page is **http://www.marketwire.com/mw/home**. From here, type "cocaine dependence" (or synonyms) into the search box, and click on "Search News." As this service is technology oriented, you may wish to use it when searching for press releases covering diagnostic procedures or tests.

Search Engines

Free-to-view news can also be found in the news section of your favorite search engines (see the health news page at Yahoo: **http://dir.yahoo.com/Health/News_and_Media/**, or use this Web site's general news search page **http://news.yahoo.com/**. Type in "cocaine dependence" (or synonyms). If you know the name of a company that is relevant to cocaine dependence, you can go to any stock trading Web site (such as **www.etrade.com**) and search for the company name there. News items across various news sources are reported on indicated hyperlinks.

BBC

Covering news from a more European perspective, the British Broadcasting Corporation (BBC) allows the public free access to their news archive located at **http://www.bbc.co.uk/**. Search by "cocaine dependence" (or synonyms).

Academic Periodicals covering Cocaine Dependence

Academic periodicals can be a highly technical yet valuable source of information on cocaine dependence. We have compiled the following list of periodicals known to publish articles relating to cocaine dependence and which are currently indexed within the National Library of Medicine's PubMed database (follow hyperlinks to view more information, summaries, etc., for each). In addition to these sources, to keep current on articles written on cocaine dependence published by any of the periodicals listed below, you can simply follow the hyperlink indicated or go to **www.ncbi.nlm.nih.gov/pubmed**. Type the periodical's name into the search box to find the latest studies published.

If you want complete details about the historical contents of a periodical, visit the Web site: **http://www.ncbi.nlm.nih.gov/entrez/jrbrowser.cgi**. Here, type in the name of the journal or its abbreviation, and you will receive an index of published articles. At **http://locatorplus.gov/** you can retrieve more indexing information on medical periodicals (e.g. the name of the publisher). Select the button "Search LOCATORplus." Then type in the name of the journal and select the advanced search option "Journal Title Search." The following is a sample of periodicals which publish articles on cocaine dependence:

- **Addiction (Abingdon, England). (Addiction)**
  http://www.ncbi.nlm.nih.gov/entrez/jrbrowser.cgi?field=0&regexp=Addiction+(Abingdon,+England)&dispmax=20&dispstart=0

- **Addictive Behaviors. (Addict Behav)**
  http://www.ncbi.nlm.nih.gov/entrez/jrbrowser.cgi?field=0&regexp=Addictive+Behaviors&dispmax=20&dispstart=0

- **American Journal of Medical Genetics. (Am J Med Genet)**
  http://www.ncbi.nlm.nih.gov/entrez/jrbrowser.cgi?field=0&regexp=American+Journal+of+Medical+Genetics&dispmax=20&dispstart=0

- **Annals of Clinical Psychiatry : Official Journal of the American Academy of Clinical Psychiatrists. (Ann Clin Psychiatry)**
  http://www.ncbi.nlm.nih.gov/entrez/jrbrowser.cgi?field=0&regexp=Annals+of+Clinical+Psychiatry+:+Official+Journal+of+the+American+Academy+of+Clinical+Psychiatrists&dispmax=20&dispstart=0

- **Annals of the New York Academy of Sciences. (Ann N Y Acad Sci)**
  http://www.ncbi.nlm.nih.gov/entrez/jrbrowser.cgi?field=0&regexp=An
  nals+of+the+New+York+Academy+of+Sciences&dispmax=20&dispstart
  =0

- **Annual Review of Medicine. (Annu Rev Med)**
  http://www.ncbi.nlm.nih.gov/entrez/jrbrowser.cgi?field=0&regexp=An
  nual+Review+of+Medicine&dispmax=20&dispstart=0

- **Archives of General Psychiatry. (Arch Gen Psychiatry)**
  http://www.ncbi.nlm.nih.gov/entrez/jrbrowser.cgi?field=0&regexp=Ar
  chives+of+General+Psychiatry&dispmax=20&dispstart=0

- **Archives of Internal Medicine. (Arch Intern Med)**
  http://www.ncbi.nlm.nih.gov/entrez/jrbrowser.cgi?field=0&regexp=Ar
  chives+of+Internal+Medicine&dispmax=20&dispstart=0

- **Behavior Modification. (Behav Modif)**
  http://www.ncbi.nlm.nih.gov/entrez/jrbrowser.cgi?field=0&regexp=Be
  havior+Modification&dispmax=20&dispstart=0

- **Biological Psychiatry. (Biol Psychiatry)**
  http://www.ncbi.nlm.nih.gov/entrez/jrbrowser.cgi?field=0&regexp=Bi
  ological+Psychiatry&dispmax=20&dispstart=0

- **Bipolar Disorders. (Bipolar Disord)**
  http://www.ncbi.nlm.nih.gov/entrez/jrbrowser.cgi?field=0&regexp=Bi
  polar+Disorders&dispmax=20&dispstart=0

- **British Journal of Addiction. (Br J Addict)**
  http://www.ncbi.nlm.nih.gov/entrez/jrbrowser.cgi?field=0&regexp=Bri
  tish+Journal+of+Addiction&dispmax=20&dispstart=0

- **Canadian Journal of Psychiatry. Revue Canadienne De Psychiatrie. (Can J Psychiatry)**
  http://www.ncbi.nlm.nih.gov/entrez/jrbrowser.cgi?field=0&regexp=Ca
  nadian+Journal+of+Psychiatry.+Revue+Canadienne+De+Psychiatrie&di
  spmax=20&dispstart=0

- **Clinical Neuropharmacology. (Clin Neuropharmacol)**
  http://www.ncbi.nlm.nih.gov/entrez/jrbrowser.cgi?field=0&regexp=Cli
  nical+Neuropharmacology&dispmax=20&dispstart=0

- **Clinical Pharmacology and Therapeutics. (Clin Pharmacol Ther)**
  http://www.ncbi.nlm.nih.gov/entrez/jrbrowser.cgi?field=0&regexp=Clinical+Pharmacology+and+Therapeutics&dispmax=20&dispstart=0

- **Comprehensive Psychiatry. (Compr Psychiatry)**
  http://www.ncbi.nlm.nih.gov/entrez/jrbrowser.cgi?field=0&regexp=Comprehensive+Psychiatry&dispmax=20&dispstart=0

- **Current Psychiatry Reports. (Curr Psychiatry Rep)**
  http://www.ncbi.nlm.nih.gov/entrez/jrbrowser.cgi?field=0&regexp=Current+Psychiatry+Reports&dispmax=20&dispstart=0

- **Drug and Alcohol Dependence. (Drug Alcohol Depend)**
  http://www.ncbi.nlm.nih.gov/entrez/jrbrowser.cgi?field=0&regexp=Drug+and+Alcohol+Dependence&dispmax=20&dispstart=0

- **Experimental and Clinical Psychopharmacology. (Exp Clin Psychopharmacol)**
  http://www.ncbi.nlm.nih.gov/entrez/jrbrowser.cgi?field=0&regexp=Experimental+and+Clinical+Psychopharmacology&dispmax=20&dispstart=0

- **Journal of Addictive Diseases : the Official Journal of the Asam, American Society of Addiction Medicine. (J Addict Dis)**
  http://www.ncbi.nlm.nih.gov/entrez/jrbrowser.cgi?field=0&regexp=Journal+of+Addictive+Diseases+:+the+Official+Journal+of+the+Asam,+American+Society+of+Addiction+Medicine&dispmax=20&dispstart=0

- **Journal of Clinical Psychopharmacology. (J Clin Psychopharmacol)**
  http://www.ncbi.nlm.nih.gov/entrez/jrbrowser.cgi?field=0&regexp=Journal+of+Clinical+Psychopharmacology&dispmax=20&dispstart=0

- **Journal of Consulting and Clinical Psychology. (J Consult Clin Psychol)**
  http://www.ncbi.nlm.nih.gov/entrez/jrbrowser.cgi?field=0&regexp=Journal+of+Consulting+and+Clinical+Psychology&dispmax=20&dispstart=0

- **Journal of Personality Assessment. (J Pers Assess)**
  http://www.ncbi.nlm.nih.gov/entrez/jrbrowser.cgi?field=0&regexp=Jo

urnal+of+Personality+Assessment&dispmax=20&dispstart=0

- **Journal of Personality Disorders. (J Personal Disord)**
  http://www.ncbi.nlm.nih.gov/entrez/jrbrowser.cgi?field=0&regexp=Jo
  urnal+of+Personality+Disorders&dispmax=20&dispstart=0

- **Journal of Psychopharmacology (Oxford, England). (J Psychopharmacol)**
  http://www.ncbi.nlm.nih.gov/entrez/jrbrowser.cgi?field=0&regexp=Jo
  urnal+of+Psychopharmacology+(Oxford,+England)&dispmax=20&disps
  tart=0

- **Journal of Substance Abuse Treatment. (J Subst Abuse Treat)**
  http://www.ncbi.nlm.nih.gov/entrez/jrbrowser.cgi?field=0&regexp=Jo
  urnal+of+Substance+Abuse+Treatment&dispmax=20&dispstart=0

- **Journal of Substance Abuse. (J Subst Abuse)**
  http://www.ncbi.nlm.nih.gov/entrez/jrbrowser.cgi?field=0&regexp=Jo
  urnal+of+Substance+Abuse&dispmax=20&dispstart=0

- **Molecular Psychiatry. (Mol Psychiatry)**
  http://www.ncbi.nlm.nih.gov/entrez/jrbrowser.cgi?field=0&regexp=M
  olecular+Psychiatry&dispmax=20&dispstart=0

- **Neuropsychopharmacology : Official Publication of the American College of Neuropsychopharmacology. (Neuropsychopharmacology)**
  http://www.ncbi.nlm.nih.gov/entrez/jrbrowser.cgi?field=0&regexp=Ne
  uropsychopharmacology+:+Official+Publication+of+the+American+Coll
  ege+of+Neuropsychopharmacology&dispmax=20&dispstart=0

- **Psychiatric Genetics. (Psychiatr Genet)**
  http://www.ncbi.nlm.nih.gov/entrez/jrbrowser.cgi?field=0&regexp=Ps
  ychiatric+Genetics&dispmax=20&dispstart=0

- **Psychiatric Services (Washington, D... (Psychiatr Serv)**
  http://www.ncbi.nlm.nih.gov/entrez/jrbrowser.cgi?field=0&regexp=Ps
  ychiatric+Services+(Washington,+D.+.+&dispmax=20&dispstart=0

- **Psychiatry Research. (Psychiatry Res)**
  http://www.ncbi.nlm.nih.gov/entrez/jrbrowser.cgi?field=0&regexp=Ps
  ychiatry+Research&dispmax=20&dispstart=0

- **Psychology of Addictive Behaviors : Journal of the Society of Psychologists in Addictive Behaviors. (Psychol Addict Behav)**
  http://www.ncbi.nlm.nih.gov/entrez/jrbrowser.cgi?field=0&regexp=Psychology+of+Addictive+Behaviors+:+Journal+of+the+Society+of+Psychologists+in+Addictive+Behaviors&dispmax=20&dispstart=0

- **Psychopharmacology Bulletin. (Psychopharmacol Bull)**
  http://www.ncbi.nlm.nih.gov/entrez/jrbrowser.cgi?field=0&regexp=Psychopharmacology+Bulletin&dispmax=20&dispstart=0

- **Public Health Reports (Washington, D.. : 1974). (Public Health Rep)**
  http://www.ncbi.nlm.nih.gov/entrez/jrbrowser.cgi?field=0&regexp=Public+Health+Reports+(Washington,+D.+.+:+1974)&dispmax=20&dispstart=0

- **Substance Use & Misuse. (Subst Use Misuse)**
  http://www.ncbi.nlm.nih.gov/entrez/jrbrowser.cgi?field=0&regexp=Substance+Use+&+Misuse&dispmax=20&dispstart=0

- **The American Journal of Drug and Alcohol Abuse. (Am J Drug Alcohol Abuse)**
  http://www.ncbi.nlm.nih.gov/entrez/jrbrowser.cgi?field=0&regexp=The+American+Journal+of+Drug+and+Alcohol+Abuse&dispmax=20&dispstart=0

- **The American Journal of Medicine. (Am J Med)**
  http://www.ncbi.nlm.nih.gov/entrez/jrbrowser.cgi?field=0&regexp=The+American+Journal+of+Medicine&dispmax=20&dispstart=0

- **The American Journal of Psychiatry. (Am J Psychiatry)**
  http://www.ncbi.nlm.nih.gov/entrez/jrbrowser.cgi?field=0&regexp=The+American+Journal+of+Psychiatry&dispmax=20&dispstart=0

- **The American Journal on Addictions / American Academy of Psychiatrists in Alcoholism and Addictions. (Am J Addict)**
  http://www.ncbi.nlm.nih.gov/entrez/jrbrowser.cgi?field=0&regexp=The+American+Journal+on+Addictions+/+American+Academy+of+Psychiatrists+in+Alcoholism+and+Addictions&dispmax=20&dispstart=0

- **The Journal of Clinical Endocrinology and Metabolism. (J Clin Endocrinol Metab)**
  http://www.ncbi.nlm.nih.gov/entrez/jrbrowser.cgi?field=0&regexp=The+Journal+of+Clinical+Endocrinology+and+Metabolism&dispmax=20&dispstart=0

- **The Journal of Clinical Psychiatry. (J Clin Psychiatry)**
  http://www.ncbi.nlm.nih.gov/entrez/jrbrowser.cgi?field=0&regexp=The+Journal+of+Clinical+Psychiatry&dispmax=20&dispstart=0

- **The Journal of Nervous and Mental Disease. (J Nerv Ment Dis)**
  http://www.ncbi.nlm.nih.gov/entrez/jrbrowser.cgi?field=0&regexp=The+Journal+of+Nervous+and+Mental+Disease&dispmax=20&dispstart=0

- **The Journal of Psychotherapy Practice and Research. (J Psychother Pract Res)**
  http://www.ncbi.nlm.nih.gov/entrez/jrbrowser.cgi?field=0&regexp=The+Journal+of+Psychotherapy+Practice+and+Research&dispmax=20&dispstart=0

- **The Nurse Practitioner. (Nurse Pract)**
  http://www.ncbi.nlm.nih.gov/entrez/jrbrowser.cgi?field=0&regexp=The+Nurse+Practitioner&dispmax=20&dispstart=0

- **The Psychiatric Clinics of North America. (Psychiatr Clin North Am)**
  http://www.ncbi.nlm.nih.gov/entrez/jrbrowser.cgi?field=0&regexp=The+Psychiatric+Clinics+of+North+America&dispmax=20&dispstart=0

- **The Western Journal of Medicine. (West J Med)**
  http://www.ncbi.nlm.nih.gov/entrez/jrbrowser.cgi?field=0&regexp=The+Western+Journal+of+Medicine&dispmax=20&dispstart=0

CHAPTER 7. PHYSICIAN GUIDELINES AND DATABASES

Overview

Doctors and medical researchers rely on a number of information sources to help patients with their conditions. Many will subscribe to journals or newsletters published by their professional associations or refer to specialized textbooks or clinical guides published for the medical profession. In this chapter, we focus on databases and Internet-based guidelines created or written for this professional audience.

NIH Guidelines

For the more common diseases, The National Institutes of Health publish guidelines that are frequently consulted by physicians. Publications are typically written by one or more of the various NIH Institutes. For physician guidelines, commonly referred to as "clinical" or "professional" guidelines, you can visit the following Institutes:

- Office of the Director (OD); guidelines consolidated across agencies available at **http://www.nih.gov/health/consumer/conkey.htm**

- National Institute of General Medical Sciences (NIGMS); fact sheets available at **http://www.nigms.nih.gov/news/facts/**

- National Library of Medicine (NLM); extensive encyclopedia (A.D.A.M., Inc.) with guidelines:
  http://www.nlm.nih.gov/medlineplus/healthtopics.html

- National Institute on Drug Abuse (NIDA); guidelines available at
  http://www.nida.nih.gov/DrugAbuse.html

NIH Databases

In addition to the various Institutes of Health that publish professional guidelines, the NIH has designed a number of databases for professionals.[25] Physician-oriented resources provide a wide variety of information related to the biomedical and health sciences, both past and present. The format of these resources varies. Searchable databases, bibliographic citations, full text articles (when available), archival collections, and images are all available. The following are referenced by the National Library of Medicine:[26]

- **Bioethics:** Access to published literature on the ethical, legal and public policy issues surrounding healthcare and biomedical research. This information is provided in conjunction with the Kennedy Institute of Ethics located at Georgetown University, Washington, D.C.: **http://www.nlm.nih.gov/databases/databases_bioethics.html**

- **HIV/AIDS Resources:** Describes various links and databases dedicated to HIV/AIDS research: **http://www.nlm.nih.gov/pubs/factsheets/aidsinfs.html**

- **NLM Online Exhibitions:** Describes "Exhibitions in the History of Medicine": **http://www.nlm.nih.gov/exhibition/exhibition.html**. Additional resources for historical scholarship in medicine: **http://www.nlm.nih.gov/hmd/hmd.html**

- **Biotechnology Information:** Access to public databases. The National Center for Biotechnology Information conducts research in computational biology, develops software tools for analyzing genome data, and disseminates biomedical information for the better understanding of molecular processes affecting human health and disease: **http://www.ncbi.nlm.nih.gov/**

- **Population Information:** The National Library of Medicine provides access to worldwide coverage of population, family planning, and related health issues, including family planning technology and programs, fertility, and population law and policy: **http://www.nlm.nih.gov/databases/databases_population.html**

- **Cancer Information:** Access to caner-oriented databases: **http://www.nlm.nih.gov/databases/databases_cancer.html**

---

[25] Remember, for the general public, the National Library of Medicine recommends the databases referenced in MEDLINE*plus* (**http://medlineplus.gov/** or **http://www.nlm.nih.gov/medlineplus/databases.html**).
[26] See **http://www.nlm.nih.gov/databases/databases.html**.

- **Profiles in Science:** Offering the archival collections of prominent twentieth-century biomedical scientists to the public through modern digital technology: **http://www.profiles.nlm.nih.gov/**

- **Chemical Information:** Provides links to various chemical databases and references: **http://sis.nlm.nih.gov/Chem/ChemMain.html**

- **Clinical Alerts:** Reports the release of findings from the NIH-funded clinical trials where such release could significantly affect morbidity and mortality: **http://www.nlm.nih.gov/databases/alerts/clinical_alerts.html**

- **Space Life Sciences:** Provides links and information to space-based research (including NASA): **http://www.nlm.nih.gov/databases/databases_space.html**

- **MEDLINE:** Bibliographic database covering the fields of medicine, nursing, dentistry, veterinary medicine, the healthcare system, and the pre-clinical sciences: **http://www.nlm.nih.gov/databases/databases_medline.html**

- **Toxicology and Environmental Health Information (TOXNET):** Databases covering toxicology and environmental health: **http://sis.nlm.nih.gov/Tox/ToxMain.html**

- **Visible Human Interface:** Anatomically detailed, three-dimensional representations of normal male and female human bodies: **http://www.nlm.nih.gov/research/visible/visible_human.html**

While all of the above references may be of interest to physicians who study and treat cocaine dependence, the following are particularly noteworthy.

The NLM Gateway[27]

The NLM (National Library of Medicine) Gateway is a Web-based system that lets users search simultaneously in multiple retrieval systems at the U.S. National Library of Medicine (NLM). It allows users of NLM services to initiate searches from one Web interface, providing "one-stop searching" for many of NLM's information resources or databases.[28] One target audience for the Gateway is the Internet user who is new to NLM's online resources and does not know what information is available or how best to search for it. This audience may include physicians and other healthcare providers,

---

[27] Adapted from NLM: **http://gateway.nlm.nih.gov/gw/Cmd?Overview.x.**
[28] The NLM Gateway is currently being developed by the Lister Hill National Center for Biomedical Communications (LHNCBC) at the National Library of Medicine (NLM) of the National Institutes of Health (NIH).

researchers, librarians, students, and, increasingly, patients, their families, and the public.[29] To use the NLM Gateway, simply go to the search site at **http://gateway.nlm.nih.gov/gw/Cmd**. Type "cocaine dependence" (or synonyms) into the search box and click "Search." The results will be presented in a tabular form, indicating the number of references in each database category.

Results Summary

Category	Items Found
Journal Articles	2433
Books / Periodicals / Audio Visual	47
Consumer Health	910
Meeting Abstracts	132
Other Collections	24
Total	3546

HSTAT[30]

HSTAT is a free, Web-based resource that provides access to full-text documents used in healthcare decision-making.[31] HSTAT's audience includes healthcare providers, health service researchers, policy makers, insurance companies, consumers, and the information professionals who serve these groups. HSTAT provides access to a wide variety of publications, including clinical practice guidelines, quick-reference guides for clinicians, consumer health brochures, evidence reports and technology assessments from the Agency for Healthcare Research and Quality (AHRQ), as well as AHRQ's Put Prevention Into Practice.[32] Simply search by "cocaine dependence" (or synonyms) at the following Web site: **http://text.nlm.nih.gov**.

---

[29] Other users may find the Gateway useful for an overall search of NLM's information resources. Some searchers may locate what they need immediately, while others will utilize the Gateway as an adjunct tool to other NLM search services such as PubMed® and MEDLINEplus®. The Gateway connects users with multiple NLM retrieval systems while also providing a search interface for its own collections. These collections include various types of information that do not logically belong in PubMed, LOCATORplus, or other established NLM retrieval systems (e.g., meeting announcements and pre-1966 journal citations). The Gateway will provide access to the information found in an increasing number of NLM retrieval systems in several phases.

[30] Adapted from HSTAT: **http://www.nlm.nih.gov/pubs/factsheets/hstat.html**.

[31] The HSTAT URL is **http://hstat.nlm.nih.gov/**.

[32] Other important documents in HSTAT include: the National Institutes of Health (NIH) Consensus Conference Reports and Technology Assessment Reports; the HIV/AIDS

Coffee Break: Tutorials for Biologists[33]

Some patients may wish to have access to a general healthcare site that takes a scientific view of the news and covers recent breakthroughs in biology that may one day assist physicians in developing treatments. To this end, we recommend "Coffee Break," a collection of short reports on recent biological discoveries. Each report incorporates interactive tutorials that demonstrate how bioinformatics tools are used as a part of the research process. Currently, all Coffee Breaks are written by NCBI staff.[34] Each report is about 400 words and is usually based on a discovery reported in one or more articles from recently published, peer-reviewed literature.[35] This site has new articles every few weeks, so it can be considered an online magazine of sorts, and intended for general background information. You can access Coffee Break at **http://www.ncbi.nlm.nih.gov/Coffeebreak/**.

Other Commercial Databases

In addition to resources maintained by official agencies, other databases exist that are commercial ventures addressing medical professionals. Here are some examples that may interest you:

- **CliniWeb International:** Index and table of contents to selected clinical information on the Internet; see **http://www.ohsu.edu/cliniweb/**.

- **Medical World Search:** Searches full text from thousands of selected medical sites on the Internet; see **http://www.mwsearch.com/**.

Treatment Information Service (ATIS) resource documents; the Substance Abuse and Mental Health Services Administration's Center for Substance Abuse Treatment (SAMHSA/CSAT) Treatment Improvement Protocols (TIP) and Center for Substance Abuse Prevention (SAMHSA/CSAP) Prevention Enhancement Protocols System (PEPS); the Public Health Service (PHS) Preventive Services Task Force's *Guide to Clinical Preventive Services*; the independent, nonfederal Task Force on Community Services *Guide to Community Preventive Services*; and the Health Technology Advisory Committee (HTAC) of the Minnesota Health Care Commission (MHCC) health technology evaluations.

[33] Adapted from **http://www.ncbi.nlm.nih.gov/Coffeebreak/Archive/FAQ.html**.

[34] The figure that accompanies each article is frequently supplied by an expert external to NCBI, in which case the source of the figure is cited. The result is an interactive tutorial that tells a biological story.

[35] After a brief introduction that sets the work described into a broader context, the report focuses on how a molecular understanding can provide explanations of observed biology and lead to therapies for diseases. Each vignette is accompanied by a figure and hypertext links that lead to a series of pages that interactively show how NCBI tools and resources are used in the research process.

CHAPTER 8. DISSERTATIONS ON COCAINE DEPENDENCE

Overview

University researchers are active in studying almost all known diseases. The result of research is often published in the form of Doctoral or Master's dissertations. You should understand, therefore, that applied diagnostic procedures and/or therapies can take many years to develop after the thesis that proposed the new technique or approach was written.

In this chapter, we will give you a bibliography on recent dissertations relating to cocaine dependence. You can read about these in more detail using the Internet or your local medical library. We will also provide you with information on how to use the Internet to stay current on dissertations.

Dissertations on Cocaine Dependence

ProQuest Digital Dissertations is the largest archive of academic dissertations available. From this archive, we have compiled the following list covering dissertations devoted to cocaine dependence. You will see that the information provided includes the dissertation's title, its author, and the author's institution. To read more about the following, simply use the Internet address indicated. The following covers recent dissertations dealing with cocaine dependence:

- **A CASE STUDY OF COCAINE USAGE BY STUDENT-ATHLETES AND SUBSTANCE ABUSE PROGRAMS FOR STUDENT-ATHLETES AT NCAA DIVISION I-A UNIVERSITIES** by ATKINSON, EVE, EDD from Temple University, 1991, 153 pages
http://wwwlib.umi.com/dissertations/fullcit/9134913

- **A COMPARATIVE STUDY OF BLACK COCAINE ADDICTS' SUCCESS PATTERNS THROUGH NATURAL RECOVERY AND/OR DRUG TREATMENT CENTER METHODS** by GATHRIGHT, WILLIAM MCKINLEY, PHD from Saint Louis University, 1991, 240 pages
http://wwwlib.umi.com/dissertations/fullcit/9130996

- **A COMPARISON OF SELF-INITIATED COPING BEHAVIORS IN PREMATURE AND LOW-BIRTHWEIGHT INFANTS-TODDLERS WITH AND WITHOUT PRENATAL COCAINE EXPOSURE (INFANTS, TODDLERS)** by TURNER, ALFREDA LYNETTE, PHD from University of California, Berkeley with San Francisco State Univ., 1995, 139 pages
http://wwwlib.umi.com/dissertations/fullcit/9621546

- **A multidimensional approach to the study of prenatal cocaine exposure** by Armbrister Edwards, Carla Denise; PhD from University of Florida, 2001, 117 pages
http://wwwlib.umi.com/dissertations/fullcit/3039760

- **A STUDY OF COGNITIVE AND BEHAVIOR MODIFICATION TECHNIQUES IN SHORT TERM AFTER CARE (CONTINUING CARE) GROUP THERAPY WITH COCAINE CRACK ADDICTS IN THE PREVENTION OF RELAPSE (ADDICTION, CHEMICAL DEPENDENCY)** by DICKERSON, LEON, PHD from New York University, 1994, 139 pages
http://wwwlib.umi.com/dissertations/fullcit/9502372

- **A STUDY OF THE EFFECTS OF FETAL COCAINE EXPOSURE ON SELECTED LANGUAGE SKILLS OF CHILDREN FROM TWELVE TO EIGHTEEN MONTHS OF AGE (DRUG EXPOSURE)** by WHITE, BARBARA ANN MORGAN, EDD from Seattle University, 1992, 142 pages
http://wwwlib.umi.com/dissertations/fullcit/9231344

- **A STUDY OF THE SOCIAL BEHAVIORS OF YOUNG CHILDREN EXPOSED TO CRACK COCAINE BEFORE BIRTH (PRENATAL DRUG EXPOSURE)** by KOSTELL, PATRICIA HOFFMAN, PHD from University of South Carolina, 1993, 200 pages
http://wwwlib.umi.com/dissertations/fullcit/9410018

- **Activator of G-protein signaling 3: A cocaine addiction gatekeeper** by Bowers, Michael Scott; PhD from Medical University of South Carolina, 2003, 141 pages
  http://wwwlib.umi.com/dissertations/fullcit/3098202

- **An analysis of urban smokable cocaine clients' perception of intensive out-patient treatment dynamics and treatment outcome** by Taylor, Christie Crews, EdD from Texas Southern University, 1998, 132 pages
  http://wwwlib.umi.com/dissertations/fullcit/9917516

- **AN EMPIRICAL STUDY OF SELECTED URBAN SCHOOL ADMINISTRATORS' PERCEPTIONS REGARDING THE BEHAVIORS OF STUDENTS PRENATALLY EXPOSED TO COCAINE (URBAN EDUCATION)** by SCALES, JOYCE MARIE WALKER, EDD from Texas Southern University, 1993, 162 pages
  http://wwwlib.umi.com/dissertations/fullcit/9433151

- **An examination of the family histories, social support systems, perceived life difficulties and role definitions of grandparents raising grandchildren who were prenatally cocaine exposed** by Katz, Lynne Feldman, EdD from University of Miami, 1999, 110 pages
  http://wwwlib.umi.com/dissertations/fullcit/9934237

- **BETWEEN A ROCK AND A HARD PLACE: CURRICULUM DEVELOPMENT IN A PRESCHOOL DEVOTED TO CHILDREN WHO HAVE BEEN PRENATALLY EXPOSED TO COCAINE AND OTHER DANGEROUS DRUGS (DRUG EXPOSURE)** by SAUDI, JAMILA KARIMA, PHD from Stanford University, 1995, 158 pages
  http://wwwlib.umi.com/dissertations/fullcit/9602953

- **DEVELOPMENTAL OUTCOMES IN TWO GROUPS OF INFANTS AND TODDLERS: PRENATAL COCAINE EXPOSED AND NON-COCAINE EXPOSED** by CHAPMAN, JOHN KEITH, PHD from The University of Alabama, 1994, 136 pages
  http://wwwlib.umi.com/dissertations/fullcit/9508487

- **EFFECTS OF A VIDEOTAPED FAMILY INTERVENTION ON THE DENIAL LEVEL OF ALCOHOLICS AND COCAINE ABUSERS** by RICHARDSON, DONALD RAY, PHD from Memphis State University, 1992, 87 pages
  http://wwwlib.umi.com/dissertations/fullcit/9239627

- **EVALUATING THE RELATIVE EFFICACY OF THREE AVERSION THERAPIES DESIGNED TO REDUCE CRAVING AMONG MALE COCAINE ABUSERS** by BORDNICK, PATRICK SHANNON, PHD from University of Georgia, 1995, 119 pages
  http://wwwlib.umi.com/dissertations/fullcit/9604021

- **FAMILY HISTORY AND PATTERNS OF ADDICTION IN AFRICAN-AMERICAN COCAINE AND ALCOHOL DEPENDENT INDIVIDUALS** by FORD, SABRINA, PHD from The University of Iowa, 1990, 215 pages
  http://wwwlib.umi.com/dissertations/fullcit/9112423

- **GLIMPSES OF HEAVEN: A PHENOMENOLOGICAL STUDY OF PERCEPTIONS OF COCAINE USE AND PERSONAL EMPOWERMENT (SELF MEDICATION)** by GLAUSER, ANN SHANKS, PHD from University of Georgia, 1992, 174 pages
  http://wwwlib.umi.com/dissertations/fullcit/9316341

- **Impaired intrinsic gating mechanisms of prefrontal cortical activity after repeated cocaine exposure** by Sidiropoulou, Kyriaki; PhD from The Herman M. Finch U. of Health Sciences - the Chicago Medical Sch., 2003, 169 pages
  http://wwwlib.umi.com/dissertations/fullcit/3102147

- **In utero exposure to crack cocaine and its behavioral outcomes among children in special education** by Washington, Curtis Dean; PhD from Walden University, 2002, 200 pages
  http://wwwlib.umi.com/dissertations/fullcit/3099948

- **Investigation of the pharmacological MRI signal induced by cocaine or heroin in rat brain** by Luo, Feng; PhD from The Medical College of Wisconsin, 2004, 142 pages
  http://wwwlib.umi.com/dissertations/fullcit/3109934

- **MODERN DRUG, MODERN MENACE: THE LEGAL USE AND DISTRIBUTION OF COCAINE IN THE UNITED STATES, 1880-1920** by SPILLANE, JOSEPH FRANCIS, PHD from Carnegie-Mellon University, 1994, 399 pages
  http://wwwlib.umi.com/dissertations/fullcit/9519035

- **Motivation for cocaine abuse treatment: Can the Addiction Severity Index be used at treatment intake to predict during-treatment outcomes?** by Linder, Paul R.; PhD from Temple University, 2003, 88 pages
  http://wwwlib.umi.com/dissertations/fullcit/3112294

- **Neurochemical mechanisms within the mesolimbic dopamine system of sensitization to the locomotor-stimulating effect of cocaine in rodents** by Licata, Stephanie Christine; PhD from Boston University, 2003, 142 pages
  http://wwwlib.umi.com/dissertations/fullcit/3084841

- **Nonlinear dynamics of the electroencephalogram of infants with prenatal cocaine exposure during sleep** by Chaicharn, Jarree; MS from University of Southern California, 2003, 36 pages
http://wwwlib.umi.com/dissertations/fullcit/1416538

- **Noradrenergic neurotransmission in the prefrontal cortex: Effects of prenatal cocaine exposure** by Mitra, Jayashree; PhD from Yale University, 2003, 185 pages
http://wwwlib.umi.com/dissertations/fullcit/3109434

- **PARENT-CHILD INTERACTION OF ONE COCAINE EXPOSED TODDLER IN A FOSTER-ADOPTIVE FAMILY** by MCCLINTON, GWENDOLYN ELAINE, EDD from University of Cincinnati, 1994, 131 pages
http://wwwlib.umi.com/dissertations/fullcit/9502573

- **PERCEIVED FAMILY DYNAMICS OF COCAINE ABUSERS, AS COMPARED TO OPIATE ABUSERS AND NON-DRUG ABUSERS** by DOUGLAS, LORRAINE JEAN, PHD from University of Florida, 1987, 168 pages
http://wwwlib.umi.com/dissertations/fullcit/8809631

- **Performance of school-age children of prenatal cocaine exposure: Five case studies** by Wallace, Susan Larson, EdD from The College of William and Mary, 1996, 292 pages
http://wwwlib.umi.com/dissertations/fullcit/9701098

- **Prenatal cocaine exposure and enduring cognitive dysfunction: Evidence from an animal model** by Gendle, Mathew Hayden; PhD from Cornell University, 2003, 167 pages
http://wwwlib.umi.com/dissertations/fullcit/3104589

- **Prenatal exposure to cocaine and other substances: Its effect on newborn behavior and subsequent attachment behavior** by Bombardier, Cynthia Lee, EdD from University of Massachusetts Amherst, 1997, 130 pages
http://wwwlib.umi.com/dissertations/fullcit/9737507

- **PROBLEM-SOLVING ABILITY OF YOUNG CHILDREN WITH PRENATAL COCAINE EXPOSURE (COCAINE, BRAIN FUNCTIONING)** by LIEBERTHAL, YOLETTA, PHD from University of California, Los Angeles, 1993, 103 pages
http://wwwlib.umi.com/dissertations/fullcit/9318749

- **Repeated cocaine administration alters medium spiny neuron excitability in the nucleus accumbens core and shell** by Basu, Somnath; PhD from The Herman M. Finch U. of Health Sciences - the Chicago Medical Sch., 2003, 126 pages
  http://wwwlib.umi.com/dissertations/fullcit/3102137

- **Role of the subicular regions of the rat hippocampus on cognitive task performance and cocaine self-administration and reinstatement behavior** by Black, Yolanda D.; PhD from Boston University, 2004, 110 pages
  http://wwwlib.umi.com/dissertations/fullcit/3101067

- **SNOW JOB? THE EFFICACY OF SOURCE COUNTRY COCAINE POLICIES (BOLIVIA, COLOMBIA, PERU)** by RILEY, KEVIN JACK, PHD from The Rand Graduate Institute, 1993, 190 pages
  http://wwwlib.umi.com/dissertations/fullcit/9332737

- **TEACHER EXPECTATIONS OF THE BEHAVIORS OF CHILDREN WITH PRENATAL COCAINE EXPOSURE** by MUMMERT, DARLOS K., EDD from Illinois State University, 1995, 118 pages
  http://wwwlib.umi.com/dissertations/fullcit/9633399

- **THE COCAINE CULTURE IN AFTER HOURS CLUBS.** by WILLIAMS, TERRY MOSES, PHD from City University of New York, 1978, 264 pages
  http://wwwlib.umi.com/dissertations/fullcit/7818825

- **The development of assays and their application in elaborating the pharmacokinetic disposition of cocaine and its metabolites in the mature dog** by Boni, Riccardo L; PhD from The University of Manitoba (Canada), 1986
  http://wwwlib.umi.com/dissertations/fullcit/NL33892

- **The effects of perinatal exposure to cocaine on the medial amygdala and sexually dimorphic nucleus of the preoptic area in rats** by Hammond, Heather Lynesse; MS from Loyola University of Chicago, 2003, 83 pages
  http://wwwlib.umi.com/dissertations/fullcit/1413566

- **THE EFFECTS OF PRENATAL COCAINE EXPOSURE ON EARLY CHILDHOOD DEVELOPMENT** by WALLACE, NANCY VIRGINIA, PHD from State University of New York at Buffalo, 1995, 75 pages
  http://wwwlib.umi.com/dissertations/fullcit/9603666

- **The impact of prenatal cocaine use on maternal reflective functioning** by Levy, Dahlia Wohlgemuth; PhD from City University of New York, 2003, 105 pages
  http://wwwlib.umi.com/dissertations/fullcit/3083680

- **The life of a cell: Managerial practice and strategy in Colombian cocaine distribution in the United States** by Fuentes, Joseph Ricardo, PhD from City University of New York, 1998, 309 pages
http://wwwlib.umi.com/dissertations/fullcit/9830708

- **The mode of action of cocaine in producing supersensitivity to noradrenaline in the human umbilical artery** by Triggle, C. R; PhD from University of Alberta (Canada), 1972
http://wwwlib.umi.com/dissertations/fullcit/NK11172

- **The neuropsychological effects of cocaine addiction with and without alcohol abuse** by Justice, Ananda K.; MA from Florida Atlantic University, 2003, 47 pages
http://wwwlib.umi.com/dissertations/fullcit/1417206

- **The war on drugs and the black female: Testing the impact of the sentencing policies for crack cocaine on black females in the federal system** by Bush-Baskette, Stephanie Regina; PhD from Rutgers the State University of New Jersey - Newark, 2000, 216 pages
http://wwwlib.umi.com/dissertations/fullcit/9967091

- **Three empirical essays on economic causes and consequences of marijuana and cocaine use** by DeSimone, Jeffrey Scott, PhD from Yale University, 1998, 135 pages
http://wwwlib.umi.com/dissertations/fullcit/9925572

- **TOWARD A BASIS FOR TREATMENT MATCHING FOR PREGNANT/POST-PARTUM CRACK COCAINE USERS: A PRELIMINARY STUDY OF CLINICAL PROFILES, PERCEIVED TREATMENT NEEDS, AND DRUG ABUSE ETIOLOGIES** by HIGGS, KERRY I., PHD from University of South Florida, 1995, 209 pages
http://wwwlib.umi.com/dissertations/fullcit/9542074

- **Wild hunger: Crack cocaine and heroin dependency in postcolonial Ghana** by Owusu-Darkwa, Lily Nana Abena; PhD from Univ. of Calif., Berkeley with the Univ. of Calif., San Francisco, 2001, 263 pages
http://wwwlib.umi.com/dissertations/fullcit/3044810

Keeping Current

As previously mentioned, an effective way to stay current on dissertations dedicated to cocaine dependence is to use the database called *ProQuest Digital Dissertations* via the Internet, located at the following Web address: **http://wwwlib.umi.com/dissertations.** The site allows you to freely access the last two years of citations and abstracts. Ask your medical librarian if the library has full and unlimited access to this database. From the library, you should be able to do more complete searches than with the limited 2-year access available to the general public.

Vocabulary Builder

The following vocabulary builder provides definitions of words used in this chapter that have not been defined in previous chapters:

Excitability: Property of a cardiac cell whereby, when the cell is depolarized to a critical level (called threshold), the membrane becomes permeable and a regenerative inward current causes an action potential. [NIH]

PART III. APPENDICES

ABOUT PART III

Part III is a collection of appendices on general medical topics which may be of interest to patients with cocaine dependence and related conditions.

APPENDIX A. RESEARCHING YOUR MEDICATIONS

Overview

There are a number of sources available on new or existing medications which could be prescribed to patients with cocaine dependence. While a number of hard copy or CD-Rom resources are available to patients and physicians for research purposes, a more flexible method is to use Internet-based databases. In this chapter, we will begin with a general overview of medications. We will then proceed to outline official recommendations on how you should view your medications. You may also want to research medications that you are currently taking for other conditions as they may interact with medications for cocaine dependence. Research can give you information on the side effects, interactions, and limitations of prescription drugs used in the treatment of cocaine dependence. Broadly speaking, there are two sources of information on approved medications: public sources and private sources. We will emphasize free-to-use public sources.

Your Medications: The Basics[36]

The Agency for Health Care Research and Quality has published extremely useful guidelines on how you can best participate in the medication aspects of cocaine dependence. Taking medicines is not always as simple as swallowing a pill. It can involve many steps and decisions each day. The AHCRQ recommends that patients with cocaine dependence take part in treatment decisions. Do not be afraid to ask questions and talk about your concerns. By taking a moment to ask questions early, you may avoid

---

[36] This section has been adapted from AHCRQ:
http://www.ahcpr.gov/consumer/ncpiebro.htm.

problems later. Here are some points to cover each time a new medicine is prescribed:

- Ask about all parts of your treatment, including diet changes, exercise, and medicines.

- Ask about the risks and benefits of each medicine or other treatment you might receive.

- Ask how often you or your doctor will check for side effects from a given medication.

Do not hesitate to ask what is important to you about your medicines. You may want a medicine with the fewest side effects, or the fewest doses to take each day. You may care most about cost, or how the medicine might affect how you live or work. Or, you may want the medicine your doctor believes will work the best. Telling your doctor will help him or her select the best treatment for you.

Do not be afraid to "bother" your doctor with your concerns and questions about medications for cocaine dependence. You can also talk to a nurse or a pharmacist. They can help you better understand your treatment plan. Feel free to bring a friend or family member with you when you visit your doctor. Talking over your options with someone you trust can help you make better choices, especially if you are not feeling well. Specifically, ask your doctor the following:

- The name of the medicine and what it is supposed to do.

- How and when to take the medicine, how much to take, and for how long.

- What food, drinks, other medicines, or activities you should avoid while taking the medicine.

- What side effects the medicine may have, and what to do if they occur.

- If you can get a refill, and how often.

- About any terms or directions you do not understand.

- What to do if you miss a dose.

- If there is written information you can take home (most pharmacies have information sheets on your prescription medicines; some even offer large-print or Spanish versions).

Do not forget to tell your doctor about all the medicines you are currently taking (not just those for cocaine dependence). This includes prescription medicines and the medicines that you buy over the counter. Then your doctor can avoid giving you a new medicine that may not work well with the medications you take now. When talking to your doctor, you may wish to prepare a list of medicines you currently take, the reason you take them, and how you take them. Be sure to include the following information for each:

- Name of medicine

- Reason taken

- Dosage

- Time(s) of day

Also include any over-the-counter medicines, such as:

- Laxatives

- Diet pills

- Vitamins

- Cold medicine

- Aspirin or other pain, headache, or fever medicine

- Cough medicine

- Allergy relief medicine

- Antacids

- Sleeping pills

- Others (include names)

Learning More about Your Medications

Because of historical investments by various organizations and the emergence of the Internet, it has become rather simple to learn about the medications your doctor has recommended for cocaine dependence. One such source is the United States Pharmacopeia. In 1820, eleven physicians met in Washington, D.C. to establish the first compendium of standard drugs for the United States. They called this compendium the "U.S. Pharmacopeia (USP)." Today, the USP is a non-profit organization consisting of 800 volunteer scientists, eleven elected officials, and 400 representatives of state associations and colleges of medicine and pharmacy. The USP is located in Rockville, Maryland, and its home page is located at **www.usp.org**. The USP currently provides standards for over 3,700 medications. The resulting USP DI® Advice for the Patient® can be accessed through the National Library of

Medicine of the National Institutes of Health. The database is partially derived from lists of federally approved medications in the Food and Drug Administration's (FDA) Drug Approvals database.[37]

While the FDA database is rather large and difficult to navigate, the Phamacopeia is both user-friendly and free to use. It covers more than 9,000 prescription and over-the-counter medications. To access this database, simply type the following hyperlink into your Web browser: **http://www.nlm.nih.gov/medlineplus/druginformation.html**. To view examples of a given medication (brand names, category, description, preparation, proper use, precautions, side effects, etc.), simply follow the hyperlinks indicated within the United States Pharmacopeia (USP).

Of course, we as editors cannot be certain as to what medications you are taking. Therefore, we have compiled a list of medications associated with the treatment of cocaine dependence. Once again, due to space limitations, we only list a sample of medications and provide hyperlinks to ample documentation (e.g. typical dosage, side effects, drug-interaction risks, etc.). The following drugs have been mentioned in the Pharmacopeia and other sources as being potentially applicable to cocaine dependence:

Antidepressants, Tricyclic

- **Systemic - U.S. Brands:** Anafranil; Asendin; Aventyl; Elavil; Endep; Norfranil; Norpramin; Pamelor; Sinequan; Surmontil; Tipramine; Tofranil; Tofranil-PM; Vivactil
  http://www.nlm.nih.gov/medlineplus/druginfo/uspdi/202055.html

Commercial Databases

In addition to the medications listed in the USP above, a number of commercial sites are available by subscription to physicians and their institutions. You may be able to access these sources from your local medical library or your doctor's office.

---

[37] Though cumbersome, the FDA database can be freely browsed at the following site: **www.fda.gov/cder/da/da.htm**.

Reuters Health Drug Database

The Reuters Health Drug Database can be searched by keyword at the hyperlink: **http://www.reutershealth.com/frame2/drug.html**.

Mosby's GenRx

Mosby's GenRx database (also available on CD-Rom and book format) covers 45,000 drug products including generics and international brands. It provides prescribing information, drug interactions, and patient information. Information can be obtained at the following hyperlink: **http://www.genrx.com/Mosby/PhyGenRx/group.html**.

PDR*health*

The PDR*health* database is a free-to-use, drug information search engine that has been written for the public in layman's terms. It contains FDA-approved drug information adapted from the Physicians' Desk Reference (PDR) database. PDR*health* can be searched by brand name, generic name, or indication. It features multiple drug interactions reports. Search PDR*health* at **http://www.pdrhealth.com/drug_info/index.html**.

Other Web Sites

A number of additional Web sites discuss drug information. As an example, you may like to look at **www.drugs.com** which reproduces the information in the Pharmacopeia as well as commercial information. You may also want to consider the Web site of the Medical Letter, Inc. which allows users to download articles on various drugs and therapeutics for a nominal fee: **http://www.medletter.com/**.

Researching Orphan Drugs

Orphan drugs are a special class of pharmaceuticals used by patients who are unaffected by existing treatments or with illnesses for which no known drug is effective. Orphan drugs are most commonly prescribed or developed for "rare" diseases or conditions.[38] According to the FDA, an orphan drug (or

---

[38] The U.S. Food and Drug Administration defines a rare disease or condition as "any disease or condition which affects less than 200,000 persons in the United States, or affects

biological) may already be approved, or it may still be experimental. A drug becomes an "orphan" when it receives orphan designation from the Office of Orphan Products Development at the FDA.[39] Orphan designation qualifies the sponsor to receive certain benefits from the U.S. Government in exchange for developing the drug. The drug must then undergo the new drug approval process as any other drug would. To date, over 1000 orphan products have been designated, and over 200 have been approved for marketing. Historically, the approval time for orphan products as a group has been considerably shorter than the approval time for other drugs. This is due to the fact that many orphan products receive expedited review because they are developed for serious or life-threatening diseases.

The cost of orphan products is determined by the sponsor of the drug and can vary greatly. Reimbursement rates for drug expenses are set by each insurance company and outlined in your policy. Insurance companies will generally reimburse for orphan products that have been approved for marketing, but may not reimburse for products that are considered experimental. Consult your insurance company about specific reimbursement policies. If an orphan product has been approved for marketing, it will be available through the normal pharmaceutical supply channels. If the product has not been approved, the sponsor may make the product available on a compassionate-use basis.[40]

Although the list of orphan drugs is revised on a daily basis, you can quickly research orphan drugs that might be applicable to cocaine dependence using the database managed by the National Organization for Rare Disorders, Inc. (NORD), located at **www.raredisease.org**. Simply go to their general search page and select "Orphan Drug Designation Database." On this page (**http://www.rarediseases.org/search/noddsearch.html**), type "cocaine dependence" or a synonym into the search box and click "Submit Query." When you see a list of drugs, understand that not all of the drugs may be relevant. Some may have been withdrawn from orphan status. Write down or print out the name of each drug and the relevant contact information.

---

more than 200,000 in the United States and for which there is no reasonable expectation that the cost of developing and making available in the United States a drug for such disease or condition will be recovered from sales in the United States of such drug." Adapted from the U.S. Food and Drug Administration: **http://www.fda.gov/opacom/laws/orphandg.htm**.

[39] The following is adapted from the U.S. Food and Drug Administration: **http://www.fda.gov/orphan/faq/index.htm**.

[40] For contact information on sponsors of orphan products, contact the Office of Orphan Products Development (**http://www.fda.gov/orphan/**). General inquiries may be routed to the main office: Office of Orphan Products Development (HF-35); Food and Drug Administration, 5600 Fishers Lane, Rockville, MD 20857; Voice: (301) 827-3666 or (800) 300-7469; FAX: (301) 443-4915.

From there, visit the Pharmacopeia Web site and type the name of each orphan drug into the search box on **http://www.nlm.nih.gov/medlineplus/druginformation.html**. Read about each drug in detail and consult your doctor to find out if you might benefit from these medications. You or your physician may need to contact the sponsor or NORD.

NORD conducts "early access programs for investigational new drugs (IND) under the Food and Drug Administration's (FDA's) approval 'Treatment INDs' programs which allow for a limited number of individuals to receive investigational drugs before FDA marketing approval." If the orphan product about which you are seeking information is approved for marketing, information on side effects can be found on the product's label. If the product is not approved, you or your physician should consult the sponsor.

The following is a list of orphan drugs currently listed in the NORD Orphan Drug Designation Database for cocaine dependence or related conditions:

- **Butyrylcholinesterase**
  http://www.rarediseases.org/nord/search/nodd_full?code=687

Contraindications and Interactions (Hidden Dangers)

Some of the medications mentioned in the previous discussions can be problematic for patients with cocaine dependence--not because they are used in the treatment process, but because of contraindications, or side effects. Medications with contraindications are those that could react with drugs used to treat cocaine dependence or potentially create deleterious side effects in patients with cocaine dependence. You should ask your physician about any contraindications, especially as these might apply to other medications that you may be taking for common ailments.

Drug-drug interactions occur when two or more drugs react with each other. This drug-drug interaction may cause you to experience an unexpected side effect. Drug interactions may make your medications less effective, cause unexpected side effects, or increase the action of a particular drug. Some drug interactions can even be harmful to you.

Be sure to read the label every time you use a nonprescription or prescription drug, and take the time to learn about drug interactions. These precautions may be critical to your health. You can reduce the risk of potentially harmful drug interactions and side effects with a little bit of knowledge and common sense.

Drug labels contain important information about ingredients, uses, warnings, and directions which you should take the time to read and understand. Labels also include warnings about possible drug interactions. Further, drug labels may change as new information becomes available. This is why it's especially important to read the label every time you use a medication. When your doctor prescribes a new drug, discuss all over-the-counter and prescription medications, dietary supplements, vitamins, botanicals, minerals and herbals you take as well as the foods you eat. Ask your pharmacist for the package insert for each prescription drug you take. The package insert provides more information about potential drug interactions.

A Final Warning

At some point, you may hear of alternative medications from friends, relatives, or in the news media. Advertisements may suggest that certain alternative drugs can produce positive results for patients with cocaine dependence. Exercise caution--some of these drugs may have fraudulent claims, and others may actually hurt you. The Food and Drug Administration (FDA) is the official U.S. agency charged with discovering which medications are likely to improve the health of patients with cocaine dependence. The FDA warns patients to watch out for[41]:

- Secret formulas (real scientists share what they know)

- Amazing breakthroughs or miracle cures (real breakthroughs don't happen very often; when they do, real scientists do not call them amazing or miracles)

- Quick, painless, or guaranteed cures

- If it sounds too good to be true, it probably isn't true.

If you have any questions about any kind of medical treatment, the FDA may have an office near you. Look for their number in the blue pages of the phone book. You can also contact the FDA through its toll-free number, 1-888-INFO-FDA (1-888-463-6332), or on the World Wide Web at **www.fda.gov**.

---

[41] This section has been adapted from **http://www.fda.gov/opacom/lowlit/medfraud.html**.

General References

In addition to the resources provided earlier in this chapter, the following general references describe medications (sorted alphabetically by title; hyperlinks provide rankings, information and reviews at Amazon.com):

- **Complete Guide to Prescription and Nonprescription Drugs 2001 (Complete Guide to Prescription and Nonprescription Drugs, 2001)** by H. Winter Griffith, Paperback 16th edition (2001), Medical Surveillance; ISBN: 0942447417;
  http://www.amazon.com/exec/obidos/ASIN/039952634X/icongroupinter na

- **The Essential Guide to Prescription Drugs, 2001** by James J. Rybacki, James W. Long; Paperback - 1274 pages (2001), Harper Resource; ISBN: 0060958162;
  http://www.amazon.com/exec/obidos/ASIN/0060958162/icongroupinter na

- **Handbook of Commonly Prescribed Drugs** by G. John Digregorio, Edward J. Barbieri; Paperback 16th edition (2001), Medical Surveillance; ISBN: 0942447417;
  http://www.amazon.com/exec/obidos/ASIN/0942447417/icongroupinter na

- **Johns Hopkins Complete Home Encyclopedia of Drugs 2nd ed.** by Simeon Margolis (Ed.), Johns Hopkins; Hardcover - 835 pages (2000), Rebus; ISBN: 0929661583;
  http://www.amazon.com/exec/obidos/ASIN/0929661583/icongroupinter na

- **Medical Pocket Reference: Drugs 2002** by Springhouse Paperback 1st edition (2001), Lippincott Williams & Wilkins Publishers; ISBN: 1582550964;
  http://www.amazon.com/exec/obidos/ASIN/1582550964/icongroupinter na

- **PDR** by Medical Economics Staff, Medical Economics Staff Hardcover - 3506 pages 55th edition (2000), Medical Economics Company; ISBN: 1563633752;
  http://www.amazon.com/exec/obidos/ASIN/1563633752/icongroupinter na

- **Pharmacy Simplified: A Glossary of Terms** by James Grogan; Paperback - 432 pages, 1st edition (2001), Delmar Publishers; ISBN: 0766828581;
  http://www.amazon.com/exec/obidos/ASIN/0766828581/icongroupinter na

- **Physician Federal Desk Reference** by Christine B. Fraizer; Paperback 2nd edition (2001), Medicode Inc; ISBN: 1563373971; http://www.amazon.com/exec/obidos/ASIN/1563373971/icongroupinterna

- **Physician's Desk Reference Supplements** Paperback - 300 pages, 53 edition (1999), ISBN: 1563632950; http://www.amazon.com/exec/obidos/ASIN/1563632950/icongroupinterna

Vocabulary Builder

The following vocabulary builder provides definitions of words used in this chapter that have not been defined in previous chapters:

Compassionate: A process for providing experimental drugs to very sick patients who have no treatment options. [NIH]

Contraindications: Any factor or sign that it is unwise to pursue a certain kind of action or treatment, e. g. giving a general anesthetic to a person with pneumonia. [NIH]

APPENDIX B. RESEARCHING NUTRITION

Overview

Since the time of Hippocrates, doctors have understood the importance of diet and nutrition to patients' health and well-being. Since then, they have accumulated an impressive archive of studies and knowledge dedicated to this subject. Based on their experience, doctors and healthcare providers may recommend particular dietary supplements to patients with cocaine dependence. Any dietary recommendation is based on a patient's age, body mass, gender, lifestyle, eating habits, food preferences, and health condition. It is therefore likely that different patients with cocaine dependence may be given different recommendations. Some recommendations may be directly related to cocaine dependence, while others may be more related to the patient's general health. These recommendations, themselves, may differ from what official sources recommend for the average person.

In this chapter we will begin by briefly reviewing the essentials of diet and nutrition that will broadly frame more detailed discussions of cocaine dependence. We will then show you how to find studies dedicated specifically to nutrition and cocaine dependence.

Food and Nutrition: General Principles

What Are Essential Foods?

Food is generally viewed by official sources as consisting of six basic elements: (1) fluids, (2) carbohydrates, (3) protein, (4) fats, (5) vitamins, and (6) minerals. Consuming a combination of these elements is considered to be a healthy diet:

- **Fluids** are essential to human life as 80-percent of the body is composed of water. Water is lost via urination, sweating, diarrhea, vomiting, diuretics (drugs that increase urination), caffeine, and physical exertion.

- **Carbohydrates** are the main source for human energy (thermoregulation) and the bulk of typical diets. They are mostly classified as being either simple or complex. Simple carbohydrates include sugars which are often consumed in the form of cookies, candies, or cakes. Complex carbohydrates consist of starches and dietary fibers. Starches are consumed in the form of pastas, breads, potatoes, rice, and other foods. Soluble fibers can be eaten in the form of certain vegetables, fruits, oats, and legumes. Insoluble fibers include brown rice, whole grains, certain fruits, wheat bran and legumes.

- **Proteins** are eaten to build and repair human tissues. Some foods that are high in protein are also high in fat and calories. Food sources for protein include nuts, meat, fish, cheese, and other dairy products.

- **Fats** are consumed for both energy and the absorption of certain vitamins. There are many types of fats, with many general publications recommending the intake of unsaturated fats or those low in cholesterol.

Vitamins and minerals are fundamental to human health, growth, and, in some cases, disease prevention. Most are consumed in your diet (exceptions being vitamins K and D which are produced by intestinal bacteria and sunlight on the skin, respectively). Each vitamin and mineral plays a different role in health. The following outlines essential vitamins:

- **Vitamin A** is important to the health of your eyes, hair, bones, and skin; sources of vitamin A include foods such as eggs, carrots, and cantaloupe.

- **Vitamin B[1]**, also known as thiamine, is important for your nervous system and energy production; food sources for thiamine include meat, peas, fortified cereals, bread, and whole grains.

- **Vitamin B[2]**, also known as riboflavin, is important for your nervous system and muscles, but is also involved in the release of proteins from nutrients; food sources for riboflavin include dairy products, leafy vegetables, meat, and eggs.

- **Vitamin B[3]**, also known as niacin, is important for healthy skin and helps the body use energy; food sources for niacin include peas, peanuts, fish, and whole grains

- **Vitamin B[6]**, also known as pyridoxine, is important for the regulation of cells in the nervous system and is vital for blood formation; food sources for pyridoxine include bananas, whole grains, meat, and fish.

- **Vitamin B¹²** is vital for a healthy nervous system and for the growth of red blood cells in bone marrow; food sources for vitamin B¹² include yeast, milk, fish, eggs, and meat.

- **Vitamin C** allows the body's immune system to fight various diseases, strengthens body tissue, and improves the body's use of iron; food sources for vitamin C include a wide variety of fruits and vegetables.

- **Vitamin D** helps the body absorb calcium which strengthens bones and teeth; food sources for vitamin D include oily fish and dairy products.

- **Vitamin E** can help protect certain organs and tissues from various degenerative diseases; food sources for vitamin E include margarine, vegetables, eggs, and fish.

- **Vitamin K** is essential for bone formation and blood clotting; common food sources for vitamin K include leafy green vegetables.

- **Folic Acid** maintains healthy cells and blood and, when taken by a pregnant woman, can prevent her fetus from developing neural tube defects; food sources for folic acid include nuts, fortified breads, leafy green vegetables, and whole grains.

It should be noted that it is possible to overdose on certain vitamins which become toxic if consumed in excess (e.g. vitamin A, D, E and K).

Like vitamins, minerals are chemicals that are required by the body to remain in good health. Because the human body does not manufacture these chemicals internally, we obtain them from food and other dietary sources. The more important minerals include:

- **Calcium** is needed for healthy bones, teeth, and muscles, but also helps the nervous system function; food sources for calcium include dry beans, peas, eggs, and dairy products.

- **Chromium** is helpful in regulating sugar levels in blood; food sources for chromium include egg yolks, raw sugar, cheese, nuts, beets, whole grains, and meat.

- **Fluoride** is used by the body to help prevent tooth decay and to reinforce bone strength; sources of fluoride include drinking water and certain brands of toothpaste.

- **Iodine** helps regulate the body's use of energy by synthesizing into the hormone thyroxine; food sources include leafy green vegetables, nuts, egg yolks, and red meat.

- **Iron** helps maintain muscles and the formation of red blood cells and certain proteins; food sources for iron include meat, dairy products, eggs, and leafy green vegetables.

- **Magnesium** is important for the production of DNA, as well as for healthy teeth, bones, muscles, and nerves; food sources for magnesium include dried fruit, dark green vegetables, nuts, and seafood.

- **Phosphorous** is used by the body to work with calcium to form bones and teeth; food sources for phosphorous include eggs, meat, cereals, and dairy products.

- **Selenium** primarily helps maintain normal heart and liver functions; food sources for selenium include wholegrain cereals, fish, meat, and dairy products.

- **Zinc** helps wounds heal, the formation of sperm, and encourage rapid growth and energy; food sources include dried beans, shellfish, eggs, and nuts.

The United States government periodically publishes recommended diets and consumption levels of the various elements of food. Again, your doctor may encourage deviations from the average official recommendation based on your specific condition. To learn more about basic dietary guidelines, visit the Web site: **http://www.health.gov/dietaryguidelines/**. Based on these guidelines, many foods are required to list the nutrition levels on the food's packaging. Labeling Requirements are listed at the following site maintained by the Food and Drug Administration: **http://www.cfsan.fda.gov/~dms/lab-cons.html**. When interpreting these requirements, the government recommends that consumers become familiar with the following abbreviations before reading FDA literature:[42]

- **DVs (Daily Values):** A new dietary reference term that will appear on the food label. It is made up of two sets of references, DRVs and RDIs.

- **DRVs (Daily Reference Values):** A set of dietary references that applies to fat, saturated fat, cholesterol, carbohydrate, protein, fiber, sodium, and potassium.

- **RDIs (Reference Daily Intakes):** A set of dietary references based on the Recommended Dietary Allowances for essential vitamins and minerals and, in selected groups, protein. The name "RDI" replaces the term "U.S. RDA."

---

[42] Adapted from the FDA: **http://www.fda.gov/fdac/special/foodlabel/dvs.html**.

- **RDAs (Recommended Dietary Allowances):** A set of estimated nutrient allowances established by the National Academy of Sciences. It is updated periodically to reflect current scientific knowledge.

What Are Dietary Supplements?[43]

Dietary supplements are widely available through many commercial sources, including health food stores, grocery stores, pharmacies, and by mail. Dietary supplements are provided in many forms including tablets, capsules, powders, gel-tabs, extracts, and liquids. Historically in the United States, the most prevalent type of dietary supplement was a multivitamin/mineral tablet or capsule that was available in pharmacies, either by prescription or "over the counter." Supplements containing strictly herbal preparations were less widely available. Currently in the United States, a wide array of supplement products are available, including vitamin, mineral, other nutrients, and botanical supplements as well as ingredients and extracts of animal and plant origin.

The Office of Dietary Supplements (ODS) of the National Institutes of Health is the official agency of the United States which has the expressed goal of acquiring "new knowledge to help prevent, detect, diagnose, and treat disease and disability, from the rarest genetic disorder to the common cold."[44] According to the ODS, dietary supplements can have an important impact on the prevention and management of disease and on the maintenance of health.[45] The ODS notes that considerable research on the effects of dietary supplements has been conducted in Asia and Europe where the use of plant products, in particular, has a long tradition. However, the overwhelming majority of supplements have not been studied scientifically. To explore the role of dietary supplements in the improvement of health care, the ODS plans, organizes, and supports conferences, workshops, and

---

[43] This discussion has been adapted from the NIH:
http://ods.od.nih.gov/showpage.aspx?pageid=46.
[44] Contact: The Office of Dietary Supplements, National Institutes of Health, Building 31, Room 1B29, 31 Center Drive, MSC 2086, Bethesda, Maryland 20892-2086, Tel: (301) 435-2920, Fax: (301) 480-1845, E-mail: ods@nih.gov.
[45] Adapted from **http://ods.od.nih.gov/showpage.aspx?pageid=2**. The Dietary Supplement Health and Education Act defines dietary supplements as "a product (other than tobacco) intended to supplement the diet that bears or contains one or more of the following dietary ingredients: a vitamin, mineral, amino acid, herb or other botanical; or a dietary substance for use to supplement the diet by increasing the total dietary intake; or a concentrate, metabolite, constituent, extract, or combination of any ingredient described above; and intended for ingestion in the form of a capsule, powder, softgel, or gelcap, and not represented as a conventional food or as a sole item of a meal or the diet."

symposia on scientific topics related to dietary supplements. The ODS often works in conjunction with other NIH Institutes and Centers, other government agencies, professional organizations, and public advocacy groups.

To learn more about official information on dietary supplements, visit the ODS site at **http://dietary-supplements.info.nih.gov/**. Or contact:

The Office of Dietary Supplements
National Institutes of Health
Building 31, Room 1B29
31 Center Drive, MSC 2086
Bethesda, Maryland 20892-2086
Tel: (301) 435-2920
Fax: (301) 480-1845
E-mail: ods@nih.gov

Finding Studies on Cocaine Dependence

The NIH maintains an office dedicated to patient nutrition and diet. The National Institutes of Health's Office of Dietary Supplements (ODS) offers a searchable bibliographic database called the IBIDS (International Bibliographic Information on Dietary Supplements). The IBIDS contains over 460,000 scientific citations and summaries about dietary supplements and nutrition as well as references to published international, scientific literature on dietary supplements such as vitamins, minerals, and botanicals.[46] IBIDS is available to the public free of charge through the ODS Internet page: **http://ods.od.nih.gov/databases/ibids.html**.

After entering the search area, you have three choices: (1) IBIDS Consumer Database, (2) Full IBIDS Database, or (3) Peer Reviewed Citations Only. We recommend that you start with the Consumer Database. While you may not find references for the topics that are of most interest to you, check back periodically as this database is frequently updated. More studies can be found by searching the Full IBIDS Database. Healthcare professionals and researchers generally use the third option, which lists peer-reviewed citations. In all cases, we suggest that you take advantage of the "Advanced

---

[46] Adapted from **http://ods.od.nih.gov**. IBIDS is produced by the Office of Dietary Supplements (ODS) at the National Institutes of Health to assist the public, healthcare providers, educators, and researchers in locating credible, scientific information on dietary supplements. IBIDS was developed and will be maintained through an interagency partnership with the Food and Nutrition Information Center of the National Agricultural Library, U.S. Department of Agriculture.

Search" option that allows you to retrieve up to 100 fully explained references in a comprehensive format. Type "cocaine dependence" (or synonyms) into the search box. To narrow the search, you can also select the "Title" field.

The following information is typical of that found when using the "Full IBIDS Database" when searching using "cocaine dependence" (or a synonym):

- **Altered HPA axis responsivity to metyrapone testing in methadone maintained former heroin addicts with ongoing cocaine addiction.**
  Author(s): Laboratory of the Biology of Addictive Diseases, The Rockefeller University, New York, NY 10021-6399, USA.
  Source: Schluger, J H Borg, L Ho, A Kreek, M J Neuropsychopharmacology. 2001 May; 24(5): 568-75 0893-133X

- **Bronchial hyperreactivity in patients who inhale heroin mixed with cocaine vaporized on aluminum foil.**
  Author(s): Seccion de Respiratorio, Hospital Juan Ramon Jimenez, Huelva, Spain.
  Source: Boto de los Bueis, Ana Pereira Vega, Antonio Sanchez Ramos, Jose Luis Maldonado Perez, Jose Antonio Ayerbe Garcia, Rut Garcia Jimenez, Domingo Pujol de la Llave, Emilio Chest. 2002 April; 121(4): 1223-30 0012-3692

- **CNS recovery from cocaine, cocaine and alcohol, or opioid dependence: a P300 study.**
  Author(s): Department of Psychiatry MC2103, University of Connecticut School of Medicine, Farmington, CT 06030-2103, USA. bauer@psychiatry.uchc.edu
  Source: Bauer, L O Clin-Neurophysiol. 2001 August; 112(8): 1508-15 1388-2457

- **Cocaine-like discriminative stimulus effects of novel cocaine and 3-phenyltropane analogs in the rat.**
  Author(s): Department of Pharmacology & Toxicology, Virginia Commonwealth University, 410 North 12th Street, Smith Building, P.O. Box 980613, Richmond, VA 23298-0613, USA. ccook@hsc.vcu.edu
  Source: Cook, C D Carroll, I F Beardsley, P M Psychopharmacology-(Berl). 2001 December; 159(1): 58-63 0033-3158

- **Corticotropin-releasing factor receptor blockade enhances conditioned aversive properties of cocaine in rats.**
  Author(s): Neurocrine Biosciences Inc., San Diego, CA 92121, USA. sheinrichs@neurocrine.com

Source: Heinrichs, S C Klaassen, A Koob, G F Schulteis, G Ahmed, S De Souza, E B Psychopharmacology-(Berl). 1998 April; 136(3): 247-55 0033-3158

- **D3 receptor test in vitro predicts decreased cocaine self-administration in rats.**
  Author(s): Department of Neuropharmacology, Scripps Research Institute, La Jolla, CA, USA.
  Source: Caine, S B Koob, G F Parsons, L H Everitt, B J Schwartz, J C Sokoloff, P Neuroreport. 1997 July 7; 8(9-10): 2373-7 0959-4965

- **Decreasing intravenous cocaine use in opiate users treated with prescribed heroin.**
  Author(s): Addiction Research Institute, Zurich. riblae@riblae.ch
  Source: Blattler, Richard Dobler Mikola, Anja Steffen, Thomas Uchtenhagen, Ambros Soz-Praventivmed. 2002; 47(1): 24-32 0303-8408

- **Dizocilpine infusion has a different effect in the development of morphine and cocaine sensitization: behavioral and neurochemical aspects.**
  Author(s): Department 'Scienze del Farmaco', University of Sassari, 07100 Sassari, Italy.
  Source: Scheggi, S Mangiavacchi, S Masi, F Gambarana, C Tagliamonte, A De Montis, M G Neuroscience. 2002; 109(2): 267-74 0306-4522

- **Does combined treatment with novel antidepressants and a dopamine D3 receptor agonist reproduce cocaine discrimination in rats?**
  Author(s): Department of Pharmacology, Institute of Pharmacology, Polish Academy of Sciences, Krakow. filip@if-pan.krakow.pl
  Source: Filip, M Papla, I Pol-J-Pharmacol. 2001 Nov-December; 53(6): 577-85 1230-6002

- **Dopamine transporter proline mutations influence dopamine uptake, cocaine analog recognition, and expression.**
  Author(s): Molecular Neurobiology Branch, NIDA-IRP, National Institutes of Health, Johns Hopkins University School of Medicine, Baltimore, Maryland 21224, USA.
  Source: Lin, Z Itokawa, M Uhl, G R FASEB-J. 2000 April; 14(5): 715-28 0892-6638

- **Drug-induced reinstatement to heroin and cocaine seeking: a rodent model of relapse in polydrug use.**
  Author(s): Center for Studies in Behavioral Neurobiology, Concordia University, Montreal, Quebec, Canada.
  Source: Leri, F Stewart, J Exp-Clin-Psychopharmacol. 2001 August; 9(3): 297-306 1064-1297

- **Effects of chronic administration of the D1 receptor partial agonist SKF 77434 on cocaine self-administration in rhesus monkeys.**
  Author(s): Harvard Medical School-McLean Hospital, Alcohol and Drug Abuse Research Center, 115 Mill Street, Belmont, MA 02478-9106, USA.
  Source: Mutschler, Nicole H Bergman, Jack Psychopharmacology-(Berl). 2002 April; 160(4): 362-70 0033-3158

- **Effects of cyclazocine on cocaine self-administration in rats.**
  Author(s): Department of Pharmacology and Neuroscience, Albany Medical College, NY 12208, USA. sglick@ccgateway.amc.edu
  Source: Glick, S D Visker, K E Maisonneuve, I M Eur-J-Pharmacol. 1998 September 11; 357(1): 9-14 0014-2999

- **Effects of dopamine D(1-like) and D(2-like) agonists on cocaine self-administration in rhesus monkeys: rapid assessment of cocaine dose-effect functions.**
  Author(s): Alcohol and Drug Abuse Research Center, McLean Hospital-Harvard Medical School, 115 Mill Street, Belmont, MA 02478, USA. barak@mclean.harvard.edu
  Source: Caine, S B Negus, S S Mello, N K Psychopharmacology-(Berl). 2000 January; 148(1): 41-51 0033-3158

- **Effects of opiates, opioid antagonists and cocaine on the endogenous opioid system: clinical and laboratory studies.**
  Author(s): Rockefeller University, New York, N.Y.
  Source: Kreek, M J NIDA-Res-Monogr. 1992; 11944-8 1046-9516

- **Effects of short-term citicoline treatment on acute cocaine intoxication and cardiovascular effects.**
  Author(s): Behavioral Psychopharmacology Research Laboratory, McLean Hospital/Havard Medical School, Belmont, MA 02478, USA. lukas@mclean.org
  Source: Lukas, S E Kouri, E M Rhee, C Madrid, A Renshaw, P F Psychopharmacology-(Berl). 2001 September; 157(2): 163-7 0033-3158

- **Enhancement of conditioned place preference response to cocaine in rats following subchronic administration of 3, 4-methylenedioxymethamphetamine (MDMA).**
  Author(s): PHS Department, College of Pharmacy and Allied Health Professions, St. John's University, Jamaica, New York 11439, USA.
  Source: Horan, B Gardner, E L Ashby, C R Synapse. 2000 February; 35(2): 160-2 0887-4476

- **Fluoxetine for cocaine abuse in methadone patients: preliminary findings.**
  Author(s): Dept. of Psychiatry, UCSF.

Source: Batki, S L Manfredi, L B Sorensen, J L Jacob, P Dumontet, R Jones, R T NIDA-Res-Monogr. 1991; 105516-7 1046-9516

- **Gender effects on persistent cerebral metabolite changes in the frontal lobes of abstinent cocaine users.**
  Author(s): Department of Neurology, UCLA School of Medicine, Harbor-UCLA Medical Center, Torrance 90509, USA. LindavChang@humc.edu
  Source: Chang, L Ernst, T Strickland, T Mehringer, C M Am-J-Psychiatry. 1999 May; 156(5): 716-22 0002-953X

- **Naltrexone treatment of comorbid alcohol and cocaine use disorders.**
  Author(s): University of Connecticut Health Center, Department of Psychiatry, Farmington CT 06030-2103, USA.
  Source: Hersh, D Van Kirk, J R Kranzler, H R Psychopharmacology-(Berl). 1998 September; 139(1-2): 44-52 0033-3158

- **Novelty seeking as a predictor of treatment retention for heroin dependent cocaine users.**
  Author(s): Research Division on Substance Abuse, Department of Psychiatry and Behavioral Neurosciences, School of Medicine, Wayne State University, 2761 E. Jefferson, Detroit, MI 48207, USA. thelmus@gopher.chem.wayne.edu
  Source: Helmus, T C Downey, K K Arfken, C L Henderson, M J Schuster, C R Drug-Alcohol-Depend. 2001 February 1; 61(3): 287-95 0376-8716

- **Prenatal exposure to morphine enhances cocaine and heroin self-administration in drug-naive rats.**
  Author(s): Department of Pharmacology, Rudolf Magnus Institute, Medical Faculty, State University of Utrecht, The Netherlands.
  Source: Ramsey, N F Niesink, R J Van Ree, J M Drug-Alcohol-Depend. 1993 June; 33(1): 41-51 0376-8716

- **Rats prefer cocaine over nicotine in a two-lever self-administration choice test.**
  Author(s): College of Medicine, Department of Pharmacology, University of California-Irvine, Irvine, CA 92697-4625, USA. manzardo@scripps.edu
  Source: Manzardo, A M Stein, L Belluzzi, J D Brain-Res. 2002 January 4; 924(1): 10-9 0006-8993

- **Relationship between extent of cocaine use and dependence among adolescents and adults in the United States.**
  Author(s): Department of Psychiatry, College of Physicians and Surgeons, Columbia University, 1051 Riverside Drive, Unit 20, New York, NY 10032, USA.
  Source: Chen, K Kandel, D Drug-Alcohol-Depend. 2002 September 1; 68(1): 65-85 0376-8716

- **Sensitization to the cardiovascular but not subject-rated effects of oral cocaine in humans.**
  Author(s): Department of Psychiatry and Behavioral Science, Duke University Medical Center, Durham, North Carolina, USA.
  Source: Kollins, Scott H Rush, Craig R Biol-Psychiatry. 2002 January 15; 51(2): 143-50 0006-3223

- **Synthesis and opioid receptor affinity of morphinan and benzomorphan derivatives: mixed kappa agonists and mu agonists/antagonists as potential pharmacotherapeutics for cocaine dependence.**
  Author(s): Department of Psychiatry, Harvard Medical School, McLean Hospital, Alcohol and Drug Abuse Research Center, Belmont, Massachusetts 02478-9106, USA. neumeyer@mclean.harvard.edu
  Source: Neumeyer, J L Bidlack, J M Zong, R Bakthavachalam, V Gao, P Cohen, D J Negus, S S Mello, N K J-Med-Chem. 2000 January 13; 43(1): 114-22 0022-2623

- **The pH dependence of cocaine interaction with cardiac sodium channels.**
  Author(s): Department of Pharmacology, Tulane University School of Medicine, New Orleans, Louisiana, USA.
  Source: Crumb, W J Clarkson, C W J-Pharmacol-Exp-Ther. 1995 September; 274(3): 1228-37 0022-3565

- **The stimulus effect of 5,6,7,8-tetrahydro-1,3-dioxolo[4,5-g]isoquinoline is similar to that of cocaine but different from that of amphetamine.**
  Author(s): Department of Medicinal Chemistry, School of Pharmacy, Virginia Commonwealth University, Box 980540 VCU, Richmond, VA 23298-0540, USA.
  Source: Young, Richard Glennon, Richard A Pharmacol-Biochem-Behavolume 2002 Jan-February; 71(1-2): 205-13 0091-3057

Federal Resources on Nutrition

In addition to the IBIDS, the United States Department of Health and Human Services (HHS) and the United States Department of Agriculture (USDA) provide many sources of information on general nutrition and health. Recommended resources include:

- healthfinder®, HHS's gateway to health information, including diet and nutrition:
  http://www.healthfinder.gov/scripts/SearchContext.asp?topic=238&page=0

- The United States Department of Agriculture's Web site dedicated to nutrition information: **www.nutrition.gov**

- The Food and Drug Administration's Web site for federal food safety information: **www.foodsafety.gov**

- The National Action Plan on Overweight and Obesity sponsored by the United States Surgeon General: **http://www.surgeongeneral.gov/topics/obesity/**

- The Center for Food Safety and Applied Nutrition has an Internet site sponsored by the Food and Drug Administration and the Department of Health and Human Services: **http://vm.cfsan.fda.gov/**

- Center for Nutrition Policy and Promotion sponsored by the United States Department of Agriculture: **http://www.usda.gov/cnpp/**

- Food and Nutrition Information Center, National Agricultural Library sponsored by the United States Department of Agriculture: **http://www.nal.usda.gov/fnic/**

- Food and Nutrition Service sponsored by the United States Department of Agriculture: **http://www.fns.usda.gov/fns/**

Additional Web Resources

A number of additional Web sites offer encyclopedic information covering food and nutrition. The following is a representative sample:

- AOL: **http://search.aol.com/cat.adp?id=174&layer=&from=subcats**

- Family Village: **http://www.familyvillage.wisc.edu/med_nutrition.html**

- Google: **http://directory.google.com/Top/Health/Nutrition/**

- Open Directory Project: **http://dmoz.org/Health/Nutrition/**

- Yahoo.com: **http://dir.yahoo.com/Health/Nutrition/**

- WebMD®Health: **http://my.webmd.com/nutrition**

- WholeHealthMD.com: **http://www.wholehealthmd.com/reflib/0,1529,,00.html**

The following is a specific Web list relating to cocaine dependence; please note that any particular subject below may indicate either a therapeutic use, or a contraindication (potential danger), and does not reflect an official recommendation:

- **Minerals**

  Manganese
  Source: Integrative Medicine Communications; www.drkoop.com

Appendix C. Finding Medical Libraries

Overview

At a medical library you can find medical texts and reference books, consumer health publications, specialty newspapers and magazines, as well as medical journals. In this Appendix, we show you how to quickly find a medical library in your area.

Preparation

Before going to the library, highlight the references mentioned in this sourcebook that you find interesting. Focus on those items that are not available via the Internet, and ask the reference librarian for help with your search. He or she may know of additional resources that could be helpful to you. Most importantly, your local public library and medical libraries have Interlibrary Loan programs with the National Library of Medicine (NLM), one of the largest medical collections in the world. According to the NLM, most of the literature in the general and historical collections of the National Library of Medicine is available on interlibrary loan to any library. NLM's interlibrary loan services are only available to libraries. If you would like to access NLM medical literature, then visit a library in your area that can request the publications for you.[47]

---

[47] Adapted from the NLM: **http://www.nlm.nih.gov/psd/cas/interlibrary.html**.

Finding a Local Medical Library

The quickest method to locate medical libraries is to use the Internet-based directory published by the National Network of Libraries of Medicine (NN/LM). This network includes 4626 members and affiliates that provide many services to librarians, health professionals, and the public. To find a library in your area, simply visit **http://nnlm.gov/members/adv.html** or call 1-800-338-7657.

Medical Libraries in the U.S. and Canada

In addition to the NN/LM, the National Library of Medicine (NLM) lists a number of libraries with reference facilities that are open to the public. The following is the NLM's list and includes hyperlinks to each library's Web site. These Web pages can provide information on hours of operation and other restrictions. The list below is a small sample of libraries recommended by the National Library of Medicine (sorted alphabetically by name of the U.S. state or Canadian province where the library is located)[48]:

- **Alabama:** Health InfoNet of Jefferson County (Jefferson County Library Cooperative, Lister Hill Library of the Health Sciences), **http://www.uab.edu/infonet/**

- **Alabama:** Richard M. Scrushy Library (American Sports Medicine Institute)

- **Arizona:** Samaritan Regional Medical Center: The Learning Center (Samaritan Health System, Phoenix, Arizona), **http://www.samaritan.edu/library/bannerlibs.htm**

- **California:** Kris Kelly Health Information Center (St. Joseph Health System, Humboldt), **http://www.humboldt1.com/~kkhic/index.html**

- **California:** Community Health Library of Los Gatos, **http://www.healthlib.org/orgresources.html**

- **California:** Consumer Health Program and Services (CHIPS) (County of Los Angeles Public Library, Los Angeles County Harbor-UCLA Medical Center Library) - Carson, CA, **http://www.colapublib.org/services/chips.html**

- **California:** Gateway Health Library (Sutter Gould Medical Foundation)

- **California:** Health Library (Stanford University Medical Center), **http://www-med.stanford.edu/healthlibrary/**

---

[48] Abstracted from **http://www.nlm.nih.gov/medlineplus/libraries.html**.

- **California:** Patient Education Resource Center - Health Information and Resources (University of California, San Francisco), **http://sfghdean.ucsf.edu/barnett/PERC/default.asp**

- **California:** Redwood Health Library (Petaluma Health Care District), **http://www.phcd.org/rdwdlib.html**

- **California:** Los Gatos PlaneTree Health Library, **http://planetreesanjose.org/**

- **California:** Sutter Resource Library (Sutter Hospitals Foundation, Sacramento), **http://suttermedicalcenter.org/library/**

- **California:** Health Sciences Libraries (University of California, Davis), **http://www.lib.ucdavis.edu/healthsci/**

- **California:** ValleyCare Health Library & Ryan Comer Cancer Resource Center (ValleyCare Health System, Pleasanton), **http://gaelnet.stmarys-ca.edu/other.libs/gbal/east/vchl.html**

- **California:** Washington Community Health Resource Library (Fremont), **http://www.healthlibrary.org/**

- **Colorado:** William V. Gervasini Memorial Library (Exempla Healthcare), **http://www.saintjosephdenver.org/yourhealth/libraries/**

- **Connecticut:** Hartford Hospital Health Science Libraries (Hartford Hospital), **http://www.harthosp.org/library/**

- **Connecticut:** Healthnet: Connecticut Consumer Health Information Center (University of Connecticut Health Center, Lyman Maynard Stowe Library), **http://library.uchc.edu/departm/hnet/**

- **Connecticut:** Waterbury Hospital Health Center Library (Waterbury Hospital, Waterbury), **http://www.waterburyhospital.com/library/consumer.shtml**

- **Delaware:** Consumer Health Library (Christiana Care Health System, Eugene du Pont Preventive Medicine & Rehabilitation Institute, Wilmington), **http://www.christianacare.org/health_guide/health_guide_pmri_health_info.cfm**

- **Delaware:** Lewis B. Flinn Library (Delaware Academy of Medicine, Wilmington), **http://www.delamed.org/chls.html**

- **Georgia:** Family Resource Library (Medical College of Georgia, Augusta), **http://cmc.mcg.edu/kids_families/fam_resources/fam_res_lib/frl.htm**

- **Georgia:** Health Resource Center (Medical Center of Central Georgia, Macon), **http://www.mccg.org/hrc/hrchome.asp**

- **Hawaii:** Hawaii Medical Library: Consumer Health Information Service (Hawaii Medical Library, Honolulu), **http://hml.org/CHIS/**

- **Idaho:** DeArmond Consumer Health Library (Kootenai Medical Center, Coeur d'Alene), **http://www.nicon.org/DeArmond/index.htm**

- **Illinois:** Health Learning Center of Northwestern Memorial Hospital (Chicago), **http://www.nmh.org/health_info/hlc.html**

- **Illinois:** Medical Library (OSF Saint Francis Medical Center, Peoria), **http://www.osfsaintfrancis.org/general/library/**

- **Kentucky:** Medical Library - Services for Patients, Families, Students & the Public (Central Baptist Hospital, Lexington), **http://www.centralbap.com/education/community/library.cfm**

- **Kentucky:** University of Kentucky - Health Information Library (Chandler Medical Center, Lexington), **http://www.mc.uky.edu/PatientEd/**

- **Louisiana:** Alton Ochsner Medical Foundation Library (Alton Ochsner Medical Foundation, New Orleans), **http://www.ochsner.org/library/**

- **Louisiana:** Louisiana State University Health Sciences Center Medical Library-Shreveport, **http://lib-sh.lsuhsc.edu/**

- **Maine:** Franklin Memorial Hospital Medical Library (Franklin Memorial Hospital, Farmington), **http://www.fchn.org/fmh/lib.htm**

- **Maine:** Gerrish-True Health Sciences Library (Central Maine Medical Center, Lewiston), **http://www.cmmc.org/library/library.html**

- **Maine:** Hadley Parrot Health Science Library (Eastern Maine Healthcare, Bangor), **http://www.emh.org/hll/hpl/guide.htm**

- **Maine:** Maine Medical Center Library (Maine Medical Center, Portland), **http://www.mmc.org/library/**

- **Maine:** Parkview Hospital (Brunswick), **http://www.parkviewhospital.org/**

- **Maine:** Southern Maine Medical Center Health Sciences Library (Southern Maine Medical Center, Biddeford), **http://www.smmc.org/services/service.php3?choice=10**

- **Maine:** Stephens Memorial Hospital's Health Information Library (Western Maine Health, Norway), **http://www.wmhcc.org/Library/**

- **Manitoba, Canada:** Consumer & Patient Health Information Service (University of Manitoba Libraries), **http://www.umanitoba.ca/libraries/units/health/reference/chis.html**

- **Manitoba, Canada:** J.W. Crane Memorial Library (Deer Lodge Centre, Winnipeg), **http://www.deerlodge.mb.ca/crane_library/about.asp**

- **Maryland:** Health Information Center at the Wheaton Regional Library (Montgomery County, Dept. of Public Libraries, Wheaton Regional Library), **http://www.mont.lib.md.us/healthinfo/hic.asp**

- **Massachusetts:** Baystate Medical Center Library (Baystate Health System), **http://www.baystatehealth.com/1024/**

- **Massachusetts:** Boston University Medical Center Alumni Medical Library (Boston University Medical Center), **http://med-libwww.bu.edu/library/lib.html**

- **Massachusetts:** Lowell General Hospital Health Sciences Library (Lowell General Hospital, Lowell), **http://www.lowellgeneral.org/library/HomePageLinks/WWW.htm**

- **Massachusetts:** Paul E. Woodard Health Sciences Library (New England Baptist Hospital, Boston), **http://www.nebh.org/health_lib.asp**

- **Massachusetts:** St. Luke's Hospital Health Sciences Library (St. Luke's Hospital, Southcoast Health System, New Bedford), **http://www.southcoast.org/library/**

- **Massachusetts:** Treadwell Library Consumer Health Reference Center (Massachusetts General Hospital), **http://www.mgh.harvard.edu/library/chrcindex.html**

- **Massachusetts:** UMass HealthNet (University of Massachusetts Medical School, Worchester), **http://healthnet.umassmed.edu/**

- **Michigan:** Botsford General Hospital Library - Consumer Health (Botsford General Hospital, Library & Internet Services), **http://www.botsfordlibrary.org/consumer.htm**

- **Michigan:** Helen DeRoy Medical Library (Providence Hospital and Medical Centers), **http://www.providence-hospital.org/library/**

- **Michigan:** Marquette General Hospital - Consumer Health Library (Marquette General Hospital, Health Information Center), **http://www.mgh.org/center.html**

- **Michigan:** Patient Education Resouce Center - University of Michigan Cancer Center (University of Michigan Comprehensive Cancer Center, Ann Arbor), **http://www.cancer.med.umich.edu/learn/leares.htm**

- **Michigan:** Sladen Library & Center for Health Information Resources - Consumer Health Information (Detroit), **http://www.henryford.com/body.cfm?id=39330**

- **Montana:** Center for Health Information (St. Patrick Hospital and Health Sciences Center, Missoula)

- **National:** Consumer Health Library Directory (Medical Library Association, Consumer and Patient Health Information Section), **http://caphis.mlanet.org/directory/index.html**

- **National:** National Network of Libraries of Medicine (National Library of Medicine) - provides library services for health professionals in the United States who do not have access to a medical library, **http://nnlm.gov/**

- **National:** NN/LM List of Libraries Serving the Public (National Network of Libraries of Medicine), **http://nnlm.gov/members/**

- **Nevada:** Health Science Library, West Charleston Library (Las Vegas-Clark County Library District, Las Vegas), **http://www.lvccld.org/special_collections/medical/index.htm**

- **New Hampshire:** Dartmouth Biomedical Libraries (Dartmouth College Library, Hanover), **http://www.dartmouth.edu/~biomed/resources.htmld/conshealth.htmld**

- **New Jersey:** Consumer Health Library (Rahway Hospital, Rahway), **http://www.rahwayhospital.com/library.htm**

- **New Jersey:** Dr. Walter Phillips Health Sciences Library (Englewood Hospital and Medical Center, Englewood), **http://www.englewoodhospital.com/links/index.htm**

- **New Jersey:** Meland Foundation (Englewood Hospital and Medical Center, Englewood), **http://www.geocities.com/ResearchTriangle/9360/**

- **New York:** Choices in Health Information (New York Public Library) - NLM Consumer Pilot Project participant, **http://www.nypl.org/branch/health/links.html**

- **New York:** Health Information Center (Upstate Medical University, State University of New York, Syracuse), **http://www.upstate.edu/library/hic/**

- **New York:** Health Sciences Library (Long Island Jewish Medical Center, New Hyde Park), **http://www.lij.edu/library/library.html**

- **New York:** ViaHealth Medical Library (Rochester General Hospital), **http://www.nyam.org/library/**

- **Ohio:** Consumer Health Library (Akron General Medical Center, Medical & Consumer Health Library), **http://www.akrongeneral.org/hwlibrary.htm**

- **Oklahoma:** The Health Information Center at Saint Francis Hospital (Saint Francis Health System, Tulsa), **http://www.sfh-tulsa.com/services/healthinfo.asp**

- **Oregon:** Planetree Health Resource Center (Mid-Columbia Medical Center, The Dalles), **http://www.mcmc.net/phrc/**

- **Pennsylvania:** Community Health Information Library (Milton S. Hershey Medical Center, Hershey), **http://www.hmc.psu.edu/commhealth/**

- **Pennsylvania:** Community Health Resource Library (Geisinger Medical Center, Danville), **http://www.geisinger.edu/education/commlib.shtml**

- **Pennsylvania:** HealthInfo Library (Moses Taylor Hospital, Scranton), **http://www.mth.org/healthwellness.html**

- **Pennsylvania:** Hopwood Library (University of Pittsburgh, Health Sciences Library System, Pittsburgh), **http://www.hsls.pitt.edu/guides/chi/hopwood/index_html**

- **Pennsylvania:** Koop Community Health Information Center (College of Physicians of Philadelphia), **http://www.collphyphil.org/kooppg1.shtml**

- **Pennsylvania:** Learning Resources Center - Medical Library (Susquehanna Health System, Williamsport), **http://www.shscares.org/services/lrc/index.asp**

- **Pennsylvania:** Medical Library (UPMC Health System, Pittsburgh), **http://www.upmc.edu/passavant/library.htm**

- **Quebec, Canada:** Medical Library (Montreal General Hospital), **http://www.mghlib.mcgill.ca/**

- **South Dakota:** Rapid City Regional Hospital Medical Library (Rapid City Regional Hospital), **http://www.rcrh.org/Services/Library/Default.asp**

- **Texas:** Houston HealthWays (Houston Academy of Medicine-Texas Medical Center Library), **http://hhw.library.tmc.edu/**

- **Washington:** Community Health Library (Kittitas Valley Community Hospital), **http://www.kvch.com/**

- **Washington:** Southwest Washington Medical Center Library (Southwest Washington Medical Center, Vancouver), **http://www.swmedicalcenter.com/body.cfm?id=72**

APPENDIX D. PRINCIPLES OF DRUG ADDICTION TREATMENT

Overview[49]

No single treatment is appropriate for all individuals. Matching treatment settings, interventions, and services to each individual's particular problems and needs is critical to his or her ultimate success in returning to productive functioning in the family, workplace, and society.

This appendix reproduces information created by the National Institute for Drug Abuse (NIDA) concerning drug abuse treatment entitled "Principles of Drug Addiction Treatment: A Research-Based Guide".

Principles of Effective Treatment

Treatment needs to be readily available. Because individuals who are addicted to drugs may be uncertain about entering treatment, taking advantage of opportunities when they are ready for treatment is crucial. Potential treatment applicants can be lost if treatment is not immediately available or is not readily accessible.

Effective treatment attends to multiple needs of the individual, not just his or her drug use. To be effective, treatment must address the individual's drug use and any associated medical, psychological, social, vocational, and legal problems.

---

[49] Adapted from the National Institute on Drug Abuse: **http://165.112.78.61/PODAT/PODATIndex.html.**

An individual's treatment and services plan must be assessed continually and modified as necessary to ensure that the plan meets the person's changing needs. A patient may require varying combinations of services and treatment components during the course of treatment and recovery. In addition to counseling or psychotherapy, a patient at times may require medication, other medical services, family therapy, parenting instruction, vocational rehabilitation, and social and legal services. It is critical that the treatment approach be appropriate to the individual's age, gender, ethnicity, and culture.

Remaining in treatment for an adequate period of time is critical for treatment effectiveness. The appropriate duration for an individual depends on his or her problems and needs. Research indicates that for most patients, the threshold of significant improvement is reached at about 3 months in treatment. After this threshold is reached, additional treatment can produce further progress toward recovery. Because people often leave treatment prematurely, programs should include strategies to engage and keep patients in treatment.

Counseling and Other Behavioral Therapies

Counseling (individual and/or group) and other behavioral therapies are critical components of effective treatment for addiction. In therapy, patients address issues of motivation, build skills to resist drug use, replace drug-using activities with constructive and rewarding non-drug-using activities, and improve problem-solving abilities. Behavioral therapy also facilitates interpersonal relationships and the individual's ability to function in the family and community.

Medications

Medications are an important element of treatment for many patients, especially when combined with counseling and other behavioral therapies. Methadone and levo-alpha-acetylmethadol (LAAM) are very effective in helping individuals addicted to heroin or other opiates stabilize their lives and reduce their illicit drug use. Naltrexone is also an effective medication for some opiate addicts and some patients with co-occurring alcohol dependence. For persons addicted to nicotine, a nicotine replacement product (such as patches or gum) or an oral medication (such as bupropion) can be an effective component of treatment. For patients with mental disorders, both behavioral treatments and medications can be critically important.

Patients with Mental Disorders

Addicted or drug-abusing individuals with coexisting mental disorders should have both disorders treated in an integrated way. Because addictive disorders and mental disorders often occur in the same individual, patients presenting for either condition should be assessed and treated for the co-occurrence of the other type of disorder.

Medical Detoxification

Medical detoxification is only the first stage of addiction treatment and by itself does little to change long-term drug use. Medical detoxification safely manages the acute physical symptoms of withdrawal associated with stopping drug use. While detoxification alone is rarely sufficient to help addicts achieve long-term abstinence, for some individuals it is a strongly indicated precursor to effective drug addiction treatment.

Patient Cooperation

Treatment does not need to be voluntary to be effective. Strong motivation can facilitate the treatment process. Sanctions or enticements in the family, employment setting, or criminal justice system can increase significantly both treatment entry and retention rates and the success of drug treatment interventions.

Possible drug use during treatment must be monitored continuously. Lapses to drug use can occur during treatment. The objective monitoring of a patient's drug and alcohol use during treatment, such as through urinalysis or other tests, can help the patient withstand urges to use drugs. Such monitoring also can provide early evidence of drug use so that the individual's treatment plan can be adjusted. Feedback to patients who test positive for illicit drug use is an important element of monitoring.

Treatment programs should provide assessment for HIV/AIDS, hepatitis B and C, tuberculosis and other infectious diseases, and counseling to help patients modify or change behaviors that place themselves or others at risk of infection. Counseling can help patients avoid high-risk behavior.

Counseling also can help people who are already infected manage their illness.

Recovery

Recovery from drug addiction can be a long-term process and frequently requires multiple episodes of treatment. As with other chronic illnesses, relapses to drug use can occur during or after successful treatment episodes. Addicted individuals may require prolonged treatment and multiple episodes of treatment to achieve long-term abstinence and fully restored functioning. Participation in self-help support programs during and following treatment often is helpful in maintaining abstinence.

What Is Drug Addiction?

Drug addiction is a complex illness. It is characterized by compulsive, at times uncontrollable, drug craving, seeking, and use that persist even in the face of extremely negative consequences. For many people, drug addiction becomes chronic, with relapses possible even after long periods of abstinence.

The path to drug addiction begins with the act of taking drugs. Over time, a person's ability to choose not to take drugs can be compromised. Drug seeking becomes compulsive, in large part as a result of the effects of prolonged drug use on brain functioning and, thus, on behavior.

The compulsion to use drugs can take over the individual's life. Addiction often involves not only compulsive drug taking but also a wide range of dysfunctional behaviors that can interfere with normal functioning in the family, the workplace, and the broader community. Addiction also can place people at increased risk for a wide variety of other illnesses. These illnesses can be brought on by behaviors, such as poor living and health habits, that often accompany life as an addict, or because of toxic effects of the drugs themselves.

Because addiction has so many dimensions and disrupts so many aspects of an individual's life, treatment for this illness is never simple. Drug treatment must help the individual stop using drugs and maintain a drug-free lifestyle, while achieving productive functioning in the family, at work, and in society. Effective drug abuse and addiction treatment programs typically incorporate many components, each directed to a particular aspect of the illness and its consequences.

Three decades of scientific research and clinical practice have yielded a variety of effective approaches to drug addiction treatment. Extensive data document that drug addiction treatment is as effective as are treatments for most other similarly chronic medical conditions. In spite of scientific evidence that establishes the effectiveness of drug abuse treatment, many people believe that treatment is ineffective. In part, this is because of unrealistic expectations. Many people equate addiction with simply using drugs and therefore expect that addiction should be cured quickly, and if it is not, treatment is a failure. In reality, because addiction is a chronic disorder, the ultimate goal of long-term abstinence often requires sustained and repeated treatment episodes.

Of course, not all drug abuse treatment is equally effective. Research also has revealed a set of overarching principles that characterize the most effective drug abuse and addiction treatments and their implementation.

Treatment varies depending on the type of drug and the characteristics of the patient. The best programs provide a combination of therapies and other services.

Frequently Asked Questions

What Is Drug Addiction Treatment?

- There are many addictive drugs, and treatments for specific drugs can differ. Treatment also varies depending on the characteristics of the patient.

- Problems associated with an individual's drug addiction can vary significantly. People who are addicted to drugs come from all walks of life. Many suffer from mental health, occupational, health, or social problems that make their addictive disorders much more difficult to treat. Even if there are few associated problems, the severity of addiction itself ranges widely among people.

- A variety of scientifically based approaches to drug addiction treatment exist. Drug addiction treatment can include behavioral therapy (such as counseling, cognitive therapy, or psychotherapy), medications, or their combination. Behavioral therapies offer people strategies for coping with their drug cravings, teach them ways to avoid drugs and prevent relapse, and help them deal with relapse if it occurs. When a person's drug-related behavior places him or her at higher risk for AIDS or other infectious diseases, behavioral therapies can help to reduce the risk of disease transmission. Case management and referral to other medical, psychological, and social services are crucial components of treatment for many patients. The best programs provide a combination of therapies and other services to meet the needs of the individual patient, which are shaped by such issues as age, race, culture, sexual orientation, gender, pregnancy, parenting, housing, and employment, as well as physical and sexual abuse.

- Treatment medications, such as methadone, LAAM, and naltrexone, are available for individuals addicted to opiates. Nicotine preparations (patches, gum, nasal spray) and bupropion are available for individuals addicted to nicotine.

- The best treatment programs provide a combination of therapies and other services to meet the needs of the individual patient.

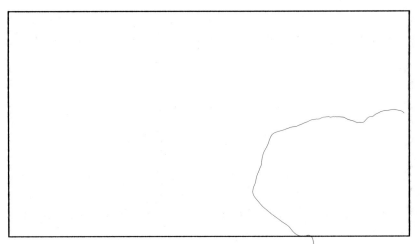

Components of Comprehensive Drug Abuse Treatment

- Medications, such as antidepressants, mood stabilizers, or neuroleptics, may be critical for treatment success when patients have co-occurring mental disorders, such as depression, anxiety disorder, bipolar disorder, or psychosis.

- Treatment can occur in a variety of settings, in many different forms, and for different lengths of time. Because drug addiction is typically a chronic disorder characterized by occasional relapses, a short-term, one-time treatment often is not sufficient. For many, treatment is a long-term process that involves multiple interventions and attempts at abstinence.

Why Can't Drug Addicts Quit on Their Own?

Nearly all addicted individuals believe in the beginning that they can stop using drugs on their own, and most try to stop without treatment. However, most of these attempts result in failure to achieve long-term abstinence. Research has shown that long-term drug use results in significant changes in brain function that persist long after the individual stops using drugs. These drug-induced changes in brain function may have many behavioral consequences, including the compulsion to use drugs despite adverse consequences. This is the defining characteristic of addiction.

Understanding that addiction has such an important biological component may help explain an individual's difficulty in achieving and maintaining abstinence without treatment. Psychological stress from work or family problems, social cues (such as meeting individuals from one's drug-using past), or the environment (such as encountering streets, objects, or even smells associated with drug use) can interact with biological factors to hinder attainment of sustained abstinence and make relapse more likely. Research studies indicate that even the most severely addicted individuals can participate actively in treatment and that active participation is essential to good outcomes.

How Effective Is Drug Addiction Treatment?

In addition to stopping drug use, the goal of treatment is to return the individual to productive functioning in the family, workplace, and community. Measures of effectiveness typically include levels of criminal behavior, family functioning, employability, and medical condition. Overall, treatment of addiction is as successful as treatment of other chronic diseases, such as diabetes, hypertension, and asthma.

Treatment of addiction is as successful as treatment of other chronic diseases such as diabetes, hypertension, and asthma. According to several studies, drug treatment reduces drug use by 40 to 60 percent and significantly decreases criminal activity during and after treatment. For example, a study of therapeutic community treatment for drug offenders demonstrated that arrests for violent and nonviolent criminal acts were reduced by 40 percent or more. Methadone treatment has been shown to decrease criminal behavior by as much as 50 percent. Research shows that drug addiction treatment reduces the risk of HIV infection and that interventions to prevent HIV are much less costly than treating HIV-related illnesses. Treatment can improve the prospects for employment, with gains of up to 40 percent after treatment.

Although these effectiveness rates hold in general, individual treatment outcomes depend on the extent and nature of the patient's presenting problems, the appropriateness of the treatment components and related services used to address those problems, and the degree of active engagement of the patient in the treatment process.

How Long Does Drug Addiction Treatment Usually Last?

Individuals progress through drug addiction treatment at various speeds, so there is no predetermined length of treatment. However, research has shown unequivocally that good outcomes are contingent on adequate lengths of treatment. Generally, for residential or outpatient treatment, participation for less than 90 days is of limited or no effectiveness, and treatments lasting significantly longer often are indicated. For methadone maintenance, 12 months of treatment is the minimum, and some opiate-addicted individuals will continue to benefit from methadone maintenance treatment over a period of years.

Good outcomes are contingent on adequate lengths of treatment. Many people who enter treatment drop out before receiving all the benefits that treatment can provide. Successful outcomes may require more than one treatment experience. Many addicted individuals have multiple episodes of treatment, often with a cumulative impact.

What Helps People Stay in Treatment?

Since successful outcomes often depend upon retaining the person long enough to gain the full benefits of treatment, strategies for keeping an individual in the program are critical. Whether a patient stays in treatment depends on factors associated with both the individual and the program. Individual factors related to engagement and retention include motivation to change drug-using behavior, degree of support from family and friends, and whether there is pressure to stay in treatment from the criminal justice system, child protection services, employers, or the family. Within the program, successful counselors are able to establish a positive, therapeutic relationship with the patient. The counselor should ensure that a treatment plan is established and followed so that the individual knows what to expect during treatment. Medical, psychiatric, and social services should be available.

Whether a patient stays in treatment depends on factors associated with both the individual and the program. Since some individual problems (such as serious mental illness, severe cocaine or crack use, and criminal involvement) increase the likelihood of a patient dropping out, intensive treatment with a range of components may be required to retain patients who have these problems. The provider then should ensure a transition to continuing care or "aftercare" following the patient's completion of formal treatment.

Is the Use of Medications Like Methadone Simply Replacing One Drug Addiction with Another?

No. As used in maintenance treatment, methadone and LAAM are not heroin substitutes. They are safe and effective medications for opiate addiction that are administered by mouth in regular, fixed doses. Their pharmacological effects are markedly different from those of heroin.

Injected, snorted, or smoked heroin causes an almost immediate "rush" or brief period of euphoria that wears off very quickly, terminating in a "crash." The individual then experiences an intense craving to use more heroin to stop the crash and reinstate the euphoria. The cycle of euphoria, crash, and craving is repeated several times a day which leads to a cycle of addiction and behavioral disruption. These characteristics of heroin use result from the drug's rapid onset of action and its short duration of action in the brain. An individual who uses heroin multiple times per day subjects his or her brain and body to marked, rapid fluctuations as the opiate effects come and go. These fluctuations can disrupt a number of important bodily functions. Because heroin is illegal, addicted persons often become part of a volatile drug-using street culture characterized by hustling and crimes for profit.

Methadone and LAAM have far more gradual onsets of action than heroin, and as a result, patients stabilized on these medications do not experience any rush. In addition, both medications wear off much more slowly than heroin, so there is no sudden crash, and the brain and body are not exposed to the marked fluctuations seen with heroin use. Maintenance treatment with methadone or LAAM markedly reduces the desire for heroin. If an individual maintained on adequate, regular doses of methadone (once a day) or LAAM (several times per week) tries to take heroin, the euphoric effects of heroin will be significantly blocked. According to research, patients undergoing maintenance treatment do not suffer the medical abnormalities and behavioral destabilization that rapid fluctuations in drug levels cause in heroin addicts.

What Role Can the Criminal Justice System Play in the Treatment of Drug Addiction?

Increasingly, research is demonstrating that treatment for drug-addicted offenders during and after incarceration can have a significant beneficial effect upon future drug use, criminal behavior, and social functioning. The case for integrating drug addiction treatment approaches with the criminal justice system is compelling. Combining prison- and community-based treatment for drug-addicted offenders reduces the risk of both recidivism to drug-related criminal behavior and relapse to drug use. For example, a recent study found that prisoners who participated in a therapeutic treatment program in the Delaware State Prison and continued to receive treatment in a work-release program after prison were 70 percent less likely than non-participants to return to drug use and incur rearrest.

Individuals who enter treatment under legal pressure have outcomes as favorable as those who enter treatment voluntarily. The majority of offenders involved with the criminal justice system are not in prison but are under community supervision. For those with known drug problems, drug addiction treatment may be recommended or mandated as a condition of probation. Research has demonstrated that individuals who enter treatment under legal pressure have outcomes as favorable as those who enter treatment voluntarily.

The criminal justice system refers drug offenders into treatment through a variety of mechanisms, such as diverting nonviolent offenders to treatment, stipulating treatment as a condition of probation or pretrial release, and convening specialized courts that handle cases for offenses involving drugs. Drug courts, another model, are dedicated to drug offender cases. They mandate and arrange for treatment as an alternative to incarceration, actively monitor progress in treatment, and arrange for other services to drug-involved offenders.

The most effective models integrate criminal justice and drug treatment systems and services. Treatment and criminal justice personnel work together on plans and implementation of screening, placement, testing, monitoring, and supervision, as well as on the systematic use of sanctions and rewards for drug abusers in the criminal justice system. Treatment for incarcerated drug abusers must include continuing care, monitoring, and supervision after release and during parole.

How Does Drug Addiction Treatment Help Reduce the Spread of HIV/AIDS and Other Infectious Diseases?

Many drug addicts, such as heroin or cocaine addicts and particularly injection drug users, are at increased risk for HIV/AIDS as well as other infectious diseases like hepatitis, tuberculosis, and sexually transmitted infections. For these individuals and the community at large, drug addiction treatment is disease prevention.

Drug injectors who do not enter treatment are up to six times more likely to become infected with HIV than injectors who enter and remain in treatment. Drug users who enter and continue in treatment reduce activities that can spread disease, such as sharing injection equipment and engaging in unprotected sexual activity. Participation in treatment also presents opportunities for screening, counseling, and referral for additional services. The best drug abuse treatment programs provide HIV counseling and offer HIV testing to their patients.

Where Do 12-Step or Self-Help Programs Fit into Drug Addiction Treatment?

Self-help groups can complement and extend the effects of professional treatment. The most prominent self-help groups are those affiliated with Alcoholics Anonymous (AA), Narcotics Anonymous (NA), and Cocaine Anonymous (CA), all of which are based on the 12-step model, and Smart Recovery®. Most drug addiction treatment programs encourage patients to participate in a self-help group during and after formal treatment.

How Can Families and Friends Make a Difference in the Life of Someone Needing Treatment?

Family and friends can play critical roles in motivating individuals with drug problems to enter and stay in treatment. Family therapy is important, especially for adolescents. Involvement of a family member in an individual's treatment program can strengthen and extend the benefits of the program.

Is Drug Addiction Treatment Worth Its Cost?

Drug addiction treatment is cost-effective in reducing drug use and its associated health and social costs. Treatment is less expensive than alternatives, such as not treating addicts or simply incarcerating addicts. For example, the average cost for 1 full year of methadone maintenance treatment is approximately $4,700 per patient, whereas 1 full year of imprisonment costs approximately $18,400 per person.

According to several conservative estimates, every $1 invested in addiction treatment programs yields a return of between $4 and $7 in reduced drug-related crime, criminal justice costs, and theft alone. When savings related to health care are included, total savings can exceed costs by a ratio of 12 to 1. Major savings to the individual and society also come from significant drops in interpersonal conflicts, improvements in workplace productivity, and reductions in drug-related accidents.

Drug Addiction Treatment in the United States

Drug addiction is a complex disorder that can involve virtually every aspect of an individual's function in the family, at work, and in the community. Because of addiction's complexity and pervasive consequences, drug addiction treatment typically must involve many components. Some of those components focus directly on the individual's drug use. Others, like employment training, focus on restoring the addicted individual to productive membership in the family and society.

Treatment for drug abuse and addiction is delivered in many different settings, using a variety of behavioral and pharmacological approaches. In the United States, more than 11,000 specialized drug treatment facilities provide rehabilitation, counseling, behavioral therapy, medication, case management, and other types of services to persons with drug use disorders.

Because drug abuse and addiction are major public health problems, a large portion of drug treatment is funded by local, State, and Federal governments. Private and employer-subsidized health plans also may provide coverage for treatment of drug addiction and its medical consequences.

Drug abuse and addiction are treated in specialized treatment facilities and mental health clinics by a variety of providers, including certified drug abuse counselors, physicians, psychologists, nurses, and social workers. Treatment is delivered in outpatient, inpatient, and residential settings. Although specific treatment approaches often are associated with particular treatment settings, a variety of therapeutic interventions or services can be included in any given setting.

General Categories of Treatment Programs

Research studies on drug addiction treatment have typically classified treatment programs into several general types or modalities, which are described in the following text. Treatment approaches and individual programs continue to evolve, and many programs in existence today do not fit neatly into traditional drug addiction treatment classifications.

Agonist Maintenance Treatment

Agonist maintenance treatment for opiate addicts usually is conducted in outpatient settings, often called methadone treatment programs. These programs use a long-acting synthetic opiate medication, usually methadone or LAAM, administered orally for a sustained period at a dosage sufficient to prevent opiate withdrawal, block the effects of illicit opiate use, and decrease opiate craving. Patients stabilized on adequate, sustained dosages of methadone or LAAM can function normally. They can hold jobs, avoid the crime and violence of the street culture, and reduce their exposure to HIV by stopping or decreasing injection drug use and drug-related high-risk sexual behavior.

Patients stabilized on opiate agonists can engage more readily in counseling and other behavioral interventions essential to recovery and rehabilitation. The best, most effective opiate agonist maintenance programs include individual and/or group counseling, as well as provision of, or referral to, other needed medical, psychological, and social services.

Narcotic Antagonist Treatment Using Naltrexone

Narcotic antagonist treatment using Naltrexone for opiate addicts usually is conducted in outpatient settings although initiation of the medication often begins after medical detoxification in a residential setting. Naltrexone is a long-acting synthetic opiate antagonist with few side effects that is taken orally either daily or three times a week for a sustained period of time.

Individuals must be medically detoxified and opiate-free for several days before Naltrexone can be taken to prevent precipitating an opiate abstinence syndrome. When used this way, all the effects of self-administered opiates, including euphoria, are completely blocked. The theory behind this treatment is that the repeated lack of the desired opiate effects, as well as the perceived futility of using the opiate, will gradually over time result in breaking the habit of opiate addiction. Naltrexone itself has no subjective effects or potential for abuse and is not addicting. Patient noncompliance is a common problem. Therefore, a favorable treatment outcome requires that there also be a positive therapeutic relationship, effective counseling or therapy, and careful monitoring of medication compliance.

Patients stabilized on Naltrexone can hold jobs, avoid crime and violence, and reduce their exposure to HIV. Many experienced clinicians have found Naltrexone most useful for highly motivated, recently detoxified patients who desire total abstinence because of external circumstances, including impaired professionals, parolees, probationers, and prisoners in work-release status. Patients stabilized on Naltrexone can function normally. They can hold jobs, avoid the crime and violence of the street culture, and reduce their exposure to HIV by stopping injection drug use and drug-related high-risk sexual behavior.

Outpatient Drug-Free Treatment

Outpatient drug-free treatment in the types and intensity of services offered. Such treatment costs less than residential or inpatient treatment and often is more suitable for individuals who are employed or who have extensive social supports. Low-intensity programs may offer little more than drug education and admonition. Other outpatient models, such as intensive day treatment, can be comparable to residential programs in services and effectiveness, depending on the individual patient's characteristics and needs. In many outpatient programs, group counseling is emphasized. Some outpatient programs are designed to treat patients who have medical or mental health problems in addition to their drug disorder.

Long-Term Residential Treatment

Long-term residential treatment provides care 24 hours per day, generally in non-hospital settings. The best-known residential treatment model is the therapeutic community (TC), but residential treatment may also employ other models, such as cognitive-behavioral therapy.

TCs are residential programs with planned lengths of stay of 6 to 12 months. TCs focus on the "resocialization" of the individual and use the program's entire "community," including other residents, staff, and the social context, as active components of treatment. Addiction is viewed in the context of an individual's social and psychological deficits, and treatment focuses on developing personal accountability and responsibility and socially productive lives. Treatment is highly structured and can at times be confrontational, with activities designed to help residents examine damaging beliefs, self-concepts, and patterns of behavior and to adopt new, more harmonious and constructive ways to interact with others. Many TCs are quite comprehensive and can include employment training and other support services on site.

Compared with patients in other forms of drug treatment, the typical TC resident has more severe problems, with more co-occurring mental health problems and more criminal involvement. Research shows that TCs can be modified to treat individuals with special needs, including adolescents, women, those with severe mental disorders, and individuals in the criminal justice system.

Short-Term Residential Programs

Short-term residential programs provide intensive but relatively brief residential treatment based on a modified 12-step approach. These programs were originally designed to treat alcohol problems, but during the cocaine epidemic of the mid-1980's, many began to treat illicit drug abuse and addiction. The original residential treatment model consisted of a 3 to 6 week hospital-based inpatient treatment phase followed by extended outpatient therapy and participation in a self-help group, such as Alcoholics Anonymous. Reduced health care coverage for substance abuse treatment has resulted in a diminished number of these programs, and the average length of stay under managed care review is much shorter than in early programs.

Medical Detoxification

Medical Detoxification is a process whereby individuals are systematically withdrawn from addicting drugs in an inpatient or outpatient setting, typically under the care of a physician. Detoxification is sometimes called a distinct treatment modality but is more appropriately considered a precursor of treatment, because it is designed to treat the acute physiological effects of stopping drug use. Medications are available for detoxification from opiates, nicotine, benzodiazepines, alcohol, barbiturates, and other sedatives. In some cases, particularly for the last three types of drugs, detoxification may be a medical necessity, and untreated withdrawal may be medically dangerous or even fatal.

Detoxification is not designed to address the psychological, social, and behavioral problems associated with addiction and therefore does not typically produce lasting behavioral changes necessary for recovery. Detoxification is most useful when it incorporates formal processes of assessment and referral to subsequent drug addiction treatment.

Treating Criminal Justice-Involved Drug Abusers and Addicts

Research has shown that combining criminal justice sanctions with drug treatment can be effective in decreasing drug use and related crime. Individuals under legal coercion tend to stay in treatment for a longer period of time and do as well as or better than others not under legal pressure. Often, drug abusers come into contact with the criminal justice system earlier than other health or social systems, and intervention by the criminal justice system to engage the individual in treatment may help interrupt and shorten a career of drug use. Treatment for the criminal justice-involved drug abuser or drug addict may be delivered prior to, during, after, or in lieu of incarceration.

Combining criminal justice sanctions with drug treatment can be effective in decreasing drug use and related crime.

Prison-Based Treatment Programs

Offenders with drug disorders may encounter a number of treatment options while incarcerated, including didactic drug education classes, self-help programs, and treatment based on therapeutic community or residential milieu therapy models. The TC model has been studied extensively and can be quite effective in reducing drug use and recidivism to criminal behavior. Those in treatment should be segregated from the general prison population, so that the "prison culture" does not overwhelm progress toward recovery. As might be expected, treatment gains can be lost if inmates are returned to the general prison population after treatment. Research shows that relapse to drug use and recidivism to crime are significantly lower if the drug offender continues treatment after returning to the community.

Community-Based Treatment for Criminal Justice Populations

A number of criminal justice alternatives to incarceration have been tried with offenders who have drug disorders, including limited diversion programs, pretrial release conditional on entry into treatment, and conditional probation with sanctions. The drug court is a promising approach. Drug courts mandate and arrange for drug addiction treatment, actively monitor progress in treatment, and arrange for other services to drug-involved offenders. Federal support for planning, implementation, and enhancement of drug courts is provided under the U.S. Department of Justice Drug Courts Program Office.

As a well-studied example, the Treatment Accountability and Safer Communities (TASC) program provides an alternative to incarceration by addressing the multiple needs of drug-addicted offenders in a community-based setting. TASC programs typically include counseling, medical care, parenting instruction, family counseling, school and job training, and legal and employment services. The key features of TASC include:

- Coordination of criminal justice and drug treatment;
- Early identification, assessment, and referral of drug-involved offenders;
- Monitoring offenders through drug testing; and
- Use of legal sanctions as inducements to remain in treatment.

Scientifically-Based Approaches to Drug Addiction Treatment

This section presents several examples of treatment approaches and components that have been developed and tested for efficacy through research supported by the National Institute on Drug Abuse (NIDA). Each approach is designed to address certain aspects of drug addiction and its consequences for the individual, family, and society. The approaches are to be used to supplement or enhance (not replace) existing treatment programs.

This section is not a complete list of efficacious, scientifically-based treatment approaches. Additional approaches are under development as part of NIDA's continuing support of treatment research.

Relapse Prevention

Relapse prevention, a cognitive-behavioral therapy, was developed for the treatment of problem drinking and adapted later for cocaine addicts. Cognitive-behavioral strategies are based on the theory that learning processes play a critical role in the development of maladaptive behavioral patterns. Individuals learn to identify and correct problematic behaviors. Relapse prevention encompasses several cognitive-behavioral strategies that facilitate abstinence as well as provide help for people who experience relapse.

The relapse prevention approach to the treatment of cocaine addiction consists of a collection of strategies intended to enhance self-control. Specific techniques include exploring the positive and negative consequences of continued use, self-monitoring to recognize drug cravings early on and to identify high-risk situations for use, and developing strategies for coping with and avoiding high-risk situations and the desire to use. A central element of this treatment is anticipating the problems patients are likely to meet and helping them develop effective coping strategies.

Research indicates that the skills individuals learn through relapse prevention therapy remain after the completion of treatment. In one study, most people receiving this cognitive-behavioral approach maintained the gains they made in treatment throughout the year following treatment.

The Matrix Model

The Matrix model provides a framework for engaging stimulant abusers in treatment and helping them achieve abstinence. Patients learn about issues critical to addiction and relapse, receive direction and support from a trained therapist, become familiar with self-help programs, and are monitored for drug use by urine testing. The program includes education for family members affected by the addiction.

The therapist functions simultaneously as teacher and coach, fostering a positive, encouraging relationship with the patient and using that relationship to reinforce positive behavior change. The interaction between the therapist and the patient is realistic and direct but not confrontational or parental. Therapists are trained to conduct treatment sessions in a way that promotes the patient's self-esteem, dignity, and self-worth. A positive relationship between patient and therapist is a critical element for patient retention.

Treatment materials draw heavily on other tested treatment approaches. Thus, this approach includes elements pertaining to the areas of relapse prevention, family and group therapies, drug education, and self-help participation. Detailed treatment manuals contain work sheets for individual sessions; other components include family educational groups, early recovery skills groups, relapse prevention groups, conjoint sessions, urine tests, 12-step programs, relapse analysis, and social support groups.

A number of projects have demonstrated that participants treated with the Matrix model demonstrate statistically significant reductions in drug and alcohol use, improvements in psychological indicators, and reduced risky sexual behaviors associated with HIV transmission. These reports, along with evidence suggesting comparable treatment response for methamphetamine users and cocaine users and demonstrated efficacy in enhancing naltrexone treatment of opiate addicts, provide a body of empirical support for the use of the model.

Supportive-Expressive Psychotherapy

Supportive-expressive psychotherapy is a time-limited, focused psychotherapy that has been adapted for heroin- and cocaine-addicted individuals. The therapy has two main components:

- Supportive techniques to help patients feel comfortable in discussing their personal experiences.

- Expressive techniques to help patients identify and work through interpersonal relationship issues.

Special attention is paid to the role of drugs in relation to problem feelings and behaviors, and how problems may be solved without recourse to drugs.

The efficacy of individual supportive-expressive psychotherapy has been tested with patients in methadone maintenance treatment who had psychiatric problems. In a comparison with patients receiving only drug counseling, both groups fared similarly with regard to opiate use, but the supportive-expressive psychotherapy group had lower cocaine use and required less methadone. Also, the patients who received supportive-expressive psychotherapy maintained many of the gains they had made. In an earlier study, supportive-expressive psychotherapy, when added to drug counseling, improved outcomes for opiate addicts in methadone treatment with moderately severe psychiatric problems.

Individualized Drug Counseling

Individualized drug counseling focuses directly on reducing or stopping the addict's illicit drug use. It also addresses related areas of impaired functioning such as employment status, illegal activity, family/social relations as well as the content and structure of the patient's recovery program. Through its emphasis on short-term behavioral goals, individualized drug counseling helps the patient develop coping strategies and tools for abstaining from drug use and then maintaining abstinence. The addiction counselor encourages 12-step participation and makes referrals for needed supplemental medical, psychiatric, employment, and other services. Individuals are encouraged to attend sessions one or two times per week.

In a study that compared opiate addicts receiving only methadone to those receiving methadone coupled with counseling, individuals who received only methadone showed minimal improvement in reducing opiate use. The addition of counseling produced significantly more improvement. The addition of onsite medical/psychiatric, employment, and family services further improved outcomes.

In another study with cocaine addicts, individualized drug counseling, together with group drug counseling, was quite effective in reducing cocaine use. Thus, it appears that this approach has great utility with both heroin and cocaine addicts in outpatient treatment.

Motivational Enhancement Therapy

Motivational enhancement therapy is a client-centered counseling approach for initiating behavior change by helping clients to resolve ambivalence about engaging in treatment and stopping drug use. This approach employs strategies to evoke rapid and internally motivated change in the client, rather than guiding the client stepwise through the recovery process. This therapy consists of an initial assessment battery session, followed by two to four individual treatment sessions with a therapist.

The first treatment session focuses on providing feedback generated from the initial assessment battery to stimulate discussion regarding personal substance use and to elicit self-motivational statements. Motivational interviewing principles are used to strengthen motivation and build a plan for change. Coping strategies for high-risk situations are suggested and discussed with the client. In subsequent sessions, the therapist monitors change, reviews cessation strategies being used, and continues to encourage commitment to change or sustained abstinence. Clients are sometimes encouraged to bring a significant other to sessions. This approach has been used successfully with alcoholics and with marijuana-dependent individuals.

Behavioral Therapy

Behavioral therapy for Adolescents incorporates the principle that unwanted behavior can be changed by clear demonstration of the desired behavior and consistent reward of incremental steps toward achieving it. Therapeutic activities include fulfilling specific assignments, rehearsing desired behaviors, and recording and reviewing progress, with praise and privileges given for meeting assigned goals. Urine samples are collected regularly to monitor drug use. The therapy aims to equip the patient to gain three types of control:

- Stimulus Control helps patients avoid situations associated with drug use and learn to spend more time in activities incompatible with drug use.

- Urge Control helps patients recognize and change thoughts, feelings, and plans that lead to drug use.

- Social Control involves family members and other people important in helping patients avoid drugs. A parent or significant other attends treatment sessions when possible and assists with therapy assignments and reinforcing desired behavior.

According to research studies, this therapy helps adolescents become drug free and increases their ability to remain drug free after treatment ends. Adolescents also show improvement in several other areas such as employment/school attendance, family relationships, depression, institutionalization, and alcohol use. Such favorable results are attributed largely to including family members in therapy and rewarding drug abstinence as verified by urinalysis.

Multidimensional Family Therapy (MDFT) for Adolescents

Multidimensional family therapy (MDFT) for adolescents is an outpatient family-based drug abuse treatment for teenagers. MDFT views adolescent drug use in terms of a network of influences (that is, individual, family, peer, community) and suggests that reducing unwanted behavior and increasing desirable behavior occur in multiple ways in different settings. Treatment includes individual and family sessions held in the clinic, in the home, or with family members at the family court, school, or other community locations.

During individual sessions, the therapist and adolescent work on important developmental tasks, such as developing decision-making, negotiation, and problem-solving skills. Teenagers acquire skills in communicating their thoughts and feelings to deal better with life stressors, and vocational skills. Parallel sessions are held with family members. Parents examine their particular parenting style, learning to distinguish influence from control and to have a positive and developmentally appropriate influence on their child.

Multisystemic Therapy (MST)

Multisystemic therapy (MST) addresses the factors associated with serious antisocial behavior in children and adolescents who abuse drugs. These factors include characteristics of the adolescent (for example, favorable attitudes toward drug use), the family (poor discipline, family conflict, parental drug abuse), peers (positive attitudes toward drug use), school (dropout, poor performance), and neighborhood (criminal subculture). By participating in intense treatment in natural environments (homes, schools, and neighborhood settings) most youths and families complete a full course of treatment. MST significantly reduces adolescent drug use during treatment and for at least 6 months after treatment. Reduced numbers of incarcerations and out-of-home placements of juveniles offset the cost of providing this intensive service and maintaining the clinicians' low caseloads.

Combined Behavioral and Nicotine Replacement Therapy for Nicotine Addiction

Combined behavioral and nicotine replacement therapy for nicotine addiction consists of two main components:

- The transdermal nicotine patch or nicotine gum reduces symptoms of withdrawal, producing better initial abstinence.

- The behavioral component concurrently provides support and reinforcement of coping skills, yielding better long-term outcomes.

Through behavioral skills training, patients learn to avoid high-risk situations for smoking relapse early on and later to plan strategies to cope with such situations. Patients practice skills in treatment, social, and work settings. They learn other coping techniques, such as cigarette refusal skills, assertiveness, and time management. The combined treatment is based on the rationale that behavioral and pharmacological treatments operate by different yet complementary mechanisms that produce potentially additive effects.

Community Reinforcement Approach (CRA)

Community reinforcement approach (CRA) plus vouchers is an intensive 24-week outpatient therapy for treatment of cocaine addiction. The treatment goals are twofold:

- To achieve cocaine abstinence long enough for patients to learn new life skills that will help sustain abstinence.

- To reduce alcohol consumption for patients whose drinking is associated with cocaine use.

Patients attend one or two individual counseling sessions per week, where they focus on improving family relations, learning a variety of skills to minimize drug use, receiving vocational counseling, and developing new recreational activities and social networks. Those who also abuse alcohol receive clinic-monitored disulfiram (Antabuse) therapy. Patients submit urine samples two or three times each week and receive vouchers for cocaine-negative samples. The value of the vouchers increases with consecutive clean samples. Patients may exchange vouchers for retail goods that are consistent with a cocaine-free lifestyle.

This approach facilitates patients' engagement in treatment and systematically aids them in gaining substantial periods of cocaine abstinence. The approach has been tested in urban and rural areas and used successfully in outpatient detoxification of opiate-addicted adults and with inner-city methadone maintenance patients who have high rates of intravenous cocaine abuse.

Voucher-Based Reinforcement Therapy in Methadone Maintenance Treatment

Voucher-based reinforcement therapy in Methadone maintenance treatment helps patients achieve and maintain abstinence from illegal drugs by providing them with a voucher each time they provide a drug-free urine sample. The voucher has monetary value and can be exchanged for goods and services consistent with the goals of treatment. Initially, the voucher values are low, but their value increases with the number of consecutive drug-free urine specimens the individual provides. Cocaine- or heroin-positive urine specimens reset the value of the vouchers to the initial low value. The contingency of escalating incentives is designed specifically to reinforce periods of sustained drug abstinence.

Studies show that patients receiving vouchers for drug-free urine samples achieved significantly more weeks of abstinence and significantly more weeks of sustained abstinence than patients who were given vouchers independent of urinalysis results. In another study, urinalyses positive for heroin decreased significantly when the voucher program was started and increased significantly when the program was stopped.

Day Treatment with Abstinence Contingencies and Vouchers

Day treatment with abstinence contingencies and vouchers was developed to treat homeless crack addicts. For the first 2 months, participants must spend 5.5 hours daily in the program, which provides lunch and transportation to and from shelters. Interventions include individual assessment and goal setting, individual and group counseling, multiple psycho-educational groups (for example, didactic groups on community resources, housing, cocaine, and HIV/AIDS prevention; establishing and reviewing personal rehabilitation goals; relapse prevention; weekend planning), and patient-governed community meetings during which patients review contract goals and provide support and encouragement to each other. Individual counseling occurs once a week, and group therapy sessions are held three times a week.

After 2 months of day treatment and at least 2 weeks of abstinence, participants graduate to a 4-month work component that pays wages that can be used to rent inexpensive, drug-free housing. A voucher system also rewards drug-free related social and recreational activities.

This innovative day treatment was compared with treatment consisting of twice-weekly individual counseling and 12-step groups, medical examinations and treatment, and referral to community resources for housing and vocational services. Innovative day treatment followed by work and housing dependent upon drug abstinence had a more positive effect on alcohol use, cocaine use, and days homeless.

Resources

The National Institute on Drug Abuse[50]

General inquiries:

- NIDA Public Information Office, Telephone: 301-443-1124.

Inquiries about NIDA's treatment research activities:

- Division of Treatment Research and Development (301) 443-6173 (for questions regarding behavioral therapies and medications);
- Division of Epidemiology, Services and Prevention Research (301) 443-4060 (for questions regarding access to treatment, organization, management, financing, effectiveness and cost-effectiveness).

Center for Substance Abuse Treatment (CSAT)

CSAT, a part of the Substance Abuse and Mental Health Services Administration, is responsible for supporting treatment services through block grants and developing knowledge about effective drug treatment, disseminating the findings to the field, and promoting their adoption. CSAT also operates the National Treatment Referral 24-hour Hotline (1-800-662-HELP) which offers information and referral to people seeking treatment programs and other assistance. CSAT publications are available through the National Clearinghouse on Alcohol and Drug Information (1-800-729-6686). Additional information can be found at CSAT's Web Site: **http://www.samhsa.gov/csat.**

---

[50] The NIDA: **http://www.nida.nih.gov.**

Selected NIDA Educational Resources on Drug Addiction Treatment

The following are available from the National Clearinghouse on Alcohol and Drug Information (NCADI), the National Technical Information Service (NTIS), or the Government Printing Office (GPO). To order, refer to the NCADI (1-800-729-6686), NTIS (1-800-553-6847), or GPO (202-512-1800) number provided with the resource description.

Manuals and Clinical Reports

- **Measuring and Improving Cost, Cost-Effectiveness, and Cost-Benefit for Substance Abuse Treatment Programs (1999).** Offers substance abuse treatment program managers tools with which to calculate the costs of their programs and investigate the relationship between those costs and treatment outcomes. NCADI # BKD340. Available online at **http://www.nida.nih.gov/IMPCOST/IMPCOSTIndex.html**.

- **A Cognitive-Behavioral Approach: Treating Cocaine Addiction (1998).** This is the first in NIDA's "Therapy Manuals for Drug Addiction" series. Describes cognitive-behavioral therapy, a short-term focused approach to helping cocaine-addicted individuals become abstinent from cocaine and other drugs. NCADI # BKD254. Available online at **http://www.nida.nih.gov/TXManuals/CBT/CBT1.html**.

- **A Community Reinforcement Plus Vouchers Approach: Treating Cocaine Addiction (1998).** This is the second in NIDA's "Therapy Manuals for Drug Addiction" series. This treatment integrates a community reinforcement approach with an incentive program that uses vouchers. NCADI # BKD255. Available online at **http://www.nida.nih.gov/TXManuals/CRA/CRA1.html**.

- **An Individual Drug Counseling Approach to Treat Cocaine Addiction: The Collaborative Cocaine Treatment Study Model (1999).** This is the third in NIDA's "Therapy Manuals for Drug Addiction" series. Describes specific cognitive-behavioral models that can be implemented in a wide range of differing drug abuse treatment settings. NCADI # BKD337. Available online at **http://www.nida.nih.gov/TXManuals/IDCA/IDCA1.html**.

- **Mental Health Assessment and Diagnosis of Substance Abusers: Clinical Report Series (1994).** Provides detailed descriptions of psychiatric disorders that can occur among drug-abusing clients. NCADI # BKD148.

- **Relapse Prevention: Clinical Report Series (1994).** Discusses several major issues to relapse prevention. Provides an overview of factors and experiences that can lead to relapse. Reviews general strategies for preventing relapses, and describes four specific approaches in detail. Outlines administrative issues related to implementing a relapse prevention program. NCADI # BKD147.

- **Addiction Severity Index Package (1993).** Provides a structured clinical interview designed to collect information about substance use and functioning in life areas from adult clients seeking drug abuse treatment. Includes a handbook for program administrators, a resource manual, two videotapes, and a training facilitator's manual. NTIS # AVA19615VNB2KUS. $150.

- **Program Evaluation Package (1993).** A practical resource for treatment program administrators and key staff. Includes an overview and case study manual, a guide for evaluation, a resource guide, and a pamphlet. NTIS # 95-167268/BDL. $86.50.

- **Relapse Prevention Package (1993).** Examines two effective relapse prevention models, the Recovery Training and Self-Help (RTSH) program and the Cue Extinction model. NTIS # 95-167250/BDL. $189; GPO # 017-024-01555-5. $57. (Sold by GPO as a set of 7 books)

Research Monographs

- **Beyond the Therapeutic Alliance: Keeping the Drug-Dependent Individual in Treatment (Research Monograph 165) (1997).** Reviews current treatment research on the best ways to retain patients in drug abuse treatment. NTIS # 97-181606. $47; GPO # 017-024-01608-0. $17. http://www.nida.nih.gov/pdf/monographs/monograph165/download165.html.

- **Treatment of Drug-Exposed Women and Children: Advances in Research Methodology (Research Monograph 166) (1997).** Presents experiences, products, and procedures of NIDA-supported Treatment Research Demonstration Program projects. NCADI # M166; NTIS # 96-179106. $75; GPO # 017-01592-0. $13. Available online at http://www.nida.nih.gov/pdf/monographs/monograph166/download.html.

- **Treatment of Drug-Dependent Individuals With Comorbid Mental Disorders (Research Monograph 172) (1997).** Promotes effective treatment by reporting state-of-the-art treatment research on individuals with comorbid mental and addictive disorders and research on HIV-related issues among people with comorbid conditions. NCADI # M172; NTIS # 97-181580. $41; GPO # 017-024-01605. $10. Available online at **http://www.nida.nih.gov/pdf/monographs/monograph172/download172 .html**

- **Medications Development for the Treatment of Cocaine Dependence: Issues in Clinical Efficacy Trials (Research Monograph 175) (1998).** A state-of-the-art handbook for clinical investigators, pharmaceutical scientists, and treatment researchers. NCADI # M175. **http://www.nida.nih.gov/pdf/monographs/monograph175/download175 .html**

Videos

- **Adolescent Treatment Approaches (1991).** Emphasizes the importance of pinpointing and addressing individual problem areas, such as sexual abuse, peer pressure, and family involvement in treatment. Running time: 25 min. NCADI # VHS40. $12.50.

- **NIDA Technology Transfer Series: Assessment (1991).** Shows how to use a number of diagnostic instruments as well as how to assess the implementation and effectiveness of the plan during various phases of the patient's treatment. Running time: 22 min. NCADI # VHS38. $12.50.

- **Drug Abuse Treatment in Prison: A New Way Out (1995).** Portrays two comprehensive drug abuse treatment approaches that have been effective with men and women in State and Federal Prisons. Running time: 23 min. NCADI # VHS72. $12.50.

- **Dual Diagnosis (1993).** Focuses on the problem of mental illness in drug-abusing and drug-addicted populations, and examines various approaches useful for treating dual-diagnosed clients. Running time: 27 min. NCADI # VHS58. $12.50.

- **LAAM: Another Option for Maintenance Treatment of Opiate Addiction (1995).** Shows how LAAM can be used to meet the opiate treatment needs of individual clients from the provider and patient perspectives. Running time: 16 min. NCADI # VHS73. $12.50.

- **Methadone: Where We Are (1993).** Examines issues such as the use and effectiveness of methadone as a treatment, biological effects of methadone, the role of the counselor in treatment, and societal attitudes toward methadone treatment and patients. Running time: 24 min. NCADI # VHS59. $12.50.

- **Relapse Prevention (1991).** Helps practitioners understand the common phenomenon of relapse to drug use among patients in treatment. Running time: 24 min. NCADI # VHS37. $12.50.

- **Treatment Issues for Women (1991).** Assists treatment counselors help female patients to explore relationships with their children, with men, and with other women. Running time: 22 min. NCADI # VHS39. $12.50.

- **Treatment Solutions (1999).** Describes the latest developments in treatment research and emphasizes the benefits of drug abuse treatment, not only to the patient, but also to the greater community. Running time: 19 min. NCADI # DD110. $12.50.

- **Program Evaluation Package (1993).** A practical resource for treatment program administrators and key staff. Includes an overview and case study manual, a guide for evaluation, a resource guide, and a pamphlet. NTIS # 95-167268/BDL. $86.50.

- **Relapse Prevention Package (1993).** Examines two effective relapse prevention models, the Recovery Training and Self-Help (RTSH) program and the Cue Extinction model. NTIS # 95-167250. $189; GPO # 017-024-01555-5. $57. (Sold by GPO as a set of 7 books)

Other Federal Resources

- **The National Clearinghouse for Alcohol and Drug Information (NCADI).** NIDA publications and treatment materials along with publications from other Federal agencies are available from this information source. Staff provide assistance in English and Spanish, and have TDD capability. Phone: 1-800-729-6686. Website: http://www.health.org.

- **The National Institute of Justice (NIJ).** As the research agency of the Department of Justice, NIJ supports research, evaluation, and demonstration programs relating to drug abuse in the contexts of crime and the criminal justice system. For information, including a wealth of publications, contact the National Criminal Justice Reference Service by telephone (1-800-851-3420 or 1-301-519-5500) or on the World Wide Web (http://www.ojp.usdoj.gov/nij).

ONLINE GLOSSARIES

The Internet provides access to a number of free-to-use medical dictionaries and glossaries. The National Library of Medicine has compiled the following list of online dictionaries:

- ADAM Medical Encyclopedia (A.D.A.M., Inc.), comprehensive medical reference: **http://www.nlm.nih.gov/medlineplus/encyclopedia.html**

- MedicineNet.com Medical Dictionary (MedicineNet, Inc.): **http://www.medterms.com/Script/Main/hp.asp**

- Merriam-Webster Medical Dictionary (Inteli-Health, Inc.): **http://www.intelihealth.com/IH/**

- Multilingual Glossary of Technical and Popular Medical Terms in Eight European Languages (European Commission) - Danish, Dutch, English, French, German, Italian, Portuguese, and Spanish: **http://allserv.rug.ac.be/~rvdstich/eugloss/welcome.html**

- On-line Medical Dictionary (CancerWEB): **http://www.graylab.ac.uk/omd/**

- Technology Glossary (National Library of Medicine) - Health Care Technology: **http://www.nlm.nih.gov/nichsr/ta101/ta10108.htm**

- Terms and Definitions (Office of Rare Diseases): **http://rarediseases.info.nih.gov/ord/glossary_a-e.html**

Beyond these, MEDLINEplus contains a very user-friendly encyclopedia covering every aspect of medicine (licensed from A.D.A.M., Inc.). The ADAM Medical Encyclopedia can be accessed via the following Web site address: **http://www.nlm.nih.gov/medlineplus/encyclopedia.html**. ADAM is also available on commercial Web sites such as Web MD (**http://my.webmd.com/adam/asset/adam_disease_articles/a_to_z/a**) and drkoop.com (**http://www.drkoop.com/**). Topics of interest can be researched by using keywords before continuing elsewhere, as these basic definitions and concepts will be useful in more advanced areas of research. You may choose to print various pages specifically relating to cocaine dependence and keep them on file. The NIH, in particular, suggests that patients with cocaine dependence visit the following Web sites in the ADAM Medical Encyclopedia:

- **Basic Guidelines for Cocaine Dependence**

  ### Cocaine intoxication
  Web site:
  http://www.nlm.nih.gov/medlineplus/ency/article/000946.htm

  ### Cocaine withdrawal
  Web site:
  http://www.nlm.nih.gov/medlineplus/ency/article/000947.htm

- **Signs & Symptoms for Cocaine Dependence**

  ### Anorexia
  Web site:
  http://www.nlm.nih.gov/medlineplus/ency/article/003121.htm

  ### Depression
  Web site:
  http://www.nlm.nih.gov/medlineplus/ency/article/003213.htm

  ### Loss of appetite
  Web site:
  http://www.nlm.nih.gov/medlineplus/ency/article/003121.htm

- **Diagnostics and Tests for Cocaine Dependence**

  ### Cocaine
  Web site:
  http://www.nlm.nih.gov/medlineplus/ency/article/003578.htm

- **Background Topics for Cocaine Dependence**

  ### Cardiovascular
  Web site:
  http://www.nlm.nih.gov/medlineplus/ency/article/002310.htm

  ### Central nervous system
  Web site:
  http://www.nlm.nih.gov/medlineplus/ency/article/002311.htm

  ### Drug abuse
  Web site:
  http://www.nlm.nih.gov/medlineplus/ency/article/001945.htm

Drug abuse first aid
Web site:
http://www.nlm.nih.gov/medlineplus/ency/article/000016.htm

Physical examination
Web site:
http://www.nlm.nih.gov/medlineplus/ency/article/002274.htm

Somatic
Web site:
http://www.nlm.nih.gov/medlineplus/ency/article/002294.htm

Online Dictionary Directories

The following are additional online directories compiled by the National Library of Medicine, including a number of specialized medical dictionaries and glossaries:

- Medical Dictionaries: Medical & Biological (World Health Organization):
  http://www.who.int/hlt/virtuallibrary/English/diction.htm#Medical

- MEL-Michigan Electronic Library List of Online Health and Medical Dictionaries (Michigan Electronic Library):
  http://mel.lib.mi.us/health/health-dictionaries.html

- Patient Education: Glossaries (DMOZ Open Directory Project):
  http://dmoz.org/Health/Education/Patient_Education/Glossaries/

- Web of Online Dictionaries (Bucknell University):
  http://www.yourdictionary.com/diction5.html#medicine

COCAINE DEPENDENCE GLOSSARY

The following is a complete glossary of terms used in this sourcebook. The definitions are derived from official public sources including the National Institutes of Health [NIH] and the European Union [EU]. After this glossary, we list a number of additional hardbound and electronic glossaries and dictionaries that you may wish to consult.

Adjustment: The dynamic process wherein the thoughts, feelings, behavior, and biophysiological mechanisms of the individual continually change to adjust to the environment. [NIH]

Alertness: A state of readiness to detect and respond to certain specified small changes occurring at random intervals in the environment. [NIH]

Anorexia: Lack or loss of appetite for food. Appetite is psychologic, dependent on memory and associations. Anorexia can be brought about by unattractive food, surroundings, or company. [NIH]

Antagonism: Interference with, or inhibition of, the growth of a living organism by another living organism, due either to creation of unfavorable conditions (e. g. exhaustion of food supplies) or to production of a specific antibiotic substance (e. g. penicillin). [NIH]

Applicability: A list of the commodities to which the candidate method can be applied as presented or with minor modifications. [NIH]

Aspartate: A synthetic amino acid. [NIH]

Attenuated: Strain with weakened or reduced virulence. [NIH]

Attenuation: Reduction of transmitted sound energy or its electrical equivalent. [NIH]

Audiologist: Study of hearing including treatment of persons with hearing defects. [NIH]

Blot: To transfer DNA, RNA, or proteins to an immobilizing matrix such as nitrocellulose. [NIH]

Catecholamine: A group of chemical substances manufactured by the adrenal medulla and secreted during physiological stress. [NIH]

Cocaethylene: Hard drug formed by cocaine and alcohol. [NIH]

Compassionate: A process for providing experimental drugs to very sick patients who have no treatment options. [NIH]

Compulsion: In psychology, an irresistible urge, sometimes amounting to obsession to perform a particular act which usually is carried out against the performer's will or better judgment. [NIH]

Consultation: A deliberation between two or more physicians concerning the diagnosis and the proper method of treatment in a case. [NIH]

Contraindications: Any factor or sign that it is unwise to pursue a certain kind of action or treatment, e. g. giving a general anesthetic to a person with pneumonia. [NIH]

Cortisol: A steroid hormone secreted by the adrenal cortex as part of the body's response to stress. [NIH]

Cytokine: Small but highly potent protein that modulates the activity of many cell types, including T and B cells. [NIH]

Deletion: A genetic rearrangement through loss of segments of DNA (chromosomes), bringing sequences, which are normally separated, into close proximity. [NIH]

Discrimination: The act of qualitative and/or quantitative differentiation between two or more stimuli. [NIH]

Dysphoric: A feeling of unpleasantness and discomfort. [NIH]

EEG: A graphic recording of the changes in electrical potential associated with the activity of the cerebral cortex made with the electroencephalogram. [NIH]

Electrode: Component of the pacing system which is at the distal end of the lead. It is the interface with living cardiac tissue across which the stimulus is transmitted. [NIH]

Enzymatic: Phase where enzyme cuts the precursor protein. [NIH]

Epitope: A molecule or portion of a molecule capable of binding to the combining site of an antibody. For every given antigenic determinant, the body can construct a variety of antibody-combining sites, some of which fit almost perfectly, and others which barely fit. [NIH]

Estrogen: One of the two female sex hormones. [NIH]

Ether: One of a class of organic compounds in which any two organic radicals are attached directly to a single oxygen atom. [NIH]

Excitability: Property of a cardiac cell whereby, when the cell is depolarized to a critical level (called threshold), the membrane becomes permeable and a regenerative inward current causes an action potential. [NIH]

Excitatory: When cortical neurons are excited, their output increases and each new input they receive while they are still excited raises their output markedly. [NIH]

Fatigue: The feeling of weariness of mind and body. [NIH]

Forearm: The part between the elbow and the wrist. [NIH]

Genetics: The biological science that deals with the phenomena and mechanisms of heredity. [NIH]

Hepatitis: Infectious disease of the liver. [NIH]

Heterogeneity: The property of one or more samples or populations which implies that they are not identical in respect of some or all of their parameters, e. g. heterogeneity of variance. [NIH]

Hybridoma: A hybrid cell resulting from the fusion of a specific antibody-producing spleen cell with a myeloma cell. [NIH]

Impairment: In the context of health experience, an impairment is any loss or abnormality of psychological, physiological, or anatomical structure or function. [NIH]

Infections: The illnesses caused by an organism that usually does not cause disease in a person with a normal immune system. [NIH]

Initiation: Mutation induced by a chemical reactive substance causing cell changes; being a step in a carcinogenic process. [NIH]

Insight: The capacity to understand one's own motives, to be aware of one's own psychodynamics, to appreciate the meaning of symbolic behavior. [NIH]

Ligands: A RNA simulation method developed by the MIT. [NIH]

Linkage: The tendency of two or more genes in the same chromosome to remain together from one generation to the next more frequently than expected according to the law of independent assortment. [NIH]

Medial: Lying near the midsaggital plane of the body; opposed to lateral. [NIH]

Mesolimbic: Inner brain region governing emotion and drives. [NIH]

Metabotropic: A glutamate receptor which triggers an increase in production of 2 intracellular messengers: diacylglycerol and inositol 1, 4, 5-triphosphate. [NIH]

Modeling: A treatment procedure whereby the therapist presents the target behavior which the learner is to imitate and make part of his repertoire. [NIH]

Modification: A change in an organism, or in a process in an organism, that is acquired from its own activity or environment. [NIH]

Morphological: Relating to the configuration or the structure of live organs. [NIH]

MRNA: The RNA molecule that conveys from the DNA the information that is to be translated into the structure of a particular polypeptide molecule. [NIH]

Myopia: Astigmatism in which one principal meridian is myopic and the other enmetropic, or in which both meridians are myopic. [NIH]

Nerve: A cordlike structure of nervous tissue that connects parts of the nervous system with other tissues of the body and conveys nervous impulses to, or away from, these tissues. [NIH]

Networks: Pertaining to a nerve or to the nerves, a meshlike structure of interlocking fibers or strands. [NIH]

Nuclei: A body of specialized protoplasm found in nearly all cells and containing the chromosomes. [NIH]

Nucleus: A body of specialized protoplasm found in nearly all cells and containing the chromosomes. [NIH]

Outpatient: A patient who is not an inmate of a hospital but receives diagnosis or treatment in a clinic or dispensary connected with the hospital. [NIH]

Patch: A piece of material used to cover or protect a wound, an injured part, etc.: a patch over the eye. [NIH]

Pediatrics: The branch of medical science concerned with children and their diseases. [NIH]

Pharmacodynamic: Is concerned with the response of living tissues to chemical stimuli, that is, the action of drugs on the living organism in the absence of disease. [NIH]

Pharmacokinetic: The mathematical analysis of the time courses of absorption, distribution, and elimination of drugs. [NIH]

Phenotypes: An organism as observed, i. e. as judged by its visually perceptible characters resulting from the interaction of its genotype with the environment. [NIH]

Physiology: The science that deals with the life processes and functions of organismus, their cells, tissues, and organs. [NIH]

Plasticity: In an individual or a population, the capacity for adaptation: a) through gene changes (genetic plasticity) or b) through internal physiological modifications in response to changes of environment (physiological plasticity). [NIH]

Polymerase: An enzyme which catalyses the synthesis of DNA using a single DNA strand as a template. The polymerase copies the template in the 5'-3'direction provided that sufficient quantities of free nucleotides, dATP and dTTP are present. [NIH]

Polymorphism: The occurrence together of two or more distinct forms in the same population. [NIH]

Postsynaptic: Nerve potential generated by an inhibitory hyperpolarizing stimulation. [NIH]

Potassium: It is essential to the ability of muscle cells to contract. [NIH]

Potentiate: A degree of synergism which causes the exposure of the organism to a harmful substance to worsen a disease already contracted. [NIH]

Probe: An instrument used in exploring cavities, or in the detection and dilatation of strictures, or in demonstrating the potency of channels; an elongated instrument for exploring or sounding body cavities. [NIH]

Prodrug: A substance that gives rise to a pharmacologically active metabolite, although not itself active (i. e. an inactive precursor). [NIH]

Promoter: A chemical substance that increases the activity of a carcinogenic process. [NIH]

Prone: Having the front portion of the body downwards. [NIH]

Protease: Any enzyme that catalyzes hydrolysis of a protein. [NIH]

Protocol: The detailed plan for a clinical trial that states the trial's rationale, purpose, drug or vaccine dosages, length of study, routes of administration, who may participate, and other aspects of trial design. [NIH]

Psychoactive: Those drugs which alter sensation, mood, consciousness or other psychological or behavioral functions. [NIH]

Refer: To send or direct for treatment, aid, information, de decision. [NIH]

Reticular: Coarse-fibered, netlike dermis layer. [NIH]

Ritalin: Drug used to treat hyperactive children. [NIH]

Sayre: A metal splint used to immobilize the hip in hip joint disease. [NIH]

Schizophrenia: A mental disorder characterized by a special type of disintegration of the personality. [NIH]

Septal: An abscess occurring at the root of the tooth on the proximal surface. [NIH]

Sequencer: Device that reads off the order of nucleotides in a cloned gene. [NIH]

Sequencing: The determination of the order of nucleotides in a DNA or RNA chain. [NIH]

Specialist: In medicine, one who concentrates on 1 special branch of medical science. [NIH]

Specificity: Degree of selectivity shown by an antibody with respect to the number and types of antigens with which the antibody combines, as well as with respect to the rates and the extents of these reactions. [NIH]

Sperm: The fecundating fluid of the male. [NIH]

Stabilizer: A device for maintaining constant X-ray tube voltage or current. [NIH]

Stimulants: Any drug or agent which causes stimulation. [NIH]

Stimulus: That which can elicit or evoke action (response) in a muscle, nerve, gland or other excitable issue, or cause an augmenting action upon any function or metabolic process. [NIH]

Striatum: A higher brain's domain thus called because of its stripes. [NIH]

Subculture: A culture derived from another culture or the aseptic division and transfer of a culture or a portion of that culture (inoculum) to fresh nutrient medium. [NIH]

Suppression: A conscious exclusion of disapproved desire contrary with repression, in which the process of exclusion is not conscious. [NIH]

Synapse: The region where the processes of two neurons come into close contiguity, and the nervous impulse passes from one to the other; the fibers of the two are intermeshed, but, according to the general view, there is no direct contiguity. [NIH]

Talcum: A native magnesium silicate. [NIH]

Temporal: One of the two irregular bones forming part of the lateral surfaces and base of the skull, and containing the organs of hearing. [NIH]

Therapeutics: The branch of medicine which is concerned with the treatment of diseases, palliative or curative. [NIH]

Threshold: For a specified sensory modality (e. g. light, sound, vibration), the lowest level (absolute threshold) or smallest difference (difference threshold, difference limen) or intensity of the stimulus discernible in prescribed conditions of stimulation. [NIH]

Transcriptase: An enzyme which catalyses the synthesis of a complementary mRNA molecule from a DNA template in the presence of a mixture of the four ribonucleotides (ATP, UTP, GTP and CTP). [NIH]

Translation: The process whereby the genetic information present in the linear sequence of ribonucleotides in mRNA is converted into a corresponding sequence of amino acids in a protein. It occurs on the ribosome and is unidirectional. [NIH]

Translational: The cleavage of signal sequence that directs the passage of the protein through a cell or organelle membrane. [NIH]

Vector: Plasmid or other self-replicating DNA molecule that transfers DNA between cells in nature or in recombinant DNA technology. [NIH]

Vitro: Descriptive of an event or enzyme reaction under experimental investigation occurring outside a living organism. Parts of an organism or microorganism are used together with artificial substrates and/or conditions. [NIH]

Vivo: Outside of or removed from the body of a living organism. [NIH]

General Dictionaries and Glossaries

While the above glossary is essentially complete, the dictionaries listed here cover virtually all aspects of medicine, from basic words and phrases to more advanced terms (sorted alphabetically by title; hyperlinks provide rankings, information and reviews at Amazon.com):

- **Dictionary of Medical Acronymns & Abbreviations** by Stanley Jablonski (Editor), Paperback, 4th edition (2001), Lippincott Williams & Wilkins Publishers, ISBN: 1560534605, http://www.amazon.com/exec/obidos/ASIN/1560534605/icongroupinterna

- **Dictionary of Medical Terms : For the Nonmedical Person (Dictionary of Medical Terms for the Nonmedical Person, Ed 4)** by Mikel A. Rothenberg, M.D, et al, Paperback - 544 pages, 4th edition (2000), Barrons Educational Series, ISBN: 0764112015, http://www.amazon.com/exec/obidos/ASIN/0764112015/icongroupinterna

- **A Dictionary of the History of Medicine** by A. Sebastian, CD-Rom edition (2001), CRC Press-Parthenon Publishers, ISBN: 185070368X, http://www.amazon.com/exec/obidos/ASIN/185070368X/icongroupinterna

- **Dorland's Illustrated Medical Dictionary (Standard Version)** by Dorland, et al, Hardcover - 2088 pages, 29th edition (2000), W B Saunders Co, ISBN: 0721662544, http://www.amazon.com/exec/obidos/ASIN/0721662544/icongroupinterna

- **Dorland's Electronic Medical Dictionary** by Dorland, et al, Software, 29th Book & CD-Rom edition (2000), Harcourt Health Sciences, ISBN: 0721694934, http://www.amazon.com/exec/obidos/ASIN/0721694934/icongroupinterna

- **Dorland's Pocket Medical Dictionary (Dorland's Pocket Medical Dictionary, 26th Ed)** Hardcover - 912 pages, 26th edition (2001), W B Saunders Co, ISBN: 0721682812, http://www.amazon.com/exec/obidos/ASIN/0721682812/icongroupinterna/103-4193558-7304618

- **Melloni's Illustrated Medical Dictionary (Melloni's Illustrated Medical Dictionary, 4th Ed)** by Melloni, Hardcover, 4th edition (2001), CRC Press-Parthenon Publishers, ISBN: 85070094X, http://www.amazon.com/exec/obidos/ASIN/85070094X/icongroupinterna

- **Stedman's Electronic Medical Dictionary Version 5.0 (CD-ROM for Windows and Macintosh, Individual)** by Stedmans, CD-ROM edition (2000), Lippincott Williams & Wilkins Publishers, ISBN: 0781726328, http://www.amazon.com/exec/obidos/ASIN/0781726328/icongroupinter na

- **Stedman's Medical Dictionary** by Thomas Lathrop Stedman, Hardcover - 2098 pages, 27th edition (2000), Lippincott, Williams & Wilkins, ISBN: 068340007X,
  http://www.amazon.com/exec/obidos/ASIN/068340007X/icongroupinter na

- **Tabers Cyclopedic Medical Dictionary (Thumb Index)** by Donald Venes (Editor), et al, Hardcover - 2439 pages, 19th edition (2001), F A Davis Co, ISBN: 0803606540,
  http://www.amazon.com/exec/obidos/ASIN/0803606540/icongroupinter na

INDEX

A

Adjustment............................107
Alertness...............................17
Antagonism.....................73, 117
Applicability 123
Aspartate 86
Attenuated.............................83
Attenuation 68, 107

B

Blot 112

C

Catecholamine 96
Cocaethylene..................19, 25, 64
Compassionate 244
Compulsion..............111, 274, 277
Consultation...............ii, iii, 3, 45
Contraindications............... ii, 245
Cortisol................................92
Cytokine 70

D

Deletion................................71
Discrimination 74, 83, 100, 116, 180, 256
Dysphoric 80

E

Electrode...............................79
Enzymatic.............................167
Estrogen 73
Ether 24
Excitability...........................234
Excitatory............................117

F

Fatigue 25

G

Genetics 93, 96, 115, 135

H

Hepatitis 20, 273, 281
Heterogeneity 59, 93, 182, 307
Hybridoma.............................189

I

Impairment.......36, 62, 74, 84, 103, 122, 307
Infections 48, 51, 281
Initiation 60, 92, 283

L

Ligands 90, 101, 114, 118, 189, 190
Linkage 93, 96, 115

M

Medial 67, 111, 172, 234
Mesolimbic 98, 110, 112, 232

Metabotropic 118
Modeling 62, 118, 122
Modification 71
Morphological 67
Myopia 62

N

Nerve 18, 61, 184, 308, 309
Networks..........................3, 293
Nuclei 63, 114
Nucleus 15, 16, 67, 98, 111, 125, 134, 137, 234

P

Patch 21, 36, 79, 292, 308
Pharmacodynamic 54, 87
Pharmacokinetic 54, 63, 87, 234
Phenotypes 93, 96
Plasticity...................67, 183, 308
Polymerase 112, 183, 308
Polymorphism........................169
Postsynaptic.........................67
Potassium............................252
Potentiate 57
Probe....................70, 112, 125
Promoter 169
Prone...........................22, 25, 54
Protocol 64, 101, 117

R

Refer.................3, 4, 40, 223, 296
Reticular 60

S

Schizophrenia 85, 96, 113, 123, 125, 174
Septal 51, 79
Sequencer.............................93
Sequencing...........................189
Specialist 38, 40, 43
Specificity..........67, 100, 109, 189, 190
Sperm................................252
Stimulants 13, 66, 121
Stimulus 74, 100, 114, 117, 119, 182, 185, 255, 259, 306, 310
Striatum..................67, 98, 101, 113
Subculture...........................292
Suppression 66
Synapse 16, 134

T

Talcum................................13
Temporal....................68, 85, 172
Therapeutics 180, 188, 243

Threshold....54, 111, 185, 236, 272, 306, 310
Transcriptase..112
Translational 133

V
Vector 94
Vitro.. 101, 122, 256
Vivo.................60, 83, 84, 101, 111, 114, 122

Printed in the United States
57283LVS00004B/96